BRUNNER/MAZEL PSYCHOSOCIAL STRESS SERIES NO. 9

STRESS
and
ADDICTION

Edited by

Edward Gottheil, M.D., Ph.D.,
Keith A. Druley, Ph.D.,
Steven Pashko, Ph.D., &
Stephen P. Weinstein, Ph.D.

BRUNNER/MAZEL *Publishers* • New York

Library of Congress Cataloging-in-Publication Data

Stress and addiction.

(Brunner/Mazel psychosocial stress series; no. 9)
Based on papers presented at the Seventh Annual
Coatesville-Jefferson Conference, held Mar. 29–30, 1984
and sponsored by the Substance Abuse Treatment Unit of
the Coatesville VA Medical Center and the Jefferson
Center for the Study of Alcoholism and Addiction of
Thomas Jefferson University.
     1. Alcoholism—Congresses.   2. Substance abuse—
Congresses.   3. Stress (Psychology)—Congresses.
I. Gottheil, Edward L.   II. Coatesville-Jefferson
Conference (7th: 1984: Coatesville VA Medical Center)
III. Coatesville VA Medical Center. Substance Abuse
Treatment Unit.   IV. Jefferson Center for the Study
of Alcoholism and Addiction.   V. Series.
[DNLM: 1. Alcoholism—congresses.   2. Stress,
Psychological—congresses.   3. Substance Dependence—
congresses.   W1 BR917TB no.9 / WM 274 S915 1984]
RC565.S77   1987   616.86   87-7987
ISBN 0-87630-463-3

Published by
BRUNNER/MAZEL, INC.
19 Union Square
New York, New York 10003

MANUFACTURED IN THE UNITED STATES OF AMERICA

10 9 8 7 6 5 4 3 2 1

STRESS
and
ADDICTION

Brunner/Mazel Psychosocial Stress Series
Charles R. Figley, Ph.D., Series Editor

1. Stress Disorders Among Vietnam Veterans
   Edited by Charles R. Figley, Ph.D.
2. Stress and the Family Vol 1: Coping with Normative Transitions
   Edited by Hamilton I. McCubbin, Ph.D., and Charles R. Figley, Ph.D.
3. Stress and the Family Vol. 2: Coping with Catastrophe
   Edited by Charles R. Figley, Ph.D., and Hamilton I. McCubbin, Ph.D.
4. Trauma and Its Wake: The Study and Treatment of Post-Traumatic Stress Disorder
   Edited by Charles R. Figley, Ph.D.
5. Post-Traumatic Stress Disorder and the War Veteran Patient
   Edited by William E. Kelly, M.D.
6. The Crime Victim's Book, Second Edition
   By Morton Bard, Ph.D., and Dawn Sangrey
7. Stress and Coping in Time of War: Generalizations from the Israeli Experience
   Edited by Norman A. Milgram, Ph.D.
8. Trauma and Its Wake Vol. 2: Traumatic Stress Theory, Research, and Intervention
   Edited by Charles R. Figley, Ph.D.

Editorial Note

The Editorial Board of the Psychosocial Stress Book Series is proud to welcome *Stress and Addiction* as the ninth book in the Series. As dedicated Series readers already know, the Series strives to develop and publish books that in some way make a significant contribution to the understanding and management of the psychosocial stress reaction paradigm. These books are designed to advance the work of clinicians, researchers, and other professionals involved in the varied aspects of human services which confront issues of psychosocial stress reactions.

The Psychosocial Stress Book Series is among the few that are "refereed." The quality and significance of the Series are guided by a nationally and internationally respected group of scholars who compose the Editorial Board. The Board must review and approve each book that is published in the Series. Like the readership, the Board represents the fields of general medicine, pediatrics, psychiatry, nursing, psychology, sociology, social work, family therapy, political science, and anthropology.

Books in the Series focus on the stress associated with a wide variety of psychosocial stressors. Collectively, the books and chapters in the Series have focused on the immediate and long-term psychosocial consequences of extraordinary stressors such as war, divorce, parenting, separation, racism, social isolation, acute illness, drug addiction, death, sudden unemployment, rape, natural disasters, incest, crime victimization, and many others.

The first volume in the Series, *Stress Disorders Among Vietnam Veterans*, published in 1978 and edited by Charles R. Figley, focused on the immediate and long-term effects of war. It alerted the nation to the difficulties of coping with one's war experiences long after the war was over. It provided a state-of-the-art source book for scholars and practitioners working in the area of war-related stress reactions and disorders. With the publication of this book and other resources, mental health professionals and policymakers began to recognize the complexity of the post-war readjustment of Vietnam veterans. Soon a national outreach program emerged within the Veterans Administration with storefront Vet Centers in every major city in the country and inpatient treatment programs in many VA Medical Centers across the country to focus on these problems. As a result, thousands of professionals have since become aware of the special circumstances of war veterans.

The next two volumes in the Series, *Stress and the Family, Volume I: Coping with Normative Transitions* and *Stress and the Family, Volume II: Coping with Catastrophe*, edited by Charles R. Figley and Hamilton I. McCubbin, provide a comprehensive summary of the available information about how families cope with psychosocial stress. The former volume attends to the typical and predictable stressors of family life, while the latter volume focuses on how families cope with extraordinary and unpredictable stressors. Each chapter follows the same outline, which first introduces the stressor, then identifies the functional and dysfunctional ways families and family members cope.

Trauma and Its Wake: The Study and Treatment of Post-Traumatic Stress Disorder, edited by Charles R. Figley, is the fourth book in the Series. It is the first attempt to generalize research and clinical findings among a wide variety of traumatic or catastrophic events toward a generalized view of traumatic and post-traumatic stress reactions. Chapters focus on the immediate and long-term psychosocial consequences of exposure to one of many types of catastrophic events: war, rape, natural disasters, incest. Other chapters focus on effective methods of treating or preventing stress reactions or disorders. It is the first in a series of books that will review the latest innovations in theory, research, and treatment of this disorder, caused by wide variety of stressful life events.

The fifth volume in the Series, *Post-Traumatic Stress Disorder and the War Veteran Patient*, edited by William E. Kelly, focuses on war veterans in general, and Vietnam war veterans in particular. Built upon the most important contributions of the past, this volume provides a specific blueprint for conceptualizing and treating war-related post-traumatic stress disorders.

The sixth volume, *The Crime Victim's Book*, written by Morton Bard and Dawn Sangrey, deals with yet another context in which individuals struggle to manage their violent life experiences. This book is written as a primer for those interested in working with victims of crime, particularly violent crime, although the authors hoped that victims themselves would read it. The book provides summaries of two important recent task force reports: one produced by the President's Task Force on Victims of Crime and the other by the American Psychological Association's Task

Force on the Victims of Crime and Violence, chaired by the book's senior author.

Stress and Coping in Time of War, edited by Norman Milgram, is the seventh volume, but the first in the Series to focus on an international issue: the special psychosocial stress of war upon not only those who fight, but the nations, communities, and social systems directly affected as well. Although the volume looks at the special circumstances faced by one country, Israel, its content has far-reaching implications for any nation that must commit its resources toward an all-out national defense. This book focuses on the *context* of war and its multilevel impact. It is the first to focus on war-related stress and coping at the levels of the individual, the group, and the nation-state.

The eighth book in the Series is the second in a series within this Series. *Trauma and Its Wake, Volume II: Traumatic Stress Theory, Research, and Intervention,* edited by Charles R. Figley, is the state of the art in theory, research, and treatment associated with the Post-Traumatic Stress Disorder (PTSD). And PTSD is the latest and most significant conceptualization of the negative consequences of extraordinary, catastrophic stressors. As with the first volume of *Trauma and Its Wake,* Volume II includes the thoughtful work of scholars—both researchers and clinicians—from all of the major mental health disciplines. They focus on the explication and application of knowledge about the psychosocial impact of traumatic experiences: how the *memories* of extraordinarily stressful life experiences invade the everyday life of those who survived them.

Stress and Addiction, the ninth in the Series, is a logical and welcomed addition. In all, 27 scholars collaborate to contribute 21 chapters to this volume. The chapters are divided equally among four sections. Section I, "Alcohol, Drug, and Stress Interactions," presents the evolution of the tension reduction hypothesis. Section II includes four chapters which evolve from a series of animal studies associated with the link between ethanol intake and changes in stress responses. Section III focuses primarily on human studies of the relationship between alcohol and stress responses. Chapters here range from carefully controlled laboratory studies focusing on biochemistry to surveys of the influence of support groups on substance use and abuse and on coping with stress. Section IV, "Newer Conceptions and Theoretical Developments," discusses such topics as substitution of a stress reduction hypothesis for the traditional tension reduction hypothesis, the role of setting or context in alcohol consumption and response to stressful events, and general theories of alcohol use and dependence.

This remarkable collection of solid, scientific work was carefully edited and crafted by four nationally known figures in addiction research. Edward Gottheil, M.D., Ph.D., is a Distinguished Professor of Psychiatry and Human Behavior at Thomas Jefferson University in Philadelphia and is Director of its Jefferson Center for Studies of Alcohol and Addictions. Keith A. Druley, Ph.D., is Associate Professor of Psychiatry and Human Behavior at Thomas Jefferson and is Chief of the Coatesville, Pennsylvania, Veterans Administration Medical Center's Substance Abuse Treatment Unit. Steven Pashko, Ph.D., works at the same treatment unit as Dr. Druley, serving as Coordinator and Social Science Analyst. The fourth editor of this collection, Stephen P. Weinstein, Ph.D., is Clinical Professor of Psychiatry and Human Behavior and is Associate Director of Thomas Jefferson University's Division of Substance Abuse Programs.

Together with this most recent volume, these Series books form a new orientation for thinking about human behavior under extraordinary conditions. They provide an integrated set of source books for scholars and practitioners interested in how and why some individuals and social systems thrive under stressful situations, while others do not.

Charles R. Figley, Ph.D.
Series Editor
Purdue University
West Lafayette, Indiana

Contents

Editors

Edward Gottheil, M.D., Ph.D.
Professor of Psychiatry and Human Behavior, Director of Jefferson Center for Studies of Alcohol and Addictions, Thomas Jefferson University, Philadelphia, Pennsylvania; Consultant, VA Medical Center, Coatesville, Pennsylvania

Keith A. Druley, Ph.D.
Chief, Substance Abuse Treatment Unit, VA Medical Center, Coatesville, Pennsylvania; Associate Professor of Psychiatry and Human Behavior, Thomas Jefferson University, Philadelphia, Pennsylvania

Steven Pashko, Ph.D.
Coordinator and Social Science Analyst, Substance Abuse Treatment Unit, VA Medical Center, Coatesville, Pennsylvania; Research Assistant Professor of Psychiatry, Thomas Jefferson University, Philadelphia, Pennsylvania

Stephen P. Weinstein, Ph.D.
Clinical Professor of Psychiatry and Human Behavior, Associate Director, Division of Substance Abuse Programs, Thomas Jefferson University, Philadelphia, Pennsylvania

Contributors

Stewart L. Baker, M.D.
Associate Director for Alcohol and Drug Dependency, Mental Health and Behavioral Sciences Service, Department of Medicine and Surgery, Veterans Administration Central Office, Washington, DC

Lisa F. Berkman, Ph.D.
Associate Professor of Epidemiology and Public Health, Yale University, School of Medicine, New Haven, Connecticut

John Brick, Ph.D.
Assistant Research Professor, Laboratory Director, Alcohol Behavior Research Laboratory, Rutgers University—Busch Campus, New Brunswick, New Jersey

Howard Cappell, Ph.D.
Addiction Research Foundation, Toronto, Canada

Kathryn H. DeTurck, Ph.D.
Center of Alcohol Studies, Rutgers University, Piscataway, New Jersey

Keith A. Druley, Ph.D.
Chief, Substance Abuse Treatment Unit, VA Medical Center, Coatesville, Pennsylvania; Associate Professor of Psychiatry and Human Behavior, Thomas Jefferson University, Philadelphia, Pennsylvania

Marc Galanter, M.D.
Professor, Department of Psychiatry, Director of Division of Alcoholism and Drug Abuse, New York University, New York, New York

Selby C. Jacobs, M.D., M.P.H.
Associate Professor of Psychiatry, Yale University, School of Medicine, New Haven, Connecticut

Stanislav V. Kasl, Ph.D.
Professor of Epidemiology, Yale University, School of Medicine, New Haven, Connecticut

Mark Edward Lender, Ph.D.
Director, Research and Sponsored Programs, Kean College of New Jersey, Union, New Jersey, Visiting Professor, Rutgers University, Center of Alcohol Studies, New Brunswick, New Jersey

Dan J. Lettieri, Ph.D.
Research Psychologist, National Institute on Alcohol Abuse and Alcoholism, Rockville, Maryland

Robert W. Levenson, Ph.D.
Professor, Department of Psychology, University of California, Berkeley, California

Stephen A. Lisman, Ph.D.
Associate Professor and Director of the Psychological Research and Training Clinic, Department of Psychology, State University of New York at Binghamton, Binghamton, New York

G. Alan Marlatt, Ph.D.
Professor of Psychology and Director of the Addictive Behaviors Research Center, Department of Psychology, University of Washington, Seattle, Washington

Jules H. Masserman, M.D.
Emeritus Professor of Psychiatry, Northwestern University School of Medicine, Chicago, Illinois; President, World Association of Social Psychiatry

Joanne Miller, B.S.
Department of Pharmacology, Thomas Jefferson University, Philadelphia, Pennsylvania

Kenneth C. Mills, Ph.D.
Profile Associates, Chapel Hill, North Carolina

Adrian M. Ostfeld, M.D.
Anna M.R. Lauder Professor of Epidemiology and Public Health, Yale University, School of Medicine, New Haven, Connecticut

Donald V. Ottenberg, M.D.
Former Executive Director, Eagleville Hospital and Rehabilitation Center, Eagleville, Pennsylvania

Steven Pashko, Ph.D.
Coordinator and Social Science Analyst, Substance Abuse Treatment Unit, VA Medical Center, Coatesville, Pennsylvania; Research Assistant Professor of Psychiatry, Thomas Jefferson University, Philadelphia, Pennsylvania

Larissa A. Pohorecky, Ph.D.
Professor, Department of Pharmacology, Rutgers University, Center of Alcohol Studies, Piscataway, New Jersey

Robert J. Powers, Ph.D.
Clinical Assistant Professor of Psychiatry, New Jersey Medical School, Newark, New Jersey; Chief, Alcohol Treatment Program, VA Medical Center, East Orange, New Jersey

Hedwig Roggendorf, B.S.
Department of Pharmacology, Thomas Jefferson University, Philadelphia, Pennsylvania

Leonard S. Rubin, Ph.D.
Professor, Physiology/Pharmacology Department, Philadelphia College of Osteopathic Medicine, Philadelphia, Pennsylvania

Jalie A. Tucker, Ph.D.
Associate Professor of Clinical Research, Department of Psychology and Center for Alcohol Studies, Wayne State University, Detroit, Michigan

Wolfgang H. Vogel, Ph.D.
Professor of Pharmacology, Professor of Psychiatry and Human Behavior, Thomas Jefferson University, Philadelphia, Pennsylvania

Marvin Zuckerman, Ph.D.
Professor, Department of Psychology, University of Delaware, Newark, Delaware

Preface

We do live in interesting times, and can only wonder whether future generations will refer to this period as the computer, star wars, cultural shock, or nuclear age. Or, more simply, the stress age. It might also come to be known as the drug age. Societal costs attributed to alcohol problems have risen steadily and are now estimated to amount to $100 billion annually. Cocaine has taken its place alongside of marijuana, sedative-hypnotics, heroin, amphetamines, and PCP. Twenty years ago there were an estimated 10,000 cocaine users. Ten years ago there were 100,000. Currently, it is estimated that there are over 20 million users buying over $30 billion worth of the drug each year.

Covariation, of course, does not imply a cause-effect relationship. Nevertheless, the possible associations of stress, drinking, and drugs have become major issues in the public mind and the scientific literature. Our purpose for the Seventh Annual Coatesville-Jefferson Conference, and for this volume, then, was to bring together leading experts from many disciplines to review what was known, what kinds of studies were being done, and what theoretical developments seemed most likely to further our understanding with respect to the interactions of "Stress and Addiction."

The image of the executive coming home to suburbia after a tense day at the office and being greeted at the door by his wife with a martini, a kiss, and the newspaper, in varying order except that the martini comes first, is part of our cultural heritage. It is common knowledge that drinking and drugs promote relaxation, reduce anxiety, improve sleep, and make it easier to relate to others. We see the camaraderie of former all-American, athletic heroes drinking together in television commercials. In our comic strips it is difficult to imagine how Andy Capp or Mr. Lockhorn would make it through the day without chemical support. We read about the peaceful and happy lotus-eaters. But the problems of drinking and drugs are also common knowledge, and in sharp contrast to the above images are those of the thirsty panhandler, the boozer being thrown out of the saloon, the nasty drunk, the opium fiend, and the speed freak. Clearly, the effects of alcohol and drugs on mood, tension, and behavior are neither simple nor consistent.

The first and still relevant laboratory studies of this complex relationship were conducted in the forties by Masserman and are described by him in Section I of this volume entitled "Alcohol, Drug, and Stress Interactions." Even though the conceptual origins of the tension reduction hypothesis (TRH), according to Lender, could have been inferred from the attitudes and drinking practices of nineteenth-century Americans, it was the classic series of experiments in which Masserman operationalized, tested, and demonstrated the tension reducing properties of alcohol that paved the way for the future scientific investigation of the area.

Not all of the subsequent studies that were done, however, supported the TRH. Druley and his coworkers, in their overview chapter, carefully trace a number of different themes regarding stress and the use of alcohol and drugs through historical as well as anthropological and cultural studies. Depending on the circumstances, stress does not always lead to drinking and drinking does not always reduce tension. Kasl et al., for example, in a large-scale community survey of elderly individuals, found little evidence to support the view that alcohol consumption was related to imputed stressors such as life events, depression, network size, neighborhood safety, functional disability, chronic illness, loss of a spouse, or having a seriously ill spouse. Lisman, following his review of laboratory and field studies of the tension reduction hypothesis, noted that there were so many inconsistencies in the findings requiring qualifications in the hypothesis as to make it almost meaningless. He concluded that TRH did not provide a systematic explanation of the available data and that we needed new questions, new approaches, and new theories. The subsequent sections of the volume, therefore, are concerned with newer animal and laboratory studies, more recent clinical and field investigations, and developing conceptions and approaches.

Section II includes four chapters deriving from animal work on "Ethanol-Induced Changes in the Stress Response." Pohorecky and Brick describe a systematic series of studies in which they examined the effects of acute and chronic administration of different doses of ethanol on corticosterone and nonesterified fatty acids (NEFA) in rats exposed to a variety of different physical and psychological stressors. The results indicated that, in general, ethanol attenuated, or protected against, stress-induced increases of blood levels of corticosterone and NEFA. There were some inconsistencies, however, related to the particular stressor, the dose level of ethanol, and the response that was being measured (corticosterone or NEFA). In the following chapter, Brick and

Pohorecky, using lesion experiments and pharmacologic manipulations, observed that different neural substrates seemed to be involved and might possibly account for some of the differences in ethanol's effects on the stress response.

Vogel et al. found that the catecholamine response of rats subjected to immobilization stress was also attenuated by low-dose ethanol. High doses of ethanol resulted in somewhat similar findings, but when the same experiments were repeated on the following day the effects were markedly changed. Part of the rationale for studying animal models is that genetic, developmental, and environmental variations can be more easily controlled. Nevertheless, the state of the animal, or previous experience, did make a difference. It was also interesting to note that even in these tightly controlled experiments using hard, objective, biochemical measures, there were wide variations in the stress response from one subject to the next and that these occurred in the rat as they do in the human.

Regarding individual differences and the effects of prior experience, DeTurck and Pohorecky studied biobehavioral responses to ethanol in rats that had been exposed to prenatal stress. The prenatally stressed rats, as compared to controls, exhibited less ethanol-induced hypothermia, more impaired swimming performance, and a reduced adrenocortical response. The authors suggest that early stress experiences may well produce persistent alterations in adult responses, neuroendocrine or otherwise, to ethanol. This approach could serve as a model for studying possible hormonal bases for individual differences in ethanol sensitivity which might influence susceptibility to dependence on the drug.

The papers included in the third section of this volume, "Contributions from Human Studies," range from descriptions of laboratory experiments similar to those reported in the previous section to clinical evaluations and naturalistic, field observations. Rubin describes a series of experiments in which he used pupillometric measurements to assess autonomic functioning in alcoholic and control subjects. Reminiscent of the findings of the animal studies, the alcoholics, as compared to controls, exhibited attenuated or deficient parasympathetic and sympathetic responses at rest, following alcohol intake, and during exposure to stress. Also, low-dose alcohol tended to normalize some of the responses of the alcoholics.

The next two chapters focus on attempts to assess the early positive and negative effects of alcohol on nonalcoholics. Using a sensitive, computerized, divided attention task, Mills was able to detect cognitive impairments in nonalcoholics given even relatively low doses of alcohol, and is currently seeking to determine whether early differences in cognitive sensitivity may be related to risk for developing alcoholism. Levenson examined short-term effects of alcohol on a range of brain, cardiovascular, mood, and behavioral variables. He suggests that many of the effects that were demonstrated could be construed as positive and beneficial and, while more complex than could be subsumed under a tension reduction hypothesis, did appear to have a stress dampening and therefore reinforcing effect. He wonders, and is currently investigating, whether these effects are greater in the children of alcoholics, and in individuals with outgoing, impulsive, antisocial, and aggressive personalities.

In a clinical study, anxiety, locus of control, and coping styles of alcoholic veterans were assessed by Pashko and Druley and examined in relation to tension reduction theory. The finding that patients who felt less able to exert control over their environments also exhibited elevated scores on measures of anxiety was interpreted as supporting such a theoretical approach and suggested a variety of avenues for further study.

The final two chapters of this section are concerned with the influence of social support groups on substance use and abuse and on coping with stress. Ottenberg describes his observations while serving as a consultant to groups of homeless street people, parents of murdered children, major league baseball, and the Peace Corps. Although the members of these groups experience distinctly different types of stress requiring different types of coping strategies, they share in common a feeling of unconnectedness and a sense of powerlessness and benefit from the intense, nurturing social support provided by mutual self-help groups. Galanter reports decreased substance abuse and anxiety in individuals joining the Divine Light Mission and Unification Church. Furthermore, he found that the stronger the feelings of affiliation to the sect the greater the benefit. Both Ottenberg and Galanter strongly recommend that professionals pay more attention and learn more about the principles governing the effectiveness of these support groups.

The fourth and last section addresses "Newer Conceptions and Theoretical Developments." Cappell, over a decade ago, in a systematic review of studies relating to the tension reduction hypothesis, was one of the first to point out the inconsistencies in the findings and question the explanatory power of the TRH. In his chapter he reviews the more recent animal and human research. While he still finds that under different conditions alcohol may either reduce or increase tension, as indicated by various physiological, biochemical, or self-report measures, accumulating knowledge now provides more satisfactory explanations of the different findings in terms of expectancies, individual differences, the type of stressor, the dose of alcohol, and the stressed or unstressed state of the subject.

Substitution of a stress reduction hypothesis (SRH) for the TRH would, according to Powers, remove a number of apparent inconsistencies in the findings. An SRH would look not only at alterations in tension, but also at other physiological, cognitive, affective, and behavioral alterations that an individual may experience either simultaneously or in close sequence to an array of internal and external, physical and mental, and conscious and unconscious stressors impacting simultaneously or in close sequence. Taking into account the overall stress response to the vectors in the overall stressor situation makes it more understandable that different individuals would drink for the relief of different forms of stress and not for others and that the same stimulus could represent distress, mesostress, or eustress to different individuals or to the same individual, depending on time and setting.

The importance of setting or context is also underlined by Tucker. Since individuals consume alcohol in response to stressful events or negative emotional states, but do not always do so, even when alcohol is available, the task, from the viewpoint of behavioral theories of choice, becomes one of distinguishing those contexts in which alcohol will or will not be a reinforcer, or in a given context what makes alcohol consumption more preferable than other behavioral alternatives. Lettieri points out that, in addition to the number and severity of stressors, one must also consider duration as the individual progresses over time from attempting to apply existing coping strategies, to a stage where these strategies do not meet the demands and attempts are made to marshall new ones, to an exhaustion stage of inability to cope and feelings of helplessness and hopelessness. Moreover, in human studies different factors come into play at different stages of the addiction cycle. Issues during initiation and escalation of substance use are not always the same as those involved in cessation and relapse.

Zuckerman also notes that the motives for drinking in the prealcoholic phase are not necessarily the same as those in the alcoholic phase. If individuals drink to reduce tension and anxiety, then, he suggests, we would expect prealcoholics to be highly anxious persons. He cites a variety of studies which do not support such a view. Instead of being anxious, prealcoholics are more likely to demonstrate psychopathic traits, to be sensation seekers, impulsive, low in platelet MAO, and augmenters of evoked potentials who are vulnerable to overstimulation.

Alcohol reduces evoked potentials and may provide protection against stressful overstimulation by substitution for endorphins, or whatever endogenous biochemicals mediate inhibition of cortical reactivity. Over time, then, prealcoholics and high sensation seekers may learn to use and rely on alcohol for stress reduction.

In the concluding chapter of the volume, Marlatt, like Zuckerman, brings together many recent findings and conceptualizations into a more unified general view. He discusses in detail the biphasic actions of alcohol, the possible mechanisms whereby individuals consume an essentially depressant drug in order to become "high" and maintain this expectancy despite contrary evidence, and the biological, cultural, experiential, and contextual factors that shape our expectancies about alcohol and determine our behavior towards it. Finally, he considers these principles in relation to the development of alcohol dependence, treatment methods, and relapse prevention.

Although stress and addiction are both complex topics, we have come a long way in this conference toward a better understanding of them and their interactions. Some of the apparent inconsistencies in previous findings are now better understood. Our theoretical constructs are more sophisticated and their explanatory powers have become more comprehensive. In addition, many ideas have been advanced which have relevance to treatment methods and implications for further, fruitful lines of investigation.

The presentation of the conference was made possible through the cooperative efforts of the Substance Abuse Treatment Unit of the Coatesville VA Medical Center and the Jefferson Center for the Study of Alcoholism and Addiction of Thomas Jefferson University. We are indebted to Mr. James Parsons, Director of the Coatesville VA Medical Center, and Dr. Daniel Lieberman, Professor and Acting Chairman of the Department of Psychiatry of Thomas Jefferson University, for their support and guidance. We wish to thank Ms. Estar Acosta for her diligence, care, and good humor in coordinating the activities of the editors and contributors and for her help in collating the material and preparing the index. The conference coordinators gratefully acknowledge the financial assistance provided to the conference by McNeil Pharmaceutical, Ciba-Geigy Corporation, Wyeth Laboratories, Mead Johnson & Company, and Merrell Dow Pharmaceuticals, Inc.

STRESS
and
ADDICTION

SECTION I

Alcohol, Drug, and Stress Interactions

1

Alcoholism: Disease or Protean Dis-Ease Syndrome?

JULES H. MASSERMAN

This paper reviews a series of studies of the effects of alcohol on animals. The studies suggest that the "neurotigenic traumata" resulting from motivational conflict can be ameliorated or treated by administering small doses of alcohol to experimental animals. In this procedure, some animals become addicted. These addicted animals can be "cured" through individual retraining, group influences, and methods analogous to those used in psychotherapy. The author suggests that this animal model helps explain the addictive process as it occurs among humans. The paper further outlines the basic elements of psychotherapy required to reestablish the addict's confidence, self-respect, communal solidarity, and belief in life's purpose, meaning, and value.

If Occam's razor, *entia non sunt multiplicanda praeter necessitatem*, is used to shave off redundant postulates, only three ultimate (Ur-) propositions about human behavior remain:

- That we have always endeavored to retain our health, prolong our lives, and expand our control over our physical environment (Ur-I).

- That we seek interpersonal relationships so as to achieve greater familial, economic, and cultural securities (Ur-II).
- That we cherish various systems of beliefs in an eternal search for philosophic or religious serenity (Ur-III).

Anyone "reasonably" successful in all these spheres is regarded in his social order as being "in good physical and mental health"; indeed, the very term *health*, as derived from the Anglo-Saxon root *hāl* or *hôl*, has the triple connotation of *hale* (physical well-being), *hail!* (friendly greeting), and *wholesome* or *holy* (philosophically acceptable). Conversely, anyone who fails in his somatic, cultural, or metapsychologic adaptations must experience discomfort and anxiety (i.e., "dis-ease"), whereas the unhyphenated term "disease" should be used only for physical incapacities. However, we are prone to apply the latter term also to sociopathies supposedly beyond the subject's control. From this stems the recent tendency also to classify as a "disease" a pattern of social irresponsibility and eventual parasitism associated with the excessive intake of ethyl spirits to the point of "addiction" or "alcoholism."[1] This is despite the fact that (unless the contrary is presented at this conference) no one has yet demonstrated any determinative genetic, constitutional, dietary, infectious, or other solely physiologic causes of "alcoholism"—although, of course, an excessive intake of this or any other drug can injure and destroy body and brain tissue, impair resistance and judgment, and thus escalate the adverse effects.[2] Addiction to drink, then, can be called a "disease" only in the sense that excessive eating, sleeping, smoking, gambling, vagrancy, or lechery may also be so classified. However, experimental, clinical, and social studies may furnish a more specific appraisal.

---

[1] Adapted from my text Principles of Dynamic Psychiatry (2nd ed) (Philadelphia, WB Saunders, 1961); from Alcohol, disease or dis-ease? Am J Ment Health 5:13–15, 1966; and from my Alcohol as a Preventive of Neurosis [film] and Neuroses and Alcohol [film] (University Park, PA, Psychological Cinema Register). These experiments were repeated at the University of Vienna and reissued in a 16-mm film in color and sound, available from Steven Pashko SATU (116A5), VA Medical Center, Coatesville, PA 19320.

[2] Pattison EM: Differential approaches to the syndrome of alcoholism, in Current Psychiatric Therapies. Edited by Masserman JH. New York, Grune & Stratton, 1984. This article presents a brilliant commentary on the inadequacies of the DSM-III classification of "alcohol dependence" in the context of the variable manifestations, therapy, and prognosis of various degrees of excessive alcohol intake.

STUDIES OF THE EFFECTS OF
ALCOHOL ON ANIMALS[3]

Series A: Effects of Alcohol on Normal Behavior

In 1944 my research associates and I began training cats and monkeys in progressively more difficult tasks, first to open a box to secure a pellet of food dropped by a mechanical feeder, and then to delay this response until various sound or light signals had been given. Next (long preceding B. F. Skinner's published work on "operant conditioning"), the animals learned to manipulate an electric switch to actuate the signals and feeder, and subsequently to solve increasingly complex problems of how to work the switch a required number of times despite changes in its position and the intervention of various barriers.

If then the animal was induced by thirst to drink a diluted alcohol solution at a dose of 0.5–1.2 cc of 95% alcohol per kilogram of body weight (equivalent to one to three cocktails for an average man), its adaptive patterns became progressively impaired. Specifically, the animal first lost its capacity to work the switch efficiently; then, the different "meanings" of the conditional sensory signals were less effectively discriminated; next, the animal could no longer find or open the foodbox, although it avidly took food offered directly; and finally, it entered into an alcoholic stupor in which all stimuli—signals, switch, food, mice, etc.—ceased to have any apparent significance. Conversely, as the drug was metabolized, the animal's responses returned in reverse order: first it began to take food from the box; then it again responded to the feeding signals; next it recovered its ability to work the switch in simple positions; and finally, it regained its capacity to solve increasingly adaptive approaches to the switch and food-box, other animals, and the experimenter.

In short, alcohol progressively disorganized external orientations and learned skills until only the most elementary remained; then, as the animal recovered, it regained its perceptions, memories, and abilities in their order of complexity and efficiency.

Series B: Production of an Experimental Neurosis

If on several irregularly spaced occasions a trained cat or dog was subjected to a mild, physiologically harmless, but unexpected air blast or electric shock at the very moment it reached for the food, or if a monkey

---

[3] Masserman JH: Biodynamic Roots of Human Behavior. Springfield, IL, Charles C Thomas, 1968.

was confronted with a psychologic deterrent such as the appearance of a toy rubber snake in the food box, the situation obviously became motivationally conflictual. In response to several repetitions of these and other experimental manipulations that induced an adaptational impasse, drastic changes in behavior occurred clearly corresponding to neurotic human patterns so that both may be subsumed under the following headings.

Manifestations of "anxiety." The animal crouched and trembled with hair erect and pupils dilated; breathed rapidly, shallowly, and irregularly; and had a fast, pounding pulse and a markedly increased blood pressure. Special physiologic and neuromuscular studies concurrently indicated the mobilization of "emergency mechanisms" for fight or flight that also paralleled those in the human.

Phobias and startle reactions. These increased markedly in response to "symbolic" stimuli associated with the traumatic experience, i.e., the formerly welcomed light or bell signals, or when, though hungry, the animal was offered food pellets similar to those previously accepted. As in human neuroses, the aversions quickly became more generalized; the animal elsewhere developed severe startle reactions to sudden lights, sounds, constricted spaces, and other stimuli reminiscent of its traumatic experiences, lost its sexual drive, and became aggressive toward other animals and the experimenter. Some monkeys also displayed substitutive "schizoid" patterns such as working nonexistent switches and chewing imaginary food, and yet refusing real food and drink to the point of physical deterioration.

Series C: Alcohol as a Preventive of Neuroses

A normal animal trained as in Series A was given 1 cc of ethyl alcohol per kilogram of body weight and, while thus mildly intoxicated, was subjected every second day for two weeks to various intensities of air blasts and/or electric shocks at the moment of taking food. These ordinarily "neurotinegic" traumata, if sufficiently severe and frequent, again induced mild and transient hesitation in feeding, but the animal developed none of the dramatic and persistent aberrations of behavior produced in Series B. Conversely, if the preventive doses of alcohol were discontinued and the animal was again subjected to the same conflictual experiences for a few more days, a full-blown neurosis usually developed.

Human analogies hardly need elaboration. As we have seen, beer and wine were long ago utilized by man to mitigate the horrors of his primeval milieu, and we still are inclined to take a "bracer" before the presumed uncertainties of asking for a raise, proposing marriage, or demanding a divorce.

Series D: Effects of Alcohol on Neurotic Behavior

If now the "neurotic" animals described in Series B were induced to drink about 1 cc of alcohol in solution per kilogram of body weight, their newly complex reactions were in turn partially disintegrated, permitting earlier, simpler goal-orientated (i.e., more "normal") responses, such as conditional feeding, to break through. Indeed, neurotic animals, when mildly intoxicated, often attempted to reassert group dominance in a manner reminiscent of what occurs at human cocktail parties.

Series E: Neurosis and Alcohol Addiction

Of all the animals who experienced repeated mild intoxicants, about half apparently associated the odor or taste of alcohol with relief from conflict and inhibition and *began to prefer food or milk containing alcohol to plain milk*—i.e., they developed an "addiction to alcohol." Moreover, this avidity persisted until their underlying neurosis was "cured" by individual retraining, group influences, or other methods analogous to those employed in human psychotherapy.

Series F: Therapy of Animal Neuroses

As described in detail elsewhere, this consisted of various combinations of environmental press, motivational resolution, individual retraining, and group rehabilitation. As normal adaptive behavior was restored, the intake of alcohol correspondingly diminished.

RELEVANCE TO HUMAN BEHAVIOR

But the question may well be asked: Do these animal experiments have any clinical relevance? Let us examine a few parallels to human behavior.

Psychiatric and psychoanalytic studies of addicts have indicated that the ingestion of alcohol or other neuroleptics clouds posttraumatic perceptions, ameliorates mnemonic tensions, partially dissolves repressions and inhibitions, and thereby permits previously repressed drives to find release in action. The alcoholic also titillates his "oral" desires and may continue to drink himself into a regressive torpor. The neurotic who has found these escapes from intrapersonal and social conflicts—however illusory and evanescent—therefore continues to use alcohol to the point of chronic addiction. Regrettably, in many cultures, including our own, intoxication is accepted to a considerable degree as a mitigating circumstance for the expression of erotic (including homosexual), aggressive, or destructive conduct that would be severely condemned in a completely sober person. Indeed, alcohol intake, sometimes to excess, is associated with many social, patriotic ("Gentleman, a toast to the Queen!") and religious rituals. Historically, men (and women) have nearly always everywhere concocted and consumed various nepenthics and substances allied to mescal, marijuana, cocaine, and opiates, as well as ethers and alcohols, to guard against or release them from real or fantasied threats of disappointment or injury. Accordingly, we as physicians also prescribe various sedative (sitting) or hynotic (sleeping) drugs to troubled patients to ease their pains, dull their perceptions, blunt their fears, and give them temporary but welcome surcease until we can help them more substantially to resolve their somatic, interpersonal, and/or existential dysfunctions.

COMPREHENSIVE TREATMENT
OF ALCOHOLISM

This is a topic upon which, with greater or less futility, billions of words have been spoken and millions written, and which presumably will again be dealt with in this symposium—a word, incidentally, derived from the Greek for "drink together." However, perhaps the rationale of integrating various modalities will be more evident because of the previous discussion.

Physicians who have taken the Hippocratic Oath have thereby pledged themselves to treat the whole patient in his unique milieu rather than merely his presenting complaints or somatic disabilities. In alcoholism there are, therefore, two patients: the "alcoholic" and the society that, also being "dis-eased," tends to condemn and outlaw rather than rehabilitate him. Comprehensive therapy (Greek *thereapeien* = service) therefore must serve them both as follows:

Individual. The physician approaches the patient not as a DSM-III "alcohol dependent" *sui generis, but as a complexly troubled human being seeking medical relief and social guidance.* Bodily dysfunctions are to be alleviated by every means available, including carefully prescribed benzodiazepines or hypnotics in small, guarded doses as a substitute for alcohol to dull painful memories, diminish apprehension, and quiet agitation, with the dangers of synergistic action and substitute addictions always being kept in mind. After three days of abstinence from alcohol, 0.5 g of Antabuse or of the milder-acting deterrent drug Stopethyl may be taken daily for several months in the *presence of the spouse* or other mentor, with the full understanding that even a single omission on any pretext undeniably signals an intent to resume drinking (Ur-I).

However, in all comprehensive therapy, such mixed suggestive and pharmacologic measures are merely the first stage of treatment. As soon as the patient's tensions and anxieties have abated sufficiently to make him more accessible and cooperative, every effort must be made to reevoke his initiative, restore his strength, renew his skills, and encourage him to regain confidence and self-respect that can come only from useful accomplishment.

Social. Concurrently, since "No man is an Island, entire of itself," the therapist, whatever his specialty, has a broader task: to recognize that his patient may be deeply concerned about sexual, marital, occupational, and other problems that can seriously affect his well-being. This involves exploration, varying in depth and duration, but always discerning and tactful, of the attitudes and values the patient has derived from his past experiences, his present goals and tribulations, his effective (normal), socially ineffective (neurotic or "sociopathic"), or bizarrely unrealistic (psychotic) conduct, the ways in which alcohol relieves or exacerbates his current difficulties, and whether they are accessible to various methods of medico-psychiatric therapy.

Retrospective reviews can be combined with gentle reasoning, personal guidance, and progressive social explorations to help the patient alter past misconceptions and prejudices, abandon childlike or escapist patterns of behavior that have long since lost their effectiveness, revise goals and values, and adopt a more realistic, productive, and lastingly rewarding ("mature") style of life. In this skillfully directed reeducation (good psychotherapy, despite recent fads to the contrary, is about as "nondirective" as good surgery), the enlightened cooperation of family, friends, employer, organizations such as Alcoholics Anonymous, or other sources of effective guidance and support may, with the patient's assent, be secured and utilized to the full. By such means the patient's second Ur-needs will be strengthened by renewed communal solidarity and security—a *sine qua non* of comprehensive treatment.

Finally, and to mitigate the third or metaphysical Ur-anxiety, the patient's philosophic or other convictions, instead of being ignored or undermined, should be respected and strengthened insofar as they furnish him with what each of us requires: a belief in life's purpose, meaning, and value. In this respect, medical and other truly humanitarian sciences can never be in conflict with philosophy or religion, since all are designed by a beneficient providence to preserve, cheer, and comfort man and thereby constitute a trinity to be respected by any therapist deeply concerned with man's health and sanity.

The milieu. Therapists must value the regard the public has for them not only as skilled technicians but also as dedicated humanitarians deserving the highest respect and confidence, if patients are to continue to come at all for the comprehensive care they need. Differences of professional opinion, as in any scientific discipline, are acceptable; but we must face the fact that, of late, public polemics, a trade-union image, and sometimes blatant economic and political partisanships have diminished and impaired the trust medical and other therapists must inspire if they are to serve both patients and society to their best advantage.

In this regard, physicians have a double duty to correct current medico-legal misconceptions as to the nature and therapy of addictions, whether to alcohol or other drugs. First, we must make clear that addicts should not be encouraged to consider themselves helpless victims of some mysterious genetic or metabolic "disease" for which they cannot be held responsible; and second, we must work to establish properly planned and staffed comprehensive health-care facilities for preventing and treating the personal and cultural causes of drug addictions in order to counter their growing threat to individual and social welfare.

2

Alcohol, Stress, and Society: The 19th-Century Origins of the Tension Reduction Hypothesis

MARK EDWARD LENDER

The Tension Reduction Hypothesis (TRH) emerged in its modern form in the late nineteenth century, reflecting early medical and social interest in the effects of stress on drinking behavior and the tensions inherent in an industrializing society. The most articulate professionals concerned with the TRH were the members (mostly physicians) of the Association for the Study and Cure of Inebriety, who linked social tensions to drinking problems. Medical comment on the TRH was frequent after the 1870s, but satisfactory explanations failed to emerge. The idea, however, was fixed in lay and professional opinion before 1900, awaiting the modern alcohol research effort.

The question of why people drink, and especially why they drink to excess or to alcoholism, has been a matter of considerable debate in American history. Any number of hypotheses on the subject have had

The author gratefully acknowledges the assistance of Penny Booth Page, Librarian at the Rutgers Center of Alcohol Studies, who commented extensively on an earlier draft of this paper. Francis Siburn, at Kean College of New Jersey, graciously provided secretarial support.

their proponents, although some ideas have proved more intriguing and enduring than others. Of these, the belief in a causal link between stress and drinking has had a particular appeal to the lay, the research, and the medical communities. Images of men and women using the bottle to escape the pressures and anxieties of the job or the difficulties of family situations have served as staples in literature, while business, industry, and professional groups generally have recognized the complications of tension-related alcohol abuse as a practical reality. Alcohol research has also accepted the likelihood of this relationship, although without being able to explain it fully. Now known as the Tension Reduction Hypothesis (TRH), the question has attracted the attention of an increasingly sophis-ticated research effort on the part of scientists in a number of disciplines (e.g., 1, 2, 3).

This research effort, however, is relatively new—or at least so it would appear from the present scientific literature on drinking and stress. Most modern authorities look to the work of Walter Cannon as the traditional beginning of TRH experimentation. Cannon (4), who conducted his in-vestigations over the first quarter of the twentieth century, was interested in the relations of stress and disease. He was the first to demonstrate that psychological stimuli could activate the adrenal medulla in experimental animals and humans, but few others followed immediately in his line of inquiry (5). With the exception of some relatively isolated studies, dec-ades elapsed before experimental reports emerged on the subject again with any frequency. Indeed, when E. M. Jellinek (6) carried out his classic reviews of the alcohol research literature in the late 1930s and early 1940s, the absence of a substantial body of stress-related reports struck him as remarkable. There was a general belief, he observed, that people drank to relieve tension, but no one had adequately tested this idea or the related question of whether alcohol actually did reduce stress in humans.

These questions defied ready answers even as research on the TRH became increasingly active over the 1950s and 1960s; in fact, the litera-ture did not expand to any major extent until the mid-1960s. At this point, work on alcohol-related conflict and neuroses lent credence to some aspects of the TRH—in particular the notion that many people did indeed drink for the purpose of relieving stress—but the precise role of alcohol in the process remained largely a mystery. In any case, despite the recent interest in the matter, and the high quality of much of the new research, the point here is that the bulk of the experimental literature on the TRH is now less than two decades old (e.g., 1).

Yet in tracing the lineage of the Tension Reduction Hypothesis, too close a focus on the experimental literature is misleading in some important respects. It has partly obscured the recognition that stress, broadly defined, has been a significant part of the medical and social reform literature of drinking and alcoholism since the last quarter of the nineteenth century—that is, for at least a generation before Cannon reported his initial results. This essay will focus on some of the more important aspects of this earlier interest in the TRH; in particular it will concentrate on the idea as it emerged in the work of a small but articulate group of physicians actively engaged in alcoholism research and treatment in the years after the Civil War, and used by them to explain the nature of drinking-related problems, both individual and social. The thinking of these individuals, while not in the experimental vein of today, arguably provided a large measure of impetus to later scientific interest in the connections between alcohol and stress. What follows, then, will shed new light on the origins of the TRH as we currently understand it, and suggest why it grew and evolved as it initially did.

THE TENSION REDUCTION HYPOTHESIS: SOME HISTORICAL BACKGROUND

We should note at the outset that stress in the nineteenth century had much the same meaning it does today. It involves anxieties and tensions engendered by the various tribulations and worries of life, as well as more serious psychological trauma. In a recent study of the TRH explanation of drinking behavior, Lisman, Keane, and Noel based their work on a typically broad understanding of stress. The term included, they emphasized, most situations calling on human adaptive resources; such specific circumstances as fear and anger, as well as affective states such as anxiety and depression, all fell under the rubric of stress (7). All of this would have made perfect sense to the medical community a century ago, and it is in this broad meaning that we will consider stress here.

By whatever definition, however, stress, at least as a reason for drinking, did not become part of the alcohol vocabulary until after the Civil War. The timing here is a significant point: The postbellum years saw the United States facing the full brunt of the industrialization process, which was in many respects a wrenching experience. The shift from a predominantly agricultural society to a nation built in great measure on business and heavy industry, with its intricate and demanding economic relationships, was a matter of concern to millions of Americans. The rising new society, at least in the minds of many, demanded clear thinking and efficient managers and workers if it was to function for the good of all. Any disruptive elements—human or otherwise—were likely to provoke a sharp response (8). This outlook clearly helped shape popular attitudes toward alcohol, which had come under heavy fire even before the sectional conflict, as a threat to industrial society.

As early as the 1840s, temperance workers decried the role of Demon Rum as productive of accidents, waste, and inefficiency in the workplaces of the nation, and many members of the rising industrial elite took up the cry. Antebellum railroad managers, for example, were almost phobic in their concerns over the potential for mayhem inherent in drunken train crews; and by the turn of the century, some of the leading industrialists of the land, including Andrew Carnegie and John D. Rockefeller, saw drinking problems as a major social and economic concern (9). But these protests focused on the results of drinking—worker absences, industrial accidents, and the like—not on why people drank in the first place.

Gradually, however, the nature of concerns over alcohol changed, and by the later 1800s it was clear that the industrialization of America had produced a new fear—many citizens came to believe that somehow, by some process that no one fully understood, life in the new society was actually driving people to drink. The demands of social interaction, as a missive of the National Temperance Society (10) explained the matter, had become "a perpetual whirl," sending the unwary to "the cordial or tonic" for relief "until the appetite" was "confirmed and, Satan . . . wound around his victim the chain of habit" (p. 20). This was a typical view, and there is simply no telling who first made this sort of observation. But we do know that it was prevalent, a public belief, as an explanation for drinking—especially problem drinking—over the last quarter of the century.

THE STRESSFUL SOCIETY

If some reformers lamented the connection between alcohol and the industrial age, the question also attracted a great deal of intelligent thought. The most sustained attention came from the medical profession, or at least that part of it concerned with the research and treatment of alcohol addiction. The chief vehicle for such opinion was the American Association for the Cure of Inebriates (a name soon changed to the Association for the Study and Cure of Inebriety), a group founded in

1870 by medical proponents of the disease conception of alcoholism and other addictions. Writing in the professional and lay press (and in their own quarterly, the *Journal of Inebriety*), members touched on virtually all aspects of alcohol problems over the late nineteenth and early twentieth centuries, and they considered at length the matter of stress as a cause of drinking problems (e.g., 11, 12).

The work of Association physicians anticipated a good deal of modern interest in the TRH, focusing both on the question of whether Americans drank to relieve the stress supposedly inherent in the industrial age and on the matter of whether alcohol actually reduced stress. On the first count, Association members were in general agreement. As civilization became more advanced and complex, wrote Dr. George Beard (13) in 1876, those enmeshed in it came under correspondingly greater stress. It was no surprise, he noted, to find drinking problems increasing as a result, along with other stress-related health complications. Beard, an early specialist in addictions, found his comments well received, and in fact they were only typical. Dr. Thomas Davidson Crothers (14), one of the leading proponents of alcoholism research and treatment in the later nineteenth century, struck a similar chord a year later in the *Journal of Inebriety*. "The severe mental strain incident to our peculiar civilization, with its struggle for wealth and power, precipitates this affection" for palliative drinking which, he warned, too frequently led to alcoholism (p. 66).

This concern over the stressful nature of industrial society led to a peculiar refinement in the early TRH. There was also an assumption that the individuals most responsible for the management of the new society were at particular risk given the anxieties inherent in business schedules, the potential for failure, and the hectic pace of economic competition. "Those who use their brains to excess," Crothers speculated, were especially vulnerable, and the pages of the *Journal of Inebriety* were interspersed with case studies that seemingly proved the point. One practitioner (15) reported two patients, "men of education and of far more than ordinary intelligence," who resorted to alcohol for relief after "any weighty business transaction . . . that brought about the unfortunate condition of weariness of brain and nervous system" (pp. 133–134). Crothers (16), writing of the patients in his asylum near Hartford, Connecticut, cited instance after instance of alcoholism among business managers and stockbrokers. All were men, he reported, "under the usual strain" inherent in risky business operations or with histories of "overwork under conditions of great excitement" (pp. 226–227). Actual business failure, Crothers (17) also noted, made matters worse, as "adversity," he claimed, "has been recognized for a long time as preceding inebriety" (pp. 258–259). All of this, the director of a Boston treatment facility (the Washingtonian Home) reported (18) after surveying his patients in 1901, was cause for national alarm. "We need to be educated as to what and how to eat and drink, how to sleep, and rest," he insisted, in order "to overcome as far as possible the restlessness and feverish anxiety of this age . . . Hurry and worry has become a national habit, and decidedly injurious to health" (p. 514).

This "hurry and worry" also had an impact on domestic life. Historians have extensively documented the tensions generated in American families during the industrialization process. The stress inherent in the changing roles of men and women in the maintenance of the home, child rearing, and the economic support of the family was arguably quite high (e.g., 19, 9). In the view of reformers, social critics, and many doctors, women in particular felt the strain of all of this, finding themselves and the security of their homes dependent on the economic fortunes of their husbands (9). While many families lived happily and prosperously during these years, others did not, and marital discord received considerable attention as a source of drinking problems in the years shortly before and after the turn of the century.

Drinking reportedly was both a cause and effect in this regard. As early as the 1850s, one dry reformer found women blaming their intemperance on their husbands; frustrated by the drunkenness of their spouses, they too found solace in the bottle (20). And while this dry crusader argued that such cases were rare before the Civil War, drunkenness in wives apparently increased—or, more likely, became more evident as temperance activity focused increasing attention on the problem—as the century drew to a close.

Decades later, the accounts were the same—only better documented. Careful investigations by such scholarly groups as the Committee of Fifty (21) found that alcoholism was more prevalent in married than in unmarried women, and that "domestic trouble" was one of the chief reasons (p. 67). Thomann's (22) statistical study of alcoholics reported similar findings. By the 1890s, Evangeline Booth (23) found that inebriate couples were common in the families aided by the Salvation Army, and a history of drinking in other family members, as well, was often a notable characteristic for alcoholic women. One study cited by Booth noted that 37% of the inebriate women had intemperate fathers, 8% had intemperate mothers, and 19% alcoholic brothers or sisters (23, p. 11). And, at the turn of the century it was also common to find physicians attributing drinking problems in women to "the worry of domestic life" or "the anxieties connected with the home and children," and particularly an unhappy marriage (24, p. 415; 25, p. 191).

Although no one was able to establish a definite causal link between family concerns and the growth of problem drinking in women (and no one has yet), modern research has at least strongly associated them. Women apparently do drink more readily than men "in response to some environmental stress"; and like men alcoholics, they often come from families having serious alcohol problems (26, pp. 808–809). It is probable, then, that these contemporary observations did indicate the prevalence of drinking by many women in order to cope with tension-related difficulties.

These observations, we should note, were not the results of experimental tests of the TRH. Rather they were built upon case studies compiled in the private practices of Association doctors or from the patient records of alcoholism treatment asylums. Moreover, judgments on why these patients drank to excess were quite subjective; indeed, in the early literature no record has come to light of an attempt to deal with the TRH beyond the use of case studies. Association doctors simply inferred from information gathered from their patients that they drank to relieve tension, an approach that fails to satisfy modern canons of science and medicine (e.g., 27, 1). To their credit, however, Association doctors never claimed that stress was solely responsible for motivating drinking behavior, which they generally attributed to a combination of biological and cultural factors (e.g., 16). The important point here is that the TRH—even if not by that name—was an established part of discussion on the etiology of drinking well before the turn of the century, and that contemporary medical professionals tied the phenomenon firmly to the nature of life in the newly industrialized America.

None of this, of course, is to argue in favor of the Association's views in this regard. One can look to other chapters of the American past and make equally convincing cases for social stress driving the citizenry to the bottle; and in fact, over the past decade a number of historians have done precisely that. While no firm conclusions have emerged from their studies, they have pursued some interesting speculations, for example, on the anxieties inherent in life on the frontier and the staggering levels of alcohol consumption that marked the years of westward expansion in the early republic (e.g., 19, 28, 9). Yet it remains a fact that no one addressed the possible links between drinking and stress in any coherent fashion prior to the work of the Association doctors. Thus, they deserve recognition at least for calling attention to the subject and for suggesting that social change could have a pronounced impact on why people drink.

DRINKING AND TENSION REDUCTION: EARLY EXPLANATIONS

There is general agreement today that, under certain circumstances, at least some people do drink to relieve tension. Why that should be, however, and under what conditions alcohol really does act to reduce stress, remain questions of considerable debate (e.g., 1, 2, 3). This situation describes the nineteenth- and early twentieth-century discussion of drinking and tension as well. For if Association doctors were agreed that the TRH was real, and even believed that alcohol afforded some relief from anxiety, they were never satisfied with explanations as to why.

Speculation in this regard generally involved theories on the effects of alcohol on humans. The prevailing wisdom of the period held that alcohol was a stimulant acting on the central nervous system, and initial hopes of explaining the TRH hinged on this belief. The logic was fairly straightforward: the stresses of modern life supposedly exhausted the nerves, which could lead to any number of neuroses, depression, or other mental disorders (e.g., 29, 15, 14, 16). A resort to alcohol led to the stimulation of the nervous system, the temporary restoration of which led to the release of anxiety. Indeed, this same view held that dealing with stress in this manner too often would lead to the eventual addiction of the drinker to the tension-reducing agent (15, 16).

Faith in alcohol as a stimulant, though, was never unanimous. As the nineteenth century drew to a close, the theory in fact came under effective attack and, by 1900, if not earlier, most of the medical community had abandoned the notion. Any stimulant effect, Association authors now insisted, existed only at very low doses, with the true nature of alcohol being that of a depressant. Citing the work of such European experimentalists as Kraepelin and Schmiedeberg, the pages of the *Journal of Inebriety* and other medical publications carried sometimes alarming warnings on the narcotic impact of alcohol on the brain and nervous system (e.g., 30, 29, 31, 18). Indeed, this new research made alcohol appear a greater threat than ever to a society concerned with keeping the wits of its citizenry sharp and their minds at peak efficiency.

The increasing evidence that alcohol was a depressant, however, while certainly reflecting better research on the actions of alcohol on the central nervous system, did not shed much additional light on the TRH. There was some speculation to the effect that feelings of relaxation and a relief from stress were manifestations of alcohol's narcotic impact. Yet all of this was quite fuzzy; for while most Association members readily agreed that alcohol was a depressant and an addictive substance, they also noted that research had not explained these matters in anything approaching a definitive manner (11). Thus few of them did much with these new insights in relation to the TRH. But given modern difficulties in pinning down the roles of alcohol in alleviating anxiety, we should not be surprised at similar frustrations almost a century ago.

SOME RESULTS AND CONCLUSIONS

The inability to fully explain the TRH, however, did not consign the work of Association physicians to obscurity. On the contrary, the fact that a recognized portion of the medical community believed at least that stress was a cause of drinking, and aired its views on the matter freely, attracted considerable public attention. This was no small thing in the late nineteenth and early twentieth centuries, for the public was acutely interested in drinking-related problems in these years. Indeed, the rise of the postbellum Temperance Movement virtually paralleled the rise of the early TRH, and dry leaders eagerly seized on any information—especially if it came from seemingly creditable medical sources—that placed alcohol in an unfavorable light. Thus for temperance purposes the TRH was made almost to order; and no matter what they thought about it, Association members saw their work and speculations drawn into the arena of social reform.

In fact, dry partisans made the place of alcohol in America's industrial society one of their chief issues as they mounted their drive for national prohibition (e.g., 9). The possibility that the stress and tensions of engaging in business or operating complex modern machinery might have a part in the initiation of drinking was therefore a natural issue for reformers (as well, we should note, as a genuine source of worry). And in voicing their protest, they drew directly from the early TRH literature. One tract, for example, authored by J. C. MacErlain, a Catholic priest (32), noted that the America of 1891 was "the most nervous nation on the globe," and that drinking might offer at least temporary relief to the weary (pp. 16, 30). But such relief was dangerous, MacErlain warned, in that it was a step toward intemperance and addiction. Citing the work of a number of studies, including some by Association authors, he assured his readers that the perils of alcohol more than cancelled any benefits allegedly received from their drinking.

In another, similar work, Timothy Shay Arthur made the point more vividly. Arthur was arguably the greatest writer of temperance fiction in American history (33) and his novel, *Strong Drink: The Curse and the Cure* (34), was a classic popularization of the TRH as medicine understood it in the 1870s. It was a fictional account of a young businessman breaking under the stresses of the office and turning to drink as a result. In composing the story, Arthur drew carefully on the ideas of the Association, the work of which he acknowledged later in the book. The accuracy of early views on tension and drinking aside, then, fears that one led to the other were taken quite seriously and clearly played a part in the national debate over the place and legitimacy of beverage alcohol in postbellum America.

If we can document the presence of the TRH in the temperance literature, however, it is more difficult to follow the ideas of the Association through the medical and scientific reports of the early 1900s. As the prohibitionist effort picked up steam, alcohol research all too frequently became submerged in the social and political battles of the period. The Association in particular (for reasons beyond the ken of this essay) felt the strains of the wet-dry wars, paying less and less attention to science while members became enmeshed in partisan reform activities. No longer a creditable medical group, it fell apart in the 1920s (12). Yet in its heyday, the Association doctors had made a legitimate contribution; they were among the first to call major attention to the connections between stress and drinking, and when the Association itself disappeared, the issue its membership had raised remained for others to pursue in another day.

REFERENCES

1. Pohorecky LA: The interaction of alcohol and stress: A review. Neurosci. Biobehav. Rev. 5:209–229, 1981
2. Cappell H: An evaluation of tension models of alcohol consumption, in Research Advances in Alcohol and Drug Problems, II. Edited by Gibbins YI, Kalant H, Popham RE, et al. New York, John Wiley & Sons, 1975
3. Lester D: Self-selection of alcohol by animals, human variation, and the etiology of alcoholism. A critical review. Q J Stud Alc 27:395–438, 1966
4. Cannon WB: Bodily Changes in Pain, Hunger, Fear and Rage: An Account of Recent Researches Into the Function of Emotional Excitement. New York, Appleton, 1929
5. McCarty R: Stress, behavior and the sympathetic-adrenal medullary system, in Stress and Alcohol Use. Edited by Pohorecky LA, Brick J. New York, Elsevier Biomedical, 1983
6. Jellinek EM: An outline of basic policies for a research program on problems of alcohol. Q J Stud Alc 3:103–124, 1942
7. Lisman SA, Keane TM, Noel NE: Feeling depressed, angry, shy, sexually aroused?—why not have a drink, in Stress and Alcohol Use. Edited by Pohorecky LA, Brick J. New York, Elsevier Biomedical, 1983

8. Wiebe RH: The Search for Order, 1877–1920. New York, Wang, 1967
9. Lender ME, Martin JK: Drinking in America. A History. New York, Free Press/Macmillan, 1982
10. National Temperance Society: Centennial Temperance Volume. New York, National Temperance Society and Publication House, 1877
11. Lender ME: Jellinek's typology of alcoholism. Some historical antecedents. J Stud Alc 40:361–375, 1979
12. Blumberg LU: The American Association for the Study and Cure of Inebriety. Alcsm: Clin Exp Res 2:234–240, 1978
13. Beard GM: Causes of the recent increase of inebriety in America. Quarterly Journal of Inebriety 1:25–48, 1876
14. Crothers TD: Duration, mortality, and prognosis of inebriety. Quarterly Journal of Inebriety 1:65–80, 1877
15. Remondino PC: A study of the causes and nature of dipsomania. Quarterly Journal of Inebriety 23:129–146, 1901
16. Crothers TD: Inebriety caused by psychical traumatism. Quarterly Journal of Inebriety 4:219–230, 1882
17. Crothers TD: Inebriety due to the direct action of alcohol. Quarterly Journal of Inebriety 4:255–259, 1882
18. Annual report of the Washingtonian Home. Quarterly Journal of Inebriety 23:513–517, 1901
19. Clark NH: Deliver Us from Evil: An Interpretation of American Prohibition. New York, Norton, 1976
20. Weld HH: Women and temperance. American Temperance Magazine 2:243–254, 1851
21. Koren J: Alcohol and Society. New York, Holt, 1916
22. Thomann G: Real and imaginary effects of intemperance: A statistical sketch. New York, 1884
23. Booth E: Some Have Stopped Drinking. Westerville, OH, American Issue, 1928
24. Staples HL: Alcoholism. Quarterly Journal of Inebriety 22:412–425, 1900
25. Smith H: Alcohol in relation to women. Quarterly Journal of Inebriety 23:190–193, 1901
26. Beckman LJ: Women alcoholics: A review of social and psychological studies. Q J Stud Alc 34:1228–1243, 1973
27. Cappell H, Herman CP: Alcohol and tension reduction. A review. Q J Stud Alc 33:33–64, 1972
28. Rorabaugh WJ: The Alcoholic Republic: An American Tradition. New York, Oxford University Press, 1979
29. Whyte JM: Some recent researches on alcohol: Their bearing on treatment. Quarterly Journal of Inebriety 23:294–308, 1901
30. Crothers TD: Editorial. Quarterly Journal of Inebriety 23:381–382, 1901
31. Perry JF: Treatment of delirium tremens. Quarterly Journal of Inebriety 23:480–491, 1901
32. MacErlain JC: Whither Goest Thou? Or Was Father Mathew Right? New York, Kennedy, 1908
33. Lender ME: Dictionary of American Temperance Biography: From Temperance Reform to Alcohol Research, the 1600s to the 1980s. Westport, CT, Greenwood, 1984
34. Arthur TS: Strong Drink: The Curse and the Cure. Philadelphia, Hubbard, 1877

3

Stress: Alcohol and Drug Interactions

KEITH A. DRULEY, STEWART L. BAKER,
AND STEVEN PASHKO

Stress and the use of alcohol/drugs is reviewed through historical, anthropological, and cultural studies. The importance of these studies and this perspective is emphasized. In addition, the interrelation of stress, alcohol/drug use, and mediating factors like social supports, coping skills, personality variables, and physiological responsiveness is conceptualized.

Eight thousand years ago our Neolithic forefathers, with their polished stone ax in hand, gave up the ways of the hunter and settled down in valleys to till the fields and herd animals (1). Neolithic man gave us wheat, beef, pork, milk, beans, pottery, wool, and weaving; he also gave us beer and wine (1). In early societies, alcoholic beverages served many purposes (2). Beer and wine were a source of quick energy. They were the best medicines available (3), especially for the relief of pain. They served to enhance religious feelings and to facilitate feelings of communion with God, the dead, and the tribe. In the midst of great and constant threat to survival, alcoholic beverages allowed the tribe to forget their troubles and to celebrate the rites of passage. Alcohol in the form of beer and wine was important; it was used frequently and sometimes in large quantities. As Mark Keller (2) points out, "It is hard to understand why the human liver should be endowed with enough alcohol dehydrogenase, the enzyme that catalyzes the first step in the oxidation of alcohol and does not seem to have much else to do, to metabolize a quart of whiskey a day, unless alcohol was amply present in the diet of man, or of his ancestors, in remote evolutionary times" (p. 2823).

Very early on Homo sapiens began their love-hate relationship with *spiritus fermenti*. The most ancient stories in the Old Testament suggest a very negative attitude toward drunkenness (4). Noah, who was the first tiller of the soil, planted a vineyard, "And he drank of the wine, and was drunken: and he was uncovered within his tent" (Gen. 9:21). This resulted in the curse on Canaan. The prophets carried on the tradition: Wine inflames (Isa. 5:11) and is treacherous (Heb. 2:5, Hos. 4:11). Excessive drinking was such a problem (Isa. 28:7) that priests of the temple were forbidden to drink wine when engaging in their duties (Lev. 10:9, Ezek. 44:21). The first temperance movement is recorded in the Book of Numbers. At the same time, Isaac's blessing of Jacob was, "May God give you dew from heaven, and the richness of the earth, abundance of grain and wine!" (Gen. 27:28). Yet along with these benefits the author of Proverbs not only warns of drunkenness, but decribes an alcoholic: "Who has woe? Who has sorrow? Who has strife? Who has complaining? Who has wounds without cause? Who has redness of eyes? They that tarry long at the wine" (Prov. 23:29–30). There is no condemnation of wine in the New Testament (4). However, excessive drinking is repeatedly condemned (Luke 21:34; I Tim. 3:3–8; I Pet. 4:3). Drunkenness was viewed as a characteristic of the Gentile culture. Consequently, Paul of Tarsus suggested that a thoughtful Christian should not drink at all as it might cause his weaker brother to fall back into pagan ways (Rom. 14:21).

This love-hate relationship is also found in ancient literature of the Greeks, Romans, Scandinavians, and Orientals (2, 5). But specifically in the Old and New Testaments, which so influenced our Western culture, integrative drinking is seen as a divine gift. At the same time, the authors of the Bible recognized the dangers of drunkenness and condemned drunken behavior.

These attitudes, beliefs, and customs were translated to the New World. Lender and Martin (6), in their book *Drinking in America*, note that the average American colonist drank about six gallons of absolute alcohol a year. The American colonists were "serious drinkers"; however, they were not for the most part problem drinkers. Yet there were problems (6, 7). As early as 1673, Increase Mather (8) published his sermon *Wo to Drunkards*, declaring that drinking in and of itself was a good activity from God and that drinking should be received with thankfulness; however, Mather claimed that the abuse of alcohol came from Satan, that wine was from God but drunkenness from the Devil. Colonials singled out the habitual drunkards who were considered addicted and habituated to drunkenness, not to liquor (7). Lists of drunkards were circulated and tavern owners who served them could lose their license (7). By the start of the nineteenth century, there was public recognition that these poor folks suffered from an "overwhelming," "overpowering," and "irresistible" urge for alcohol (7). However, these urges were a fault of the will, a choice made for pleasure. Benjamin Rush, in his "Inquiry Into the Effects of Ardent Spirits" (9), turned the table. He recognized that the would-be drunkard used alcohol as a free agent. Unfortunately, there occurred "a disease of the will" resulting in an "inability to refrain" and "loss of control." Rush saw the causal agent as spiritous liquors, and he termed the loss of control a disease. Further, he saw abstinence from distilled alcohol as the only cure. Rush did not see a problem with beer, wine, and cider, rather with distilled substances of any kind (9).

Rush (9) woke America up to the awful results which follow from the drinking of "ardent spirits"—poverty, disease, insanity, crime, and broken homes. Rush saw the drunkard as a victim of a socially approved custom. The temperance movement of the nineteenth century expanded on Dr. Rush's theories and translated his ideas into an action program. The drunkard was seen as the victim of the disease which was allowed to incubate and flourish in the social atmosphere of the moderate drinker. Some temperance literature suggested that moderate drinkers were the criminals and the drunkards the victims (7). The leaders of this movement were also deeply concerned about their own fine citizenry, lest they fall victim to this dreaded disease.

In the latter part of the nineteenth century, the focus shifted to the Anti-Saloon League and the drive for prohibition. The focus shifted from addictive behavior to the evil effects of alcohol. Liquor was viewed as a dangerous chemical capable of undercutting the fabric of the Republic. The saloon was seen as a breeding place for all forms of corruption including labor unrest. The liquor trust and the saloon became the enemy of good citizens and the drunk became a pest if not a menace. The impact of prohibition was at first quite dramatic, but short-lived (6).

The concept of alcoholism as a disease was rediscovered in the 1930s and 1940s through the joint efforts of Alcoholics Anonymous and the Yale Center for Alcohol Studies (7). This new look recognized alcohol as a domestic drug and not as a source of evil as was the case with the temperance and prohibition movements. Levin (7) indicates "it was recognized that for some unknown reason a specific group of people became addicted to the drug and generally suffered painful consequences. Alcoholism became the only popular and scientifically accepted person-specific drug addiction" (7, p. 162). This new concept set the stage for what has been a most productive half century dedicated towards better understanding alcohol and its role in society.

CULTURAL DETERMINANTS OF DRINKING

In an attempt to understand the importance of alcohol in preliterate and modern societies (13, 14), attention was directed to the study of the cultural determinants of drinking. In the late 1930s, Horton noted that members of most cultures drink alcoholic beverages and that drinking patterns were persistent in the face of competing customs and attempts at prohibitions (10, 11). Using the Yale Cross-Cultural Survey, he studied 57 preliterate cultures in an attempt to understand what appeared to be an almost universal need, a need satisfied primarily by drinking alcoholic beverages. A consistent and popular idea related alcohol drinking to anxiety reduction. Horton's results suggested a strong correlation between what he labeled "subsistence insecurity" and drunkenness. This association was even stronger when the degree of acculturation was included.

Field (12) disputed Horton's results. Although his criticisms did not necessarily hold up, he did suggest that levels of social organization should be taken into account. In addition, he examined the relationship between certain child-training variables and drunkenness. Bacon, Barry, and Child (13, 14) reviewed the work by Horton and Field using an extended data base of 139 preliterate tribes. For the most part, they confirmed Horton's positive association between drinking/drunkenness and tribal anxiety. In the process of reevaluating Field's conclusions, they confirmed his finding of a positive association between frequency of drunkenness and a more primitive hunting economy. This positive association appeared, in part, to be related to differences in child-rearing practices. The hunting/gathering economy pressured children toward obedience and responsibility. The Bacon, Barry, and Child Studies (13, 14, 15, 16) highlighted the wide variation in degree to which preliterate societies responded to the dependency needs of infants, children, and adolescents. This variation in the degree of dependency-independency conflict could now be evaluated as a causal agent affecting the amount of drinking and drunkenness tolerated by a primitive culture. To quote Bacon et al.:

> It was hypothesized that adequate indulgence of the dependency needs of infants, mild and nonpunitive socialization pressures towards self-reliance and achievement and the acceptance of help-seeking behavior in adulthood would be associated with a low level of conflict over dependency and with relative sobriety. Conversely high levels of drinking and drunkenness would be associated with the reverse conditions. It was hypothesized further that the drinking situation might permit the temporary resolution of such conflict by simultaneously permitting these effects: satisfying of the dependency or help-seeking motives, the enjoyments of fantasies of achievement and success, and a reduction in anxiety associated with the state of conflict. This resolution of conflict might then operate as a reinforcement of drinking behavior. (14, p. 864)

Studies by Bacon in 1974 (15) and 1976 (16) yielded substantial evidence to support these hypotheses.

In a more recent cross-cultural study, Straton, Zeiner, and Parades (17) suggest that American Indian tribes with a hunting/gathering tradition have more serious drinking problems than do tribes which emphasize communal values and ceremonies within an agricultural economy. Also, Western tribes that have become more acculturated have less serious problems with alcohol than those which have maintained ceremonies and values of their hunting tradition.

Current literature on the interaction of stress, drugs, and alcohol pays little attention to and seldom makes use of cross-cultural, historical, and anthropological studies. The importance of these approaches to the understanding of drinking, drunkenness, and problem drinking cannot be overemphasized. Early on, these approaches suggested:

1. The importance of anxiety/stress as determinants.
2. The role of integrative drinking.
3. The dependency/independency conflict.
4. The importance of social supports.
5. The role of aggression/assertiveness.

Finally, cross-cultural studies, by their power to explain drinking/drug-taking behavior in preliterate societies, allow us to evaluate our concepts about alcohol/drug use, which tend to be very time/culture bound.

PSYCHO/SOCIAL/PHARMACO DYNAMICS

We have been conducting a review of the current literature on stress, drugs, and alcohol for the past four years. Our review suggests that there are three major ways of conceptualizing alcohol, drug, and stress interactions. These focus on:

1. Interaction of stress, drinking, and drug taking.
2. Mediators of stress and the failure of adaptation.
3. The physiological interaction of drugs, alcohol, and stress.

Track I—Interaction of Stress, Drinking, and Drug Taking

The studies of drinking as a response to the stresses of aging have been reviewed by Berkman (18), Nowak (19), and Finney and Moos (20). Overall, these reviews support the hypothesis that life stressors trigger drinking among younger and older populations. Review articles also suggest that there may be an increase in drug use due to the stresses of aging (21–24). A recent study (25) suggests that first time, older DWI (Driving-While-Intoxicated) offenders had experienced stressful events, especially the loss of a significant other. Likewise, Dudley et al. (26) have suggested a high frequency and magnitude of life changes (stressors) among heroin and alcohol addicts.

A series of studies (27, 28, 29) and a review article (30) outline the following constellation of characteristics as describing alcoholics and DWI offenders. As a group, alcoholics and DWI offenders have generally experienced recent stressful events which they personally consider more upsetting than normals. In addition, they are more aggressive and depressed, less responsible, and have lower self-esteem. In contrast to normals, they use more projection, are more fatalistic, and use more tranquilizers. This group has a very high rate of divorce and arrests. Alcoholics and subjects with DWI convictions report that they drink to relieve tension, and for social relaxation and comfort; however, they also report that drinking causes them serious problems. In general, they spend the majority of their leisure time drinking with friends and are less involved in church, reading, and family activity.

Literature in this area suggests that the stresses and strains of daily living are associated with the problem drinker under certain conditions and with certain populations. Literature also suggests that heavy drinking is associated with other high risk behaviors (e.g., driving, poor use of leisure time, aggressive acting out) (31–39).

Track II—Mediators of the Stress, Failure of Adaptation

The general public, clinicians, and scientists have been comfortable with the idea that there is a causal connection between life's stresses and strains and problems of adaptation.

There is a robust body of literature dealing with the interrelationship of stressors and failures to adapt (40, 41, 42, 53, 54). This literature includes not only major life events but also the compounding effects of strains, discords, and annoyances (43, 44). Data from these studies suggest that there is some evidence for a causal relationship not only between major events but also between strains, discords, and annoyances and a variety of physical illnesses. In these studies, the dependent variable—illness—covers medical/physical symptoms (45), general illness (46, 47), prognosis of pregnancy (48), health status (49, 50), myocardial infarction (51), cancer in children (52), and cardiovascular illness (42, 53).

Another category of research has assessed the relationship between life events/life experiences and a variety of mental health problems. The latter include psychological impairment (55), depression (41, 43, 54, 56, 57), neurosis (58, 59), psychiatric symptoms (60–62), psychological symptoms (63, 64), and mental distress (65).

Some of the work listed above allows us to consider the interaction of life crises and discord on a number of physical and psychological problems. As an example, Thorell (42), in a two-year prospective study, evaluated the effects of discords and life changes on blood pressure, serum lipids, serum transaminases, illness patterns, and neuroses in a population consisting of over 5,000 male building construction workers.

Another cluster of studies has focused on specific stressful events as they affect mental/physical health. These include the association between disruptive relocation experiences and cancer in children (52), behavioral and perceived stress on the health status of new mothers (66), health consequences of unemployment (67), migration and mental illness (68), and the effects of maternal stress on the course and outcome of pregnancy (69). A most important area of research focuses on stress (splashdown in Skylab, loss of a spouse) and a measurable related dysfunction in the immune system (70, 71).

To round out the picture, there are a number of studies dealing with the negative health consequences of such high stress professions as medicine (72), clergy (73), and law enforcement (74). Social scientists and epidemiologists have pursued this connection vigorously (40, 41, 47, 50, 54, 80). However, when researchers have considered a simple and direct relationship, one which assumes that stress is a sufficient cause for failures in adaptation, they have been disappointed. This has resulted in more sophisticated models that include other variables which may either enhance, modulate, or mediate the association. The factors that have been studied in detail are social supports (75, 77), sex differences (15, 28, 81), coping skills (47, 50, 82–86), the interaction of life's stresses and strains/discords and hassles (41, 44), personality factors (47, 49, 86–90), deviant perception of both the impact of an event and one's perceived reaction (25, 65, 89), and mediating physiological factors (84, 87–90).

A better understanding of the way these mediators, modulators, and enhancers work is critical to our developing more effective prevention and treatment programs. Research focusing specifically on the interaction of stress, social systems, and failures of adaptation has become very sophisticated. Reviews (20, 44, 77, 91, 92, 93) suggest that these associations are highly complex and that, for the most part, previous results need to be reviewed in the light of these outlined methodological problems. However, all of the reviewers suggest that there is sufficient evidence of an association to proceed with research in the area. Future research should focus on the dimension of social support along the lines of quantity/quality (94), satisfaction/dissatisfaction (41), and structure (77, 95).

Track III—Physiological Interaction of Alcohol and the Stress Response

The third track focuses on the physiological interaction of alcohol and the stress response. Related research is reviewed by Pohorecky, Masserman, Vogel, and Brick in this volume. However, we will briefly review one key fact about alcohol as a pharmacological agent and tie this into our historical perspective.

Alcohol is a psychoactive drug that works on higher mental centers affecting mood, feeling, anxiety, and so on. Alcohol does have very specific effects (96) on the physiological components of a number of systems (e.g., nervous, cardiovascular, hormonal, gastrointestinal). However, irrespective of these *specific* effects, it has broad-ranging, nonspecific effects. In your imagination, compare the mood resulting from administration of alcohol in a research setting to the mood effect resulting from a double vodka and collins before a banquet. The resulting moods would most likely be quite different. However, the physiological effects—the specific effects—would be almost identical (97). These nonspecific effects, directed by expectancy, setting, and belief systems, can greatly influence the specific drug effect responses.

Alcohol and other psychoactive drug effects are, to say the least, very complicated in the context of human/social consumption. Consequently, in alcohol, we have a mind-altering drug capable of serving as a reinforcing, discriminating, and conditioned stimulus. Nonspecific factors are important in influencing drug response. Personal belief systems about the drug and its use are built in from childhood, regularly reinforced within the context of social networks and, of course, in advertising and the media. The quality of belief systems surrounding the value—"good effects"—of this chemical meet the standards set by Festinger (98) for a belief that will survive strong contradictory evidence. Now, if at a purely biochemical level these cultural beliefs are supported, then the pervasiveness of alcohol consumption and the resistance to prohibition among the cultures of the world should come as no surprise.

Many up-to-date and excellent reviews are available (99–104) on the physiological system that underlies the stress response. The physiochemical stress response has been carefully measured in reaction to a variety of stressors ranging from military training for parachute jumping (100) to the chronic stress of living on Three Mile Island (84). Related studies also provide sophisticated controls for personality factors. In attempting to assess the effects of stressors, the most widely studied physiological parameters have been the activity of the pituitary-adrenal system (90). The question is: Can it be demonstrated that the psychoactive drug in question specifically reduces the (physiological parameters used to measure) response of the pituitary-adrenal system to a stressful stimulus? Research by Pohorecky (105, 106) and Vogel (107) suggests that alcohol has a specific stress-dampening effect on the pituitary-adrenal system in rats. Their work also suggests that there is a wide individual variability among rats as to their responsiveness to alcohol's dampening effect. Levenson (108), in a series of studies at the University of Indiana, and Lipscom, Nathan, and Wilson (109), at the Rutgers Center of Alcohol Studies, have demonstrated similar results using human nonalcoholic subjects. Of special interest in the works of Levenson and Nathan is the finding that specific clusters of subjects (e.g., those with high MacAndrew scores and high tolerance) were more susceptible to the tension-dampening effect of alcohol.

CATASTROPHIC STRESS, DRUGS, AND ALCOHOL

In conclusion and summary, we will briefly review issues relating to traumatic stress disorders, the interaction of drugs, alcohol, and the stressors of the Vietnam conflict, and the interaction of drugs, alcohol, and Post-Traumatic Stress Disorders (PTSD).

Mental health professionals have struggled with theoretical issues of post-traumatic stress from the time Freud published his Repetition Compulsion Theory in *Beyond the Pleasure Principle*. By the early 1960s, studies and theory moved from a focus on development/premorbid personality issues to a focus on the stressors and the resulting post-traumatic cluster of symptoms (110, 111). The stressors studied during this period included World War II combat (112–114), the atomic bombing of Hiroshima (115), marine disasters (116), persecution (117), and the holocaust and concentration camps (118–120). The stressors varied as did the patient samples. Work in this general area allowed Archibald (121), in his 1965 study of VA outpatients, to conclude: "A clear cut picture emerged of the combat veteran's chronic stress syndrome. A severely disabling, but non-schizophrenic condition involving startle reactions, sleep difficulties, dizziness, blackouts, avoidance of activities similar to combat experience and internalization of feelings" (121, p. 579). Archibald further points out that "a picture of restlessness, irritability, tension, headaches, sleep disturbances, overreactive startle reflex, feelings of isolation and distrust, sense of inadequacy and restriction of social contact and activities" (121, p. 580) is common across stressors and across patient samples.

The conflict in Vietnam added many new and novel elements. A significant factor in the conflict was the easy availability of what was then called dangerous drugs. A number of studies have assessed the use of drugs by the military in Vietnam.

Robins' study (122), sponsored by the Special Action Office for Drug Abuse Prevention, has been of utmost value as she compared preservice use with in-country and postdischarge use of drugs. This and other studies (123–127) show a significant increase in drug use by men in the lower military ranks. This use was a response to being "In-Country," to the stress of war/conflict, to availability, and to general acceptance of the behavior at a line level. That this cluster of factors had a positive causal effect on use is unquestionable. This is borne out by the finding that the greater majority of veterans on returning home readjusted their drug use behavior to conform with the standards of their home community. As an example, the reduction of narcotic use in the general sample went from 43% to 10% (preservice use was 8%). Veterans with drug-positive urines in Vietnam showed a reduction from 97% to 33% in the use of narcotics (122). From this we can conclude that within the context of a highly stressful situation, with ready availability and subgroup support, drugs and alcohol play a functional role in helping military personnel cope.

The interaction of alcohol/drugs and post-traumatic stress is a complex problem that we are in the process of attempting to unravel. Studies conducted at this medical center indicate that 60% to 75% of all veterans with a primary diagnosis of Post-Traumatic Stress Disorder also receive the diagnosis of Substance Use Disorder. These studies note that substances used almost exclusively fall into the category of "downers" (e.g., alcohol, sedative hypnotics, tranquilizers, and opiate analgesics). With the exception of marijuana (a minor hallucinogen), this patient sample shies away from psychostimulants and major hallucinogens.

Archibald and others (123–127) have noted that the post-traumatic stress disorders are unlike the schizophrenias or major mood disorders. Likewise, the results of the work at this center suggest that this population does not fall into the categories of street addicts and/or alcoholics. It is important to note that the drugs used would be just about what the doctor would prescribe.

In conclusion, our review of the literature, as well as our own work, leads us to suggest that the following populations are at risk:

1. In-country veterans.
2. Those who saw combat and/or were under fire.
3. Those who perceived that they were caught up in an unpopular conflict.
4. Those who were not welcomed home.
5. Those who lacked an intimate social support network along with the resources or opportunity to find meaningful work.

This group, on returning home, continue to use "downers" to treat their stress-related disorder, only to find themselves confronted with a PTSD disorder compounded by drug and/or alcohol dependency.

CONCLUSION

There appears to be a consistent correlation between levels of stress and the use/abuse of drugs and alcohol. This correlation exists across time and cultures. There is also solid experimental evidence that alcohol and some other drugs have a physiological dampening effect. This is not to imply that stress is the sufficient cause of drug and alcohol consumption. There is certainly evidence that drugs are taken for a variety of reasons. To assume that we eat only to reduce the pangs of hunger would be an oversimplification. To assume that the tension/stress reduction hypothesis explains in full the effects and continued use of psychoactive drugs is equally simplistic.

To summarize, our review leads us to cautiously conclude that some of the data gathered provide support for the hypothesis that life stressors/strains/discords trigger episodes of mental/physical illness and drug and alcohol use/abuse. We also infer that some people are at high risk for developing a substance use disorder because of the tension-reducing effects of alcohol/drug consumption. Finally, we cautiously conclude that social supports may mediate this relationship.

REFERENCES

1. Coon CS: The Story of Man. New York, Knopf, 1955
2. Keller M: A historical overview of alcohol and alcoholism. Cancer Research 39:2822–2829, 1979
3. Leake CD, Silverman M: Alcoholic Beverages in Clinical Medicine. Chicago, Year Book Medical Publishers, 1966
4. The Interpreters Dictionary of the Bible. Nashville, Abington, 1981
5. Heath DB: A critical review of ethnographic studies of alcohol use, in Research Advances in Alcohol and Drug Problems VII. Edited by Gibbins R. New York, Wiley, 1975
6. Lender ME, Martin JK: Drinking in America: A History. New York, The Free Press, 1982
7. Levine HG: The discovery of addiction. Journal of Studies on Alcohol 39:143–173, 1978
8. Mather I: Wo to Drunkards. Cambridge MA:1673 (2nd ed, 1712)
9. Rush B: An inquiry into the effects of ardent spirits . . . (8th ed, 1814), in A New Deal in Liquor: A Plea for Dilution. Edited by Henderson VA. New York, Doubleday, 1934
10. Horton D: The functions of alcohol in primitive societies: A cross-cultural study. Quart J of Stud Alc 4:199–203, 1943
11. Horton D: Primitive societies, in Drinking and Intoxication. Edited by McCorthy R. Glencoe, IL, Free Press, 1959
12. Field PB: A new cross-cultural study of drunkness, in Society, Culture and Drinking Patterns. Edited by Pittman DJ, Snyder CR. New York, Wiley, 1945
13. Bacon MD, Barry H III, Child IL: Cross-cultural study of drinking, II Relationship to other features of culture. Quart J Stud Alc Suppl No 3:29, 1965a
14. Bacon MK, Barry H III, Child IL, et al: Cross-cultural study of drinking, V Detailed definitions and data. Quart J Stud Alc Suppl No 3-78, 1965b
15. Bacon MK: The dependency conflict hypothesis and the frequency of drunkenness: Further evidence from a cross-cultural study. Quart J Stud Alc 35:863–865, 1974
16. Bacon MK: Alcohol use in tribal societies, in Social Aspects of Alcoholism. Edited by Kissin B, Begleiter H. New York, Plenum Press, 1976
17. Straton R, Zeiner A, Paredes A: Tribal affiliation and prevalence of alcohol problems. Journal of Studies on Alcohol 39:1166–1177, 1978
18. Berkman LF: Stress social networks and aging, in Drugs, Alcohol and Aging. Edited by Gottheil E, Druley KA, Skoloda TE, et al. Springfield, IL, Charles C Thomas, 1984
19. Nowak CA: Life events and drinking behavior in later life, in Drugs, Alcohol and Aging. Edited by Gottheil E, Druley KA, Skoloda TE, et al. Springfield, IL, Charles C Thomas, 1984
20. Finney JW, Moos RH: Life stressors and problem drinking among older adults, in Recent Developments in Alcoholism. Edited by Galanter M. New York, Plenum, 1983
21. Lamy PP: The aging: Drug use and misuse, in Alcohol, Drugs and Aging. Edited by Gottheil E, Druley KA, Skoloda TE, et al. Springfield, IL, Charles C Thomas, 1984

22. Baker W: Psychopharmacology of aging: Use, misuse and abuse of psychotropic drugs, in Alcohol, Drugs and Aging. Edited by Gottheil E, Druley KA, Skoloda TE, et al. Springfield, IL, Charles C Thomas, 1984
23. Glantz MD: The detection, identification and differentiation of elderly drug misuse and abuse in a research survey, in Alcohol, Drugs and Aging. Edited by Gottheil E, Druley KA, Skoloda TE, et al. Springfield, IL, Charles C Thomas, 1984
24. DeJarlais DC, Joseph H, Courtwright DT: Old age and addiction: A study of elderly patients in methadone maintenance treatment, in Alcohol, Drugs and Aging. Edited by Gottheil E, Druley KA, Skoloda TE, et al. Springfield, IL, Charles C Thomas, 1984
25. Wells-Parker E, Miles S, Spencer B: Stress experiences and drinking histories in elderly drunken driving offenders. Journal of Studies on Alcohol 44(3):429–437, 1983
26. Dudley DL, Mules JE, Roszell DK, et al: Frequency and magnitude distribution of life change in heroin and alcohol addicts. The International Journal of the Addictions 11(6): 977–987, 1976
27. Yoder RD, Moore RA: Characteristics of convicted drunken drivers. Quart J Stud Alc 34:927–936, 1973
28. Mulford HA, Fitzgerald JL: Changes in the climate of attitudes toward drinking in Iowa, 1961–1979. Journal of Studies on Alcohol 44(4):645–687, 1983
29. Selzer ML, Vinokur A, Wilson TD: A psychosocial comparison of drunken drivers and alcoholics. Journal of Studies on Alcohol 38(7):1294–1312, 1977
30. Donovan DM, Marlatt GA, Salzberg PM: Drinking behavior, personality factors and high risk driving. Journal of Studies on Alcohol 44:395–428, 1983
31. Goodwin D: Alcohol in suicide and homicide. Quarterly Journal of Studies on Alcohol 34:144–156, 1973
32. Evans CM: Alcohol, violence and aggression. British Journal of Alcohol and Alcoholism 15:104–117, 1980
33. Gilies H: Homicide in the west of Scotland. British Journal of Psychiatry 128:105–127, 1976
34. Gerson LW: Alcohol-related acts of violence. Journal of Studies on Alcohol 39:1294–1296, 1978
35. Parker N: Murderers: A personal series. Medical Journal of Australia 1:36–39, 1979
36. Gottheil E, Druley KA, Skoloda TE, et al: Alcohol, Drug Abuse and Aggression. Springfield, IL, Charles C Thomas, 1983
37. MacAndrew C: An examination of the individual differences (A-Trait) formulation of alcohol abuse in young males. Addictive Behaviors 7:39–45, 1982
38. Marlatt GA, Kosturn CF, Lang AR: Provocation to anger and opportunity for retaliation as determinants of alcohol consumption in social drinkers. Journal of Abnormal Psychology 84(6):652–659, 1975
39. Marlatt GA, Gordon RA: Determinants of relapse, implication for the maintenance of behavior change, in Behavioral Medicine: Changing Health Life Styles. Edited by Davidson PO, Davidson, SM. New York, Brunner/Mazel, 1980
40. Cassel J: The contribution of the social environment to host resistance. Am J Epidemiol 104:107–123, 1976
41. Blake R: Social supports, psychological stressors and risk of depression: A study of independent and interactive effects. Presented at the 133rd Annual Meeting of the American Psychiatric Association, San Francisco, May 3–9, 1980
42. Thorell T: Selected illness and somatic factors in relation to two psychosocial stress indices—A prospective study on middle-aged construction workers. Journal of Psychosomatic Research 39:7–20, 1976
43. Billings AC, Moos RF: Stressful life events and symptoms. Health Psychology 1(2):99–177, 1982
44. DeLongis A, Coyne JC, Dakof G, et al: Relationship of daily hassles, uplifts, and major life events to health status. Health Psychology 1(2):119–136, 1982
45. Miller P McC, Ingham JG, Davidson S: Life events, symptoms and social support. J Psychosom Res 20:515–522, 1976a
46. Lin N, Simeone RS, Ensel WM, et al: Social support, stressful life events and illness:

A model and an empirical test. J Health Soc Behav 20:108–119, 1979
47. Brown GW: Life events, psychiatric disorder and physical illness. Journal of Psychosomatic Research 25:461–473, 1981
48. Nuckalls KB, Cassel J, Kaplan BH: Psychosocial aspects, life crisis and the prognosis of pregnancy. American Journal of Epidemiology 95:431–441, 1972
49. McFarlane AH, Norman GR, Streiner DL, et al: A longitudinal study of the influences of the psychosocial environment on health status: A preliminary report. Journal of Health and Social Behavior 21:124–133, 1980
50. McFarlane AH, Norman GR, Streiner DL, et al: The process of social stress: Stable, reciprocal, and mediating relationships. Journal of Health and Social Behavior 24:160–173, 1983
51. Byrne DG, Whyte HM: Life events and myocardial infarction revisited: The role of measures of individual impact. Psychosomatic Medicine 42:1–10, 1980
52. Jacobs TJ, Charles E: Life events and the occurrence of cancer in children. Psychosomatic Medicine 42:11–24, 1980
53. Homes TH, Rahe RH: The social readjustment rating scale. Journal of Psychosomatic Research 11:213–218, 1967
54. Sarason IG, Johnson JH, Siegle JM: Assessing the impact of life changes: Development of a life experiences survey. Journal of Consulting and Clinical Psychology 46:932–946, 1978
55. Andrews G, Tennant C, Hewson DM, et al: Life events stress, social support, coping style, and risk of psychological impairment. J Nerv Ment Dis 166:307–316, 1978
56. Warheit GJ: Life events, coping, stress and depressive symptomatology. Am J Psychiatry 136:502–507, 1979
57. Surtees PG: Social support, residual adversity and depressive outcome. Soc Psychiatry 15:71–80, 1980
58. Henderson S, Byrne DG, Duncan-Jones P, et al: Social relationships, adversity and neurosis: A study of association in a general population sample. Brit J Psychiat 136:574–583, 1980
59. Henderson S: Social relationships, adversity and neurosis: An analysis of prospective observations. Brit J Psychiat 138:391–398, 1981
60. Frydman MI: Social support, life events and psychiatric symptoms: A study of direct, conditional and interaction effects. Soc Psychiatry 16:69–78, 1981
61. Brown GW, Bhrolchain MN, Harris T: Social class and psychiatric disturbance among women in an urban population. Sociology 9:225–54, 1975
62. Brown GW: Life events, psychiatric disorder and physical illness. Journal of Psychosomatic Research 25:461–473, 1981
63. Miller P McC, Ingham JG: Friends, confidants and symptoms. Social Psychiatry 11:51–58, 1976
64. Miller P McC, Ingham JG: Life events, symptoms and social supports. Journal of Psychosomatic Research 20:515–522, 1976
65. Vinokur A, Selzer ML: Desirable versus undesirable life events: Their relationship to stress and mental distress. Journal of Personality and Social Psychology 32:115–122, 1975.
66. Carveth WB, Gottlieb BH: The measurement of social support and its relationship to stress. Canad J Behav Sci/Rev Canad Sci Comp 11(3):179–188, 1979
67. Gore S: The effect of social support in moderating the health consequences of unemployment. Journal of Health and Social Behavior 19:157–165, 1978
68. Hitch PJ, Rack PH: Mental illness among Polish and Russian refugees. British Journal of Psychiatry 137:206–211, 1980
69. Reading AE: The influences of maternal anxiety on the course and outcome of pregnancy: A review. Health Psychology 2(2):187–202, 1983
70. Bartrop RW, Lazarus L, Luckhurst E, et al: Depressed lymphocyte function in bereavement. Lancet 1:834–836, 1977
71. Stein M: Stress, brain and immune function. The Gerontologist 22:203, 1982
72. Krakowski AJ: Stress and the practice of medicine. Journal of Psychosomatic Research 26:91–98, 1982

73. Sorenson AA: Alcoholic Priests: A Sociological Study. New York, Seabury, 1976
74. Maslach C, Jackson SE: Burned-out cops and their families. Psychology Today 12:59–62, 1979
75. Berkman LF, Syme SL: Social networks, host resistance, and mortality: A nine-year follow-up study of Alameda County Residents. Am J Epidemiol 109:186–204, 1979
76. Kimbal CP: Stress and psychosomatic illness. Journal of Psychosomatic Research 26(1):63–67, 1982
77. Moos RH, Mitchel RF: Social network resources and adaptation: A conceptual framework, in Basic Processes in Helping Relationships. Edited by Wills TA. New York, Academic Press, 1982
78. Shuckit MA: Geriatric alcoholism and drug abuse. Gerontologist 17:168–174, 1977
79. Cassel J: The contribution of the social environment to host resistance. Am J Epidemiol 104:107–123, 1976
80. Rabkin JG, Struening EL: Life events, stress and illness. Science 194:1013–1020, 1976
81. Fortin MT, Evans SB: Correlates of loss of control over drinking in women alcoholics. Journal of Studies on Alcohol 44(5):787–796, 1983
82. Andrews G, Tennant C, Newson DM, et al: Life event stress, social support, coping style, and risk of psychological impairment. Journal of Mental and Nervous Disease 166(5):307–316, 1978
83. Caplan G: Mastery of stress. American Journal of Psychiatry 138(4):413–420, 1981
84. Collins DL, Baum A, Singer JE: Coping with chronic stress and Three Mile Island: Psychological and biochemical evidence. Health Psychology 2(2):149–166, 1983
85. Levy SM: Host differences in neoplastic risk: Behavioral and social contributions to disease. Health Psychology 2(1):21–44, 1983
86. Vickers RR, Hervig LK, Rahe RH, et al: Type-A behavior pattern and coping and defense. Psychosomatic Medicine 43:381–396, 1981
87. Jenkins CD: Recent events supporting psychologial and social risk factors for coronary disease (first of two parts). The New England Journal of Medicine 294:987–994, 1976
88. Jenkins CD: Recent evidence supporting psychological and social risk factors for coronary heart disease (second of two parts). The New England Journal of Medicine 294:1033–1038, 1976
89. Suls J, Gastorf JW, Witenberg SH: Life events, psychological distress and the Type-A coronary-prone behavior pattern. Journal of Psychosomatic Research 23:315–319, 1979
90. Manuch SB, Corse CD, Winkelman PA: Behavioral correlates of individual differences in blood pressure reactivity. Journal of Psychosomatic Research 23:281–288, 1979
91. Wallstan BS, Alagna SW, DeVellis B McE, et al: Social support and physical health. Health Psychology 2(4):367–391, 1983
92. Kasl SV: Pursuing the link between life experiences and disease: A time for reappraisal, in Stress Research: Issues for the Eighties. Edited by Cooper CL. New York, John Wiley & Sons, 1983
93. Moos RH, Finney JW, Chan DA: The process of recovery from alcoholism in comparing controls. Journal of Alcohol Studies 42:383–402, 1981
94. Porritt D: Social support in crisis: Quantity or quality? Soc Sci Med 13A(6):715–721, 1979
95. Wellman B: Applying network analysis to the study of support, in Social Networks and Social Support. Edited by Gottlieb BH. Beverly Hills, Sage, 1981
96. Mills KC: A stimulus theory of intoxication to account for the association between stress and drinking: Findings with rats and young adult drinkers, in Stress and Alcohol Use. Edited by Pohorecky LA, Brick J. New York, Elsevier Biomedical, 1983
97. Ray OS: Drugs, Society and Human Behavior. St Louis, Mosby, 1972
98. Festinger L: Conflict, Decision and Dissonance. Stanford, Stanford University Press, 1964
99. Cox T: Stress. Baltimore, University Park Press, 1980
100. Ursin H, Baacle E, Levine S: Psychobiology of Stress: A Study of Coping Men. New York, Academic Press, 1978

101. Baum A, Grunberg NE, Singer JE: The use of psychological and neuroendocrinological measurements in the study of stress. Health Psychology 1(3):217-236, 1982
102. Glass DC, Lake CR, Contrade RJ, et al: Stability of individual responses to stress. Health Psychology 2(4):317-341, 1983
103. Pohorecky LA, Brick J: Stress and Alcohol Use. New York, Elsevier Biomedical, 1983
104. Cooper CL: Stress Research: Issues for the Eighties. New York, John Wiley & Sons, 1983
105. Pohorecky LA, Rassi E, Weiss JM, et al: Biochemical evidence for an interaction of ethanol and stress: Preliminary studies. Alcoholism: Clin Exp Res 4:423-426, 1980
106. Brick J, Pohorecky LA: The neuroendocrine response to stress and the effects of ethanol, in Stress and Alcohol Use. Edited by Pohorecky LA, Brick J. New York, Elsevier Biomedical, 1983
107. DeTurck H, Vogel WH: Effects of acute plasma and brain catecholamine levels in stressed and unstressed rats: Evidence for an ethanol-stress interaction. Journal of Pharmacology and Experimental Therapeutics 223:348-354, 1982
108. Sher KJ, Levenson RW: Alcohol and Tension Reduction: The importance of individual differences, in Stress and Alcohol Use. Edited by Pohorecky LA, Brick J. New York, Elsevier Biomedical, 1983
109. Lipscom TR, Nathan PE, Wilson T, et al: Effects of tolerance on the anxiety-reducing function of alcohol. Arch Gen Psychiatry 37:577-582, 1980
110. Kardiner A: Traumatic neuroses of war, in American Handbook of Psychiatry, vol 1. Edited by Arieti S. New York, Basic Books, 1959
111. Archibald HC: Gross stress reaction in combat: 15-year follow-up (WW II and Korean veterans). Am J Psychiat 119:317-322, 1962
112. Dobbs D, Wilson WP: Observations on persistence of war neurosis. Dis Nerv Syst 21:686-691, 1960
113. Futterman S, Pumpian-Mindlin E: Traumatic war neuroses five years later. Am J Psychiat 108:401, 1951
114. Kalinowsky LB: Problems of war neuroses in light of experiences in other countries. Am J Psychiat 107:340-346, 1950
115. Lifton RJ: Death in Life: Survivors of Hiroshima. New York, Simon & Schuster, 1967
116. Leopold RL, Dillon H: Psycho-anatomy of disaster: Long-term study of post-traumatic neuroses in survivors of marine explosion. Am J Psychiat 119:913-921, 1963
117. Niederland WG: Psychiatric disorders among persecution victims. Journal of Nervous and Mental Diseases 139:453-474, 1964
118. Niederland WG: Clinical observation on the survivor syndrome, in Massive Psychic Trauma. Edited by Krystal H. New York, International Universities Press, 1968
119. Chodoff P: Late effects of concentration camp syndrome. Arch Gen Psychiat 8:323-333, 1963
120. Strom A, et al: Examination of Norwegian ex-concentration camp prisoners. J Neuropsychiat 4:43-62, 1962
121. Archibald HC, Tuddenham RD: Persistent stress reaction after combat. Arch Gen Psychiat 12:475-581, 1965
122. Robins LN: The Vietnam Drug User Returns. Special Action Office Monograph 2 Series A. Washington, DC, US Government Printing Office, 1974
123. Helzer JE, Robins LN, Wish E, et al: Depression in Vietnam veterans and civilian controls. Am J Psychiatry 136:526-529, 1979
124. Penk WE, Rabonowitz WR, Patterson ET, et al: Adjustment differences among male substance abusers varying in degree of combat experience in Vietnam. Journal of Clinical and Consulting Psychology 49:426-437, 1981
125. Sanders CR: Doper's wonderland: Functional drug use by military personnel in Vietnam. Journal of Drug Issues 6:65-78, 1973
126. Stanton DM: Drug use in Vietnam. Arch of Gen Psychiat 26:279-286, 1972
127. Lacoursiere RB, Godfrey KE, Ruby LM: Traumatic neurosis in the etiology of alcoholism: Vietnam combat and other trauma. Am J Psychiatry 137:966-968, 1980

4

Stress and Alcohol Consumption: The Role of Selected Social and Environmental Factors

STANISLAV V. KASL, ADRIAN M. OSTFELD,
LISA F. BERKMAN, and SELBY C. JACOBS

This paper presents data on psychosocial and environmental influences on alcohol consumption. Data are drawn from large epidemiological studies of elderly community residents. Health effects of life-threatening illness and of the death of a marital partner are examined.

The findings from these two studies provide scant comfort for those who believe that the amount of alcohol consumption is sensitive to those environmental conditions and experiences which can be broadly designated as "stressful." However, a number of possibilities are listed which could lead to the argument that the stress-alcohol connection does exist, even though it was not detected in these two studies.

INTRODUCTION

If the boundaries of the topic "stress and alcohol" are defined by a computerized Medline search for references (1), one will find that a great variety of studies are thereby pulled in. This is, in part, due to the fact

Data presented in this report came from two studies, supported by Grant No. NO1 AG-O-2105 from the National Institute on Aging and Grant No. 1 RO1 MH 32260 from the National Institute on Mental Health.

that stress has a multiplicity of meanings (2), including: (a) a condition of environmental exposure; (b) an appraisal of an environmental situation; (c) a response to the environmental exposure or to the appraisal; (d) a state of distress, the stimulus conditions for which are not specified; and (e) an interactive term indicating the relationship between environmental demands and the person's capacity to meet these demands. However, there are other reasons as well. Another is that "alcohol" may show up in such studies as either a dependent or an independent variable, and it may be operationalized in a variety of ways on a variety of subjects, ranging from diagnosis of alcoholism in a sample of patients under treatment to asking about reasons for drinking (but not drinking itself) in an unselected community sample. Studies may also vary greatly with respect to the setting and the temporal dimension of the stress-alcohol dynamics, such as acute changes in alcohol consumption in response to short-lived experimental laboratory manipulation versus relating well-established levels of alcohol consumption to life-long social circumstances or stable traits.

In the present paper, we focus on psychosocial and environmental influences on alcohol consumption in adult community residents. After briefly considering relevant evidence from previous studies, we will present results from two separate studies, one a community survey of the elderly and the other a longitudinal study of the health effects of bereavement. Throughout, our perspective is that of psychosocial epidemiology.

THE LIMITED EVIDENCE FOR A
STRESS-ALCOHOL ASSOCIATION

When reviewing the evidence from quasi-experimental (observational) study designs, it is well to keep muttering to oneself that "correlation is not necessarily causation." The one exception to this advice is when there is an absence of an association in the first place; then, one need not go through the struggle of considering alternative explanations. Such appears to be the predominant trend of the evidence with respect to stress and alcohol consumption. This general conclusion may be rather surprising since most of us would tend to agree with Peyser's (3) comment that "Everyday observation and popular opinion agree that alcohol relieves tension and enables one to cope with stress" (p. 587). In fact, however, Peyser comes up with very little evidence to cite, as does another recent review of social factors in the etiology of alcohol consumption (4).

In broad-based surveys, the strongest correlates of alcohol consumption tend to be sociodemographic factors, religious variables, smoking and drug use habits, one's own specific attitudes towards drinking, and drinking behavior of significant others (e.g., 5–7). These are not readily interpreted as indicators of stress. Alcohol consumption may also relate to such trait-like variables as impulsivity and rigidity (7, 8), but again these are difficult to link up to notions of stress. Other correlates, however, such as neurotic tendencies or powerlessness (9, 10), may justify invoking the term "stress," at least in its one meaning as "nonspecific distress." But these correlations are of a modest magnitude, and other studies that have used similar indicators of distress, such as anxiety (11) and low self-esteem and worries (12), did not obtain significant associations with alcohol consumption. Of course, when one has to speculate about the linkages of study variables to stress, then the proper interpretation of findings is more difficult to discern. For example, two studies (10, 11) have reported higher alcohol consumption with higher social integration and social support. Since the latter variables are generally seen as buffers against stress, this finding appears unexpected from a stress-alcohol perspective. Alternately, the result could be a simple reflection of the broad social aspects of drinking behavior, in which case stress should not be brought into the interpretation at all.

It is likely that bivariate associations are inadequate to represent the stress-alcohol dynamics. For example, Pearlin and Radabaugh (13) argue that distress such as anxiety is likely to result in the use of alcohol as tranquilizer if a sense of control is lacking and self-esteem is low. Their data do support this argument. However, the problem is that their dependent variable was Cahalan's distress control question, not an actual measure of alcohol consumption, and a cognitive consistency interpretation is a reasonable alternative explanation of the results. In fact, the results from the national Quality of Employment Survey (14) clearly reveal that a variety of distress indicators (e.g., low self-esteem, depressed mood) are associated with "escapist drinking" (i.e., with type of reasons for drinking) but not with amount of drinking, even though the two measures of drinking are modestly correlated ($r = .30$).

The occupational literature perhaps gives the most consistent picture of a lack of association between alcohol consumption and a variety of job stress-distress-dissatisfaction measures (10, 14–18). In fact, traditional specific occupational stress measures (such as role ambiguity, overload) do not even appear to correlate with "escapist drinking" (17), even though the more general distress measures, such as depressed mood, do show an association (14), as noted above. There is a certain amount of irony in these consistently negative results on job stress and alcohol consumption, since the alcoholism treatment programs in industry appear to be set up as if problems with drinking had their primary etiology in the work setting.

There has also been some interest in looking at the association between stressful life events and alcohol consumption (18, 19), and the impression is that the expected positive association does exist for both frequency of events and ratings of impact of such events. However, the meaning of this association must be questioned. In their summary of many studies, Masuda and Holmes (20) showed that alcoholics and drug addicts report 4–5 times as many life events as, say, medical students, football players, and pregnant mothers. This strongly leads to the suggestion that (a) heavy alcohol consumption may precipitate many types of stressful life events, and/or (b) frequent life events and higher alcohol consumption may both be a reflection of a particular life style. The possibility of complicated dynamics (both causal and self-selection) is also hinted at by the finding (19) that the association between depression and stressful life events was stronger for either abstainers or heavy drinkers and weaker for moderate drinkers.

The evidence regarding the relationship of alcohol consumption to specific individual stressful experiences (as opposed to the summation of a large list of diverse events and quasi-events on one of the typical stressful life events measures) offers a mixed and inconclusive picture. With respect to *unemployment*, for example, Buss and Redburn (21) used community archival data to monitor liquor sales. No changes were detected after plant shutdowns and a sharp rise in unemployment. Individual instances of alcohol abuse were higher only among those who continued to be unemployed for a long time. This suggests either (a) that alcohol consumption is sensitive only to severe umemployment, or (b) that those who drink more heavily will have a harder time finding a new job. Another study (22) noted that 18% of unemployed workers reported "increased drinking," but there was no control group and the data were retrospective, asking the subjects to make direct before-after comparisons.

Results from a *bereavement* study (23) were also somewhat confusing. The bereaved were more likely than controls to admit to increased alcohol consumption over the post-bereavement period, but there were no differences in drinking "more than is good for you."

With respect to *war* experience, it would appear that veteran status alone is not associated with increased alcohol consumption, once one adjusts for a variety of socio-demographic factors (24). Exposure to heavy combat may lead to higher rates of drinking (3, 25, 26), but the results may apply only to white veterans and the measurement procedures were rather soft, involving recall over a long period of time.

Exposure to manmade *disasters* does not seem to increase alcohol consumption. For instance, workers at the Three Mile Island accident site, in comparison to those at a control nuclear plant (27), did not appear to increase their alcohol consumption as a way of coping with the stress.

Longitudinal data on stress and alcohol consumption are as scarce as they are important. They not only may help us to begin to disentangle causal relationships, but they may also indicate the length of the time cycles over which stress and alcohol may covary. In a design which utilized daily logs (11), no significant association was detected between frequency or intensity of daily moods and drinking rates or intoxication frequency (either concurrently or with time lags). In a study of occupational stress among U.S. Navy petty officers (28), daily records revealed less alcohol consumption on days of objectively defined high stress; over the total period of training, stress perceptions and chronic alcohol consumption were found unrelated. Finally, in a study of adult community residents interviewed four times during one year (28), the results appeared to suggest a relatively short-term effect of depression on increased alcohol use and long-term effect of alcohol use on heightened depression.

The cumulative impression from this brief review of evidence is that the stress-alcohol association is weak, unclear, and evanescent. Alcohol consumption is likely to be complexly and multiply determined and strong individual differences in etiological dynamics are probable. In the remainder of this paper we present selected results from two studies. As the reader will find, our findings do not call for a drastic revision of this general impression.

SOME SOCIAL AND ENVIRONMENTAL CORRELATES OF ALCOHOL CONSUMPTION AMONG ELDERLY COMMUNITY RESIDENTS

The findings to be reported in this section come from the initial cross-sectional wave of data collection in the Yale Health and Aging Project (YHAP). Yale is one of three sites funded by the Establishment of Populations for Epidemiological Study of the Elderly Program in the National Institute on Aging. The aim of this program is to assess the general level of physical and mental health in a heterogeneous population of older individuals, specifically with regard to the prevalence and incidence of selected chronic conditions, functional ability, level of depressive symptomatology, and cognitive impairment. The prospective goals are to determine which behaviors, socioenvironmental conditions, and biologic variables are predictive of future declines in health status, as indexed by morbid conditions, hospitalization, institutionalization, and death.

The target population of the YHAP are all New Haven community residents aged 65 and over; institutionalized elderly were not eligible. Three separate sampling frames were developed for the three types of housing in which the elderly live: (a) public elderly housing, which is age and income restricted; (b) private elderly housing, which is age restricted; and (c) houses and private apartments. Because the New Haven elderly are less likely to be males and to live in public housing, these two groups were oversampled in order to achieve adequate numbers. Overall, the YHAP enrolled some 2,800 subjects: 724 in the public housing stratum, 865 in the private housing stratum, and 1,213 in the community stratum. The participation rates in these three strata were 89%, 83%, and 77%, respectively; men and women had virtually identical participation rates overall and within each stratum.

The measurement of alcohol consumption is based on 12 questions, three groups of 4, which asked for identical information about beer or ale, wine, and liquor (with specific examples of the last). Respondents who did not drink any alcoholic beverages during the past year and/or the past month were classified as nondrinkers. The remainder were asked about consumption during the past month; first, how often they "had . . . [beer or ale, etc.]" and then "how many . . . [cans, glasses, etc.] did you usually have at one time?" Frequencies were multiplied by number of drinks per occasion and then summed over the three types of alcoholic beverages. Thus, for example, a person who drank a can of beer every day, a glass of wine once a week, and no liquor, would receive a total score of 34.

The results in Table 1 are presented separately for men and women and are further broken down by age. The results in Tables 1-3 are not weighted. Since the weighted data would reflect primarily the different sampling frames for the three residential strata, the major associations with alcohol consumption were also examined by the residential strata. And since the findings remained basically the same, we feel that the unweighted data (especially when presented separately for the four age-sex subgroups) in no way distort the broad findings.

The top of Table 1 reveals that about 49% of the respondents can be classified as drinkers (i.e., had at least one drink during the month

TABLE 1
Alcohol Consumption Among the Elderly:
Basic Frequencies and Association with
Social Network Variables

		Men		Women	
	Age N	65–74 675	75 + 479	65–74 870	75 + 754
% Drink last month	%	64.3	58.2	42.5	38.5
Alcohol index	$\overline{X}$	31.8	17.5	6.7	4.5
(all persons)	S.D.	73.3	40.4	22.5	11.7
Alcohol index	$\overline{X}$	49.8	30.2	15.9	11.7
(drinkers only)	S.D.	86.7	49.4	32.6	16.6
Marital status					
Married	%	66.6	60.4	52.2	43.1
Separated/divorced	%	58.1	54.5	39.3	27.5
Widowed ≤ 2 yrs.	%	58.3	64.0	38.2	37.3
Widowed ≥ 3 yrs.	%	62.7	57.8	35.6	38.4
Single	%	63.9	45.9	48.4	38.7
Married	$\overline{X}$*	−.07	−.10	+.07	−.05
Separated/divorced	$\overline{X}$*	+.31	+.23	+.32	−.10
Widowed ≤ 2 yrs.	$\overline{X}$*	+.06	+.04	−.17	+.02
Widowed ≥ 3 yrs.	$\overline{X}$*	+.05	+.07	−.16	+.03
Single	$\overline{X}$*	−.04	+.38	−.07	−.08
Network size					
0–4	%	56.5	56.5	42.3	38.1
5–8	%	68.7	52.8	39.8	38.3
9–12	%	66.4	68.2	48.7	38.1
13 +	%	70.5	61.2	41.1	40.4
0–4	$\overline{X}$*	+.07	+.07	+.17	+.11
5–8	$\overline{X}$*	−.06	−.17	−.09	−.07
9–12	$\overline{X}$*	+.11	+.10	−.09	−.07
13 +	$\overline{X}$*	−.10	−.04	−.13	−.14

*Based on drinkers only; scale in standard scores ($\overline{X}$ = 0, S.D. = 1.0), comput-
ed separately within each age-sex subgroup.

preceding the interview). The higher proportions of drinkers among
men and the younger respondents are completely in line with previous
findings. The next four lines give the means and standard deviations for
the index of alcohol consumption when it is computed on all respondents (with a zero score for nondrinkers), and then only for the drinkers.
Clearly, the distribution of scores is skewed and the standard deviations

are large. About half of the drinkers received a score between 1 and 8; the top 10% of the drinkers had a score of 65 or more.

Tables 1-3 present data on selected correlates of alcohol consumption. Social isolation, poor health, functional impairment, an unsafe residential environment, exposure to specific life events, and depression were chosen as variables because the general social gerontological literature (e.g., 30–32) suggests that they are major influences on the well-being of the elderly. They may be seen as indicators of stress for the elderly; however, we feel it is not really necessary to introduce the term stress into the discussion.

The findings are presented in two ways: (a) as prevalence of drinkers, and (b) as mean scores on the continuous index of alcohol consumption, presented for drinkers only. The latter values are given in standard scores (mean of zero, standard deviation of one) so that the reader can have a good estimate of the magnitude of the differences within each sex-age subgroup. We assume that the continuous index for drinkers is the measure that should be more sensitive to the social-environmental conditions examined, while the dichotomous measure reflects a rather stable habit of drinking vs. abstaining. These conditions presumably may affect the quantity of drinking among drinkers, but it would seem less likely that they would lead abstainers to drink.

The data on marital status show only nonsignificant variation in alcohol consumption, except in the group of women aged 65–74. Here, the prevalence of drinkers varies by marital status ($p < .01$), and the quantity of drinking among drinkers also varies by marital status ($p < .05$). Analysis of variance in the latter case reveals that marital status accounts for 2.6% of the total variance. The pattern of results with the two indices is not entirely consistent. For example, the two groups of widowed women, aged 65–74, have fewer drinkers and drinkers who drink less. The separated/divorced group has fewer drinkers, but those fewer drinkers drink more. And, of course, these are cross-sectional findings where direction of causality is difficult to pin down. Thus, for example, it is hardly a secret that alcohol consumption may lead to separation/divorce. And even the widowed category (especially those widowed ≥ 3 years) involves the possibility of self-selection, since these are women who have failed to remarry.

The next variable in Table 1, network size, extends the concept of social isolation beyond marriage. The concept of social network, together with the notion of social support, is coming into its own as a possible major influence on health (33, 34), including the health of the elderly (35). The index is a simple summation of the number of children, relatives, and friends who comprise the respondent's network in the area where they live. Of the eight significance tests which were run, only one was significant: among men 65–74, greater size of network is associated with greater prevalence of drinkers ($p < .01$ for monotonic trend). However, this does not support the notion that relative social isolation is associated with more drinking. The data on female drinkers do show this expected trend in both age groups, but it is not significant. Only about 1.2% of the variance is accounted for by the difference between means when both groups of women are combined.

Table 2 presents findings for the association of alcohol consumption with three indicators of health status. Health is a major influence on quality of life among the elderly, and poor health is a major source of distress (e.g., 36, 37). The first measure represents a global subjective evaluation, much used in gerontological research. With respect to prevalence of drinkers, the direction of association is for more drinkers to be found among those with more positive evaluation of their health; the association is significant for older men and younger elderly women. Regarding alcohol consumption among drinkers, one association is significant: younger elderly women who evaluate their health more negatively report more consumption ($r = .24$).

The second index is based on the presence of any disability (i.e., having at least some difficulty) in a number of Activities of Daily Living (ADL), such as eating, walking, bathing, and grooming. The results reveal that drinkers are less likely to be found among those with some disability; the association is significant in all groups except the older women. The data on amount of consumption among drinkers do not reveal any significant associations. The third index in Table 2 reflects the presence of chronic conditions detected in the health history section of the interview; the relevant conditions include heart disease, stroke, diabetes, cancer, arthritis, hypertension, and so on. Again, we can see the lower prevalence of drinkers among those with more chronic conditions (significant among the younger elderly women), and no significant association with amount of consumption among the drinkers.

The overall picture in Table 2 is to find more abstainers among those in poorer health; this is particularly true among the younger elderly women. However, with respect to alcohol consumption among the drinkers, only 1 of the 12 associations was found significant. These results do not support the notion that poor health leads to distress which leads to more drinking. The results are compatible with several other possibilities: (a) those in poor health become abstainers; (b) abstaining leads to poor health; and (c) abstaining leads to a sense of poor health. Cahalan et al. (6) found similarly complex results. Regarding questions about good and

TABLE 2
Alcohol Consumption Among the Elderly:
Associations With Indicators of Health Status

		Men		Women	
	Age	65–74	75 +	65–74	75 +
	N	669	475	864	751
Health rating					
Excellent	%	63.4	50.0	49.0	37.5
Good	%	66.4	66.5	47.9	42.1
Fair	%	63.2	55.0	37.1	38.2
Poor, bad	%	61.3	36.4	24.6	25.0
Excellent	$\overline{X}$*	+.04	+.01	−.09	+.13
Good	$\overline{X}$*	.00	+.01	+.01	−.05
Fair	$\overline{X}$*	−.07	−.01	−.02	+.02
Poor, bad	$\overline{X}$*	+.11	−.16	+.26	+.17
Functional disability					
None	%	65.5	60.5	44.7	38.7
Some	%	49.0	46.1	25.3	37.3
None	$\overline{X}$*	−.01	+.02	−.02	−.01
Some	$\overline{X}$*	+.11	−.14	+.31	+.03
Chronic conditions					
0 or 1	%	66.5	61.6	48.7	39.3
2 +	%	61.4	53.7	37.6	37.8
0 or 1	$\overline{X}$*	.00	+.02	−.02	−.07
2 +	$\overline{X}$*	.00	−.03	+.02	+.06

*Based on drinkers only; in standard scores.

bad things that happened in the past year, abstainers were more likely to report health among *both* the good things and the bad things, compared to the heavy drinkers.

Table 3 presents results for three additional possible sources of distress among the elderly. The first concerns perceived safety of the neighborhood and of the building where the respondents live. The results suggest that drinkers are more likely to evaluate their neighborhood as less safe; the associations are significant in all groups except the older men. However, perceptions of building safety are not significantly related to prevalence of drinkers. The associations with quantity of drinking among drinkers reveal only one of the eight associations as significant:

that for building safety among the younger elderly men. However, this association is curvilinear and thus most difficult to interpret.

The next variable in Table 3 concerns life events and it is based on an inquiry concerning a number of "objective" events for the past year: victim of crime, death of a close relative or friend, separation from close relative or friend, and serious illness or accident of spouse or a family member. The table reveals no significant associations, either with prevalence of drinkers or with frequency of drinking among drinkers.

The last variable in Table 3 involves depression, as measured by the CES-D scale (38). The positive group are those elderly who scored 16+ on the scale, a commonly accepted cutoff from validation studies (39). The results do not show a significant association with prevalence of drinkers. However, the data with amount of drinking among drinkers do show a significant effect for both groups of men: depressed men drink more. Of course, in these cross-sectional data, the direction of causality is unclear and the influence of alcohol consumption on depression is not likely to be negligible.

It is interesting to note that in additional analyses with the depression scale (not shown), the variable functional disability proved to be by far the strongest influence on depression. Yet the data in Table 2 showed no association of functional disability with amount of drinking among the drinkers. Thus depression cannot be seen as an intervening variable between functional disability and alcohol consumption, since the overall association was not observed. Similarly, life events were also substantially related to depression but not to alcohol consumption (Table 3). In short, these analyses did suggest an impact of environmental stressors on depression but not on alcohol consumption. This might make it more likely that (a) alcohol consumption is another influence on depression (among the men particularly) rather than the reverse, or (b) if depression influences alcohol consumption, it is only the stable trait-like component of it that does so.

The results in Tables 1-3 may be *summarized* as follows. With respect to the dichotomous measure, drinker-abstainer, 11 of the 36 runs were significant. Seven involved an index of health and all were opposite to expectation from a simple stress-alcohol hypothesis—fewer drinkers among those in poorer health. Another involved size of social networks and here, too, the unexpected association was fewer drinkers among the more socially isolated. With regard to marital status (women 65-74), the highest prevalence of drinkers was among the married, again unexpected. Only the two significant associations with neighborhood safety were in the expected direction. With respect to the continuous measure of

TABLE 3
Alcohol Consumption Among the Elderly:
Associations With Residential Variables, Selected
Life Events, and Depression

		Men		Women	
Age		65–74	75+	65–74	75+
N		669	475	864	751
Neighborhood safety					
Very safe	%	55.8	54.3	34.1	29.6
Fairly safe	%	68.8	64.0	45.9	40.0
Somewhat . . . not at all	%	64.5	56.6	43.6	45.5
Very safe	$\overline{X}$*	+.13	+.18	+.05	+.18
Fairly	$\overline{X}$*	−.09	−.05	−.01	−.06
Somewhat . . . not at all	$\overline{X}$*	+.04	−.07	−.01	.00
Building safety					
Very safe	%	61.6	57.8	43.4	35.9
Fairly safe	%	66.2	63.1	43.6	42.3
Somewhat . . . not at all	%	67.5	53.3	39.6	39.8
Very safe	$\overline{X}$*	+.07	+.09	+.03	−.02
Fairly safe	$\overline{X}$*	−.18	−.15	+.06	+.01
Somewhat . . . not at all	$\overline{X}$*	+.16	+.06	−.17	+.07
Life events					
0	%	61.2	57.1	40.2	34.6
1	%	65.4	54.1	41.7	41.8
2+	%	66.1	62.5	45.0	40.1
0	$\overline{X}$*	−.08	+.10	+.12	+.03
1	$\overline{X}$*	+.07	−.07	+.03	−.02
2+	$\overline{X}$*	+.01	−.04	−.10	−.01
Depressed					
No	%	64.9	60.3	43.8	39.0
Yes	%	58.9	53.6	38.3	39.7
No	$\overline{X}$*	−.04	−.04	−.03	−.04
Yes	$\overline{X}$*	+.27	+.29	+.18	+.11

*Based on drinkers only; in standard scores.

alcohol consumption computed on drinkers, only 5 of the 36 runs were significant. Three were in the expected direction and two were ambiguous. The three involved depression in both groups of men and self-rated health for women 65–74. The association with building safety was curvilinear, and the association with marital status (women 65–74) was expected for higher values among the separated/divorced but unexpected for the lower values among the widowed.

ALCOHOL CONSUMPTION CHANGES AS A RESULT OF SERIOUS ILLNESS OR DEATH OF SPOUSE

The results from this second study represent a much more focused examination of the alcohol-stress hypothesis. Specifically, we will offer findings from an ongoing prospective epidemiological study designed to examine the health effects of two major stressful experiences—life-threatening illness and, in some cases, death of a marital partner. The NIMH-funded study is entitled, "Effect of Spousal Illness and Death in Older Families" (A. M. Ostfeld, principal investigator).

The site of the study is the greater metropolitan area of New Haven, which is served by two general hospitals. We regularly screened admissions to these two hospitals to identify married patients with life-threatening illness. If the nonhospitalized spouse of the screened patient was the appropriate age (46–80), we enumerated and invited him or her to take part in the longitudinal study and, if they accepted, they were interviewed as soon as possible. During follow-up, death of the hospitalized spouse occurred in a large proportion of cases which thus subdivided this part of our sample into bereaved and nonbereaved groups. Death might occur at any time during follow-up and, therefore, the bereaved group was further subdivided into "earlier" and "later" bereaved groups. The nonbereaved group were those for whom hospitalization of a spouse with life-threatening illness was followed by recovery over the period of observation. Another group of nonbereaved participants, whose spouses were hospitalized with benign illness (e.g., hernia, psoriasis, lipoma, phlebitis, benign tumor), were also enumerated. We consider them a low stress, nonbereaved group, with a "healthy" spouse.

Follow-up was of two types. One was face-to-face interviews, lasting about an hour, by a trained interviewer at the time of hospitalization (intake), 6 weeks later (first follow-up interview), 6 months later, 13 months later, and 25 months later. Most of these interviews were done in the home of the participant. The other type of follow-up involved telephone interviews of about 10 minutes at 6 months, 13 months, and 25 months after enumeration. The data presented in this report are based on the face-to-face interviews and include the first three contacts with the subjects (through the 6th month).

The study is still in progress and findings are presented on some 343 subjects. The participation rates are as follows: (a) Among subjects who were enumerated and eligible for participation, 25% were refusals. Almost half of these are refusals because the attending physician of the critically ill, hospitalized spouse (not our eligible subject) refused access to the family. The 25% refusals did not differ significantly from the participants on age, sex, and race. (b) Among the participants, 47% entered the follow-up involving face-to-face interviews. The remainder were willing to agree only to a less intensive data collection procedure. The more cooperative subjects were comparable on sex and race but were younger and less likely to be bereaved than those participants in follow-up by telephone interview. (c) Among those who agreed to face-to-face interviews, 28% were lost by attrition over the course of the three interviews. Most of them, however, are continuing to participate in the study on a less intensive basis. The 28% lost to intensive follow-up did not differ from the remainder on age, sex, race, or socioeconomic status. It can be seen that this is a most difficult study to carry out and that recruiting and maintaining subjects, no matter how conscientiously carried out, leads to substantial attrition of eligibles.

The measure of alcohol consumption used in this study is based on the questions used in the Alameda County Study (33). Two sets of questions were asked: "How often do you drink . . . wine, beer, liquor?" and "When you drink . . . wine, beer, liquor, how many drinks do you usually have at a sitting?" Numerical codes for frequency and volume were applied to represent consumption per month; the numbers were multiplied for each of the three types of drink and then summed. Since the codes grouped actual frequencies and volume, the highest score for each drink was 90, 15 for frequency multiplied by 6 for volume. Thus the theoretical range of scores for the total index of alcohol consumption was 0 to 270.

Table 4 presents the data on the four groups of interest: (a) The 115 bereaved subjects for whom the death of spouse came mostly within a week or so of the initial interview; (b) the 34 "late" bereaved for whom the spouse's death took place between 6 weeks and 6 months after intake; (c) the 127 subjects with a "recovering" spouse, that is, a spouse with life-threatening illness who survived the hospitalization and was alive throughout the first 6 months of follow-up; and (d) the 67 subjects with a "healthy" spouse who had been hospitalized with a benign illness. Of the total group of 343, 65.6% are women, 33.5% are 65 or older, 33.7% have education beyond high school, and 86.2% have been married only once. The four groups are not significantly different from each other on sex, first marriage, health status (days in bed, doctor's visits, hospital-

TABLE 4
Alcohol Consumption Among Married Adults
Experiencing Bereavement or Serious Illness of Spouse

		Mean Alcohol Consumption				
	Bereaved	"Late" bereaved	"Recovering" spouse	"Healthy" spouse	Total Mean & S.D.	Signif. of differences
N	115	34	127	67		
Men	N					
	44	13	41	20		
Initial interview	29.6	22.2	14.9	15.9	21.5 ± 35.7	n.s.
Six weeks later	28.3	18.0	16.4	14.7	20.8 ± 21.2	n.s.
Six months later	30.4	18.2	19.4	15.9	22.8 ± 23.5	n.s.
Women	N					
	71	21	86	47		
Initial interview	13.6	9.4	11.5	17.6	13.2 ± 13.5	n.s.
Six weeks later	11.6	9.6	9.9	17.7	12.0 ± 12.8	n.s.
Six months later	12.2	11.3	13.9	14.9	13.3 ± 13.1	n.s.

izations, self-rating), religiousness, number of relatives, and number of close friends. On two variables, the controls ("healthy" spouse) were different from the other groups: they were somewhat younger and somewhat better educated. Both variables are related to higher alcohol consumption in other population studies.

In presenting the alcohol consumption data in Table 4, we offer the group means separately for men and women. The means are calculated on all subjects, including the nondrinkers who naturally receive a score of 0. The overall mean for men is approximately 22 ($\pm$25) and for women 13 ($\pm$13). The standard deviations are high, as in all other population studies which construct a similar index of consumption.

There is only one story these findings tell: alcohol consumption is completely insensitive to the experience of severe illness in spouse or death of spouse. There were no significant results, either when means are examined cross-sectionally (within each of three waves of data collection) or as changes over time. The analysis of variance with repeated measures shows no significant effects of group, time, or group by time interaction. The group of 44 bereaved men look slightly higher, but this is not significant and the values obviously do not change over time. Statistical adjustments for the slightly lower age and higher education of the subjects with a "healthy" spouse do not alter these conclusions at all.

Table 5 presents the results for three psychological outcome variables. We offer these findings only to demonstrate that we have a sensitive study design and that the experience of severe illness and/or death of a spouse is, indeed, related to differences in distress, across groups and over time. The first measure is the CES-D scale (38), already described for the first study. The second measure is a 4-item index from the PERI (Psychiatric Epidemiology Research Interview) instrument developed by Dohrenwend (40). The last measure is a 12-item index developed specifically for this study by one of the authors (S. C. J.). The items deal with such symptoms as preoccupation with thoughts of spouse, experiencing vivid mental images of spouse, feeling a need to call spouse's name, dreaming of spouse, and feeling upset when thinking about spouse. This scale was not administered during the first interview, nor was it given to the controls.

Analysis of variance with repeated measures revealed highly significant effects for all three variables: due to group, due to time, and due to group by time interactions. For the first measure—depression—these effects were particularly strong. During the initial interview, there is a strong effect due to hospitalization of spouse for life-threatening illness

TABLE 5

Affective Reactions Among Married Adults
Experiencing Bereavement or Serious Illness of Spouse

			Means on Selected Scales			
	Bereaved	"Late" bereaved	"Recovering" spouse	"Healthy" spouse	Total Mean & S.D.	Signif. of differences
N	115	34	127	67		
Depression						
Initial	19.17	17.92	18.32	9.66	16.87 ± 10.3	<.01
Six weeks later	16.17	14.26	10.36	5.36	11.72 ± 10.5	<.01
Six months later	9.87	15.34	5.98	4.26	7.87 ± 10.7	<.01
Hopelessness-helplessness						
Initial	4.34	4.26	4.08	2.31	3.84 ± 3.8	<.01
Six weeks later	2.94	3.73	3.01	1.52	2.77 ± 2.6	<.01
Six months later	2.62	4.68	2.91	2.12	2.83 ± 3.6	<.05
Separation anxiety						
Initial	—	—	—	—	—	—
Six weeks later	13.08	10.07	5.87	—	9.39 ± 7.6	<.01
Six months later	9.28	12.00	4.15	—	7.25 ± 7.4	<.01

(i.e., the first three groups vs. the controls with "healthy" spouse); the magnitude of this difference is about one standard deviation. Over time, the bereaved group shows a steady decline, but even at 6 months they are about ½ standard deviation above the controls. The "late" bereaved group begins to decline (less so than the recovering spouse group), but goes up again at 6 months, since the death of the spouse occurred between the second and third interview. The recovering spouse group shows the steepest decline overall and at 6 months they are nearly at the same level as the controls. The changes over time in the "healthy" spouse group suggest that even the benign hospitalization of the spouse had some impact, however short-lived.

The data on hopelessness-helplessness do not show changes of the magnitude seen for the depression scale, but the pattern is reasonably similar. Some of the differences are: (a) relatively little impact on the "healthy" spouse group; (b) the recovering spouse group remains elevated even at 6 months, compared to the controls; and (c) there seems to be a particularly strong impact in the "late" bereaved group. The data on separation anxiety are more limited (three groups, two occasions) but all the effects are again highly significant. The means for the acutely bereaved (at 6 weeks for the bereaved and at 6 months for the "late" bereaved) are over 1 standard deviation above the mean for the recovering spouse group at 6 months. The bereaved group at 6 months is still ⅔ of a standard deviation above the mean for the recovering spouse group. Also worth noting is the difference at 6 weeks between the "late" bereaved (10.07) and the recovering spouse (5.87) groups. This would suggest that the separation anxiety scale is also sensitive to the differential course of recovery in the spouses, since no deaths have taken place in either group thus far.

The contrast in the findings for alcohol consumption (Table 4) and psychological distress (Table 5) is unmistakable and reinforces the conclusion that alcohol consumption is not sensitive to the experience of severe illness or death of spouse. We also examined the correlations of alcohol consumption with the three measures of psychological distress. We chose the second interview as indicative of the acute reaction for the bereaved and thus more likely to reveal an effect. The data were run separately for men and women, and for the bereaved vs. the combined group of recovering and "healthy" spouses (omitting the small group of "late" bereaved). None of the 12 correlations reached statistical significance; the highest was for the 44 bereaved men with separation anxiety ($r = .228$). Thus, our overall conclusion remains unchanged.

CONCLUDING COMMENTS

The findings which have been presented from the two studies provide scant comfort for those who believe that amount of alcohol consumption is sensitive to those environmental conditions and experiences which can be broadly designated as "stressful." This is our own conclusion regarding these findings. However, we wish to list a number of possibilities which could lead to the argument that the stress-alcohol connection does exist but was not detectible because of the design and methods of the two studies. The first two are the most obvious ones:

1. Self-reports of alcohol consumption in field surveys are invalid.
2. Alcohol consumption is sensitive to other stressors which were not examined in the two studies.
3. The subjects in these two studies were mature adults, in whom alcohol consumption habits are well-established and no longer responsive to stressful experiences; different results would have been obtained for younger subjects.
4. The measure of alcohol consumption was based on summated consumption for a whole month; stress and alcohol do covary, but it is on shorter time cycles, such as days or weeks.
5. There are major individual differences in responding to stress with alcohol; as stress goes up, some persons increase alcohol consumption, others decrease (not unlike the putative association between stress and eating). When all individuals are lumped together, no effect is detected.

REFERENCES

1. Friis R: Stress and Substance Abuse: A Bibliography. Irvine, CA, Human Behavior Research Group, 1979
2. Kasl SV: Stress and health. Ann Rev Public Health 5:319–341, 1984
3. Peyser H: Stress and alcohol, in Handbook of Stress: Theoretical and Clinical Aspects. Edited by Goldberger L, Breznitz S. New York, The Free Press, 1982
4. McQueen DV, Celentano DD: Social factors in the etiology of multiple outcomes: The case of blood pressure and alcohol consumption patterns. Soc Sci Med 16:397–418, 1982
5. Bachman JG, Johnston LD, O'Malley PM: Smoking, drinking, and drug use among American high school students. Correlates and trends, 1975–1979. Am J Pub Hlth 71:59–69, 1981
6. Cahalan D, Cisin JH, Crossley HM: American Drinking Practices. New Brunswick, Rutgers Center of Alcohol Studies, 1969
7. Cahalan D, Room R: Problem drinking among American men aged 21–59. Am J Pub Hlth 62:1473–1482, 1972

8. Cisin IH, Cahalan D: Comparison of abstainers and heavy drinkers in a national survey. Psychiat Res Rep 24:10–21, 1968
9. Cahalan D, Cisin IH: American drinking practices: Summary of findings from a national probability sample. II. Measurement of massed versus spaced drinking. Quart J Stud Alc 29:642–656, 1968
10. Seeman M, Anderson CS: Alienation and alcohol: The role of work, mastery, and community in drinking behavior. Am Sociol Rev 48:60–77, 1983
11. Rohsenow DJ: Social anxiety, daily moods, and alcohol use over time among heavy social drinking men. Addict Behav 7:311–315, 1982
12. Rodin MB, Morton DR, Shimkin DB: Beverage preference, drinking and social stress in an urban community. Int J Addict 17:315–328, 1982
13. Pearlin LI, Radabaugh CW: Economic strains and the coping functions of alcohol. Am J Sociol 82:652–663, 1976
14. Quinn RP, Shepard LJ: The 1972–73 Quality of Employment Survey. Ann Arbor, Survey Research Center, The University of Michigan, 1974
15. Hingson R, Mangione T, Barrett J: Job characteristics and drinking practices in the Boston Metropolitan area. J Stud Alc 42:725–738, 1981
16. Kasl SV: Epidemiological contributions to the study of work stress, in Stress at Work. Edited by Cooper CL, Payne R. New York, Wiley, 1978
17. Margolis BL, Kroes WH, Quinn RP: Job stress: An unlisted occupational hazard. J Occup Med 16:659–661, 1974
18. Sadawa SW, Thistle R, Forsyth R: Stress, escapism, and patterns of alcohol and drug use. J Stud Alcohol 39:725–736, 1974
19. Neff JA, Husaini BA: Life events, drinking patterns and depressive symptomatology. J Stud Alc 43:301–318, 1982
20. Masuda M, Holmes TH: Life events: Perceptions and frequencies. Psychosom Med 40:236–269, 1978
21. Buss TF, Redburn FS: Shutdown at Youngstown: Public Policy for Mass Unemployment. Albany, State University of New York Press, 1983
22. Rayman PM, Bluestone B: Out of Work: The Consequences of Unemployment in the Hartford Aircraft Industry. Boston, Social Welfare Research Institute, Boston College, 1982
23. Parkes CM, Brown RJ: Health after bereavement. A controlled study of young Boston widows and widowers. Psychosom Med 34: 449–461, 1972
24. Boscarino J: Patterns of alcohol use among veterans and nonveterans: A confirmation of previous findings. Am J Pub Hlth 71:85–88, 1981
25. Egendorf A, Kadushin C, Laufer RS, et al: Legacies of Vietnam: Comparative Adjustment of Veterans and Their Peers, vol I. Summary of Findings. New York, The Center for Policy Research, 1981
26. Yager T, Laufer RS, Gallops M: Some problems associated with war experience in men of the Vietnam generation. Arch Gen Psychiat 41:327–333, 1984
27. Kasl SV, Chisholm RF, Eskenazi B: The impact of the accident at the Three Mile Island on the behavior and well-being of nuclear workers. Am J Pub Hlth 71: 472–483, 484–495, 1981
28. Conway TL, Vickers RR Jr, Ward HW, et al: Occupational stress and variation in cigarette, coffee, and alcohol consumption. J Hlth Soc Behav 22:155–165, 1981
29. Anenhensel CS, Huba GJ: Depression, alcohol use and smoking over one year: A four-wave longitudinal causal model. J Abnorm Psychol 92:134–150, 1983
30. Birren JE, Sloane RB (eds): Handbook of Mental Health and Aging. Englewood Cliffs, NJ, Prentice-Hall, 1980
31. McGaugh JL, Kiesler SB (eds): Aging: Biology and Behavior. New York, Academic Press, 1981
32. Parron DL, Solomon F, Rodin J (eds): Health, Behavior and Aging. Washington, DC, National Academy Press, 1981
33. Berkman, LF, Breslow L: Health and Ways of Living. New York, Oxford University

Press, 1983
34. Wallston BS, Alagna SW, DeVellis BM, DeVellis RF: Social support and physical health. Health Psychol 2:367–391, 1983
35. Kasl SV, Berkman LF: Some psychosocial influences on the health status of the elderly, in Aging: Biology and Behavior. Edited by McGaugh JL, Kiesler SB. New York, Academic Press, 1981
36. Kaplan GA, Camacho T: Perceived health and mortality: A nine-year follow-up of the Human Population Laboratory cohort. Am J Epidemiol 117: 292–304, 1983
37. Larson R: Thirty years of research on the subjective well-being of older Americans. J Gerontol 33:109–125, 1978
38. Radloff LS: The CES-D scale: A self-report depression scale for research in the general population. Appl Psychol Measurement 1:385–401, 1977
39. Weissman MM, Sholomskas D, Pottenger M, Prusoff BA, Locke BZ: Assessing depressive symptoms in five psychiatric populations: A validation study. Am J Epidemiol 106:203–214, 1977
40. Dohrenwend BP, Shrout PE, Egri G, Mendelsohn FS: Nonspecific psychological distress and other dimensions of psychopathology: Measures for use in the general population. Arch Gen Psychiatry 37:1229–1236, 1980

5

Alcohol and Human Stress: Closer to the Truth or Time to Ask Some New Questions?

STEPHEN A. LISMAN

In this paper I highlight studies generated by the major research approaches to the Tension Reduction Hypothesis (TRH) of drinking. I argue that the TRH, as it now stands, cannot encompass a broad array of negative and contradictory findings. What is needed are new questions and new theories; some recent directions in our own laboratory are noted.

As I have intimated in the title, the purpose of this paper is to argue that it is time to ask some new questions about alcohol and human stress. To establish such an argument, I shall present a deliberately selective overview of the research in this area and what I feel are some safe conclusions concerning alcohol and stress in humans. Many of my conclusions will stem from reasoning involving disconfirmation, a position which, over the years, has been frequently endorsed as providing the strongest tests of theories and hypotheses (1). (I shall return to this point in my final comments.) Given the emphasis on negative and contradicto-

Support for some of the research described was provided by grants from the SUNY Research Foundation and from NIAAA (No. 5-R01-AA03141). The editorial assistance of Pat Rourke is greatly appreciated.

ry results that necessarily accompanies disconfirmation, I run the risk that you may find my posture pessimistic, extreme, or too much like creating straw men. Therefore, in an effort to soften this negativism, I shall also offer a brief glimpse at some of the recent directions in which these conclusions have led me, and about which I feel rather optimistic.

My overview will proceed by summarily examining what we have learned about the reciprocal relationships between alcohol and human stress, as derived from the major strategies which have characterized research into the elusive Tension Reduction Hypothesis (TRH) of drinking (2). Simply stated, the TRH is defined by two basic corollaries: (a) alcohol reduces stress; and (b) people will drink in order to benefit from this effect.

CROSS-CULTURAL APPROACHES

One of the earliest and most widely cited investigations in this area was completed by Horton (3), who concluded that "the primary function of alcoholic beverages in all societies is the reduction of anxiety" (p. 223). Horton examined information which detailed the drinking habits of 77 societies. He focused on the degree of insobriety commonly reached by adult male drinkers and related this to different indices of "subsistence anxiety." For example, the more primitive a society's food-gathering techniques, the greater the danger of food shortages and, therefore, the more difficult are life conditions. As Horton predicted, consistent with the idea that such primitive conditions are conducive to high levels of anxiety, such societies were found to have a high level of insobriety, compared to that commonly reached by adult male drinkers in less primitive societies.

However, correlational research lends itself to many alternative explanations. Thus, Field (4) reexamined 56 of these same societies and, like Horton, noted more drunkenness in primitive hunting and gathering economies than in those based on agriculture. Nevertheless, using a different measure of insobriety than Horton, Field reached an alternative conclusion: levels of insobriety seemed best explained by focusing on the social organization of the society, since many of the more primitive societies and tribes were also characterized by an absence of kin groups and formal structure, as well as poorly defined roles and functions. When Field assessed fear levels by examining tales of sorcerers and ghosts, he found no relationship of drinking to anxiety.

"IN VIVO" APPROACHES

Here I have noted several recent studies that bear directly on the second corollary of the TRH—that people will consume alcohol for its tension-reducing properties. These studies comprise reports of alcohol intake among distinctly different populations undergoing the daily stresses of their natural environments. Like cross-cultural studies, they lack the degree of experimental control characteristic of those developed in the laboratory. However, they take advantage of relatively long time periods to monitor the onset and offset of stress—analogous to experiments of nature—and reports of drinking during those times.

An example of this approach is the study by Conway, Vickers, Ward, and Rahe (5), who examined the relationships between occupational stress and variations in cigarette, coffee, and alcohol consumption during an 8-month period in which the subjects were being trained to be Naval Company Commanders. During the several training cycles involved, there are apparently clearly and consensually defined stressful periods. Conway et al.'s results indicate that habitual cigarette smoking and coffee drinking were positively associated with chronic tendencies to perceive high stress, but alcohol consumption was not. Also, high stress days led to increased cigarette and coffee intake; increased alcohol intake was more likely to occur on days of low stress.

Counterintuitive as these findings may appear, they are completely consistent with the recent report of Rohsenow (6), who adopted a similar research strategy. She asked college males, who were classified as heavy social drinkers, to record their mood and drinking on a daily basis for about 4 months. The results were,

> No significant correlations were found between the frequency and intensity of any of the daily moods and drinking rates or intoxication frequency, either concurrently or within a few days or weeks. Drinking was also unrelated to general trait anxiety, depression, stressful life experiences, and locus of control. (p. 311)

Mulford (7) interviewed more than 700 Iowans during two periods over a 6-month span. He assessed what life stressors had occurred during that time, how much people reported that they had drunk, and how subjects perceived alcohol, i.e., its personal meaning and expected effects. Mulford concluded that some people increased and some decreased their heavy drinking in response to life stress. Also, it was more likely to be men than women that increased consumption in response to undesirable and to desirable events. Finally, he stated, " . . . not everyone who believes that alcohol reduces stress actually uses it for that purpose, and not everyone who so uses it does so to the point of becoming a problem drinker or even a normal drinker" (p. 333).

The second corollary of the TRH receives stronger and more consistent support, however, from investigations of the victims of natural disasters and the prolonged and extreme stress with which they must cope. Thus, Gleser, Green, and Winget (8) reported that over a 2-year period following the flood at Buffalo Creek, West Virginia, 30% of families reported an increase in alcohol consumption. Several years later, Adams and Adams (9) assessed the residents of a small town in the vicinity of Mt. Saint Helens, Washington. They compared behaviors during the 7 months preceding and 7 months following the volcano's eruption, and found clear social indicators of alcohol problems which had emerged among the residents. These problems included an increase in court cases of all sorts (other than driving) involving alcohol, an increase in referrals to a community alcoholism center, and an increase in police arrests for violation of liquor laws.

QUESTIONNAIRES

Because of the methodological and logistic problems confronting the researcher enamored of "in vivo" approaches, many have taken the intuitively appealing route of simply asking people why they drink and what happens to them when they do. While numerous additional problems inhere in this strategy, it does offer a means for developing hypotheses and for understanding the phenomenology of alcohol use.

Results from these questionnaire studies seem unequivocally to indicate that people claim alcohol will reduce stress—both for themselves and for others (10). This simple assertion derives from the responses of clinicians (11), college students (12), social drinkers (13), alcoholic men and women (14), and adolescents—even adolescents who have not yet begun to drink (15). Admittedly, these same studies reveal that people acknowledge that alcohol has other effects too, but the idea that alcohol will diminish stress is firmly rooted in popular consensus.

LABORATORY EXPERIMENTS

The controlled laboratory experiment is often an analogue study with a nonpatient population. Nevertheless, as Berkowitz and Donnerstein (16) and Levis (17) have so elegantly explained, it still remains, within limits, the best way to establish cause and effect, to subject theoretical ideas to critical test, to rule out alternative explanations, and to systematically accumulate knowledge in the manner of the evolution of science. With the development of experimental drinking tasks (18, 19) and laboratories in which subjects are administered intoxicating amounts of alcohol (20), behavioral scientists have produced a large number of studies to test the TRH. I shall highlight several of our own studies as examples of the laboratory approach and where it has led.

A. Stress-Induced Drinking

The second corollary of the TRH is typically explored by manipulating subjects' stress levels in the laboratory and observing subsequent drinking in any of several analogue drinking situations. Illustrative of this strategy is the study by Noel and Lisman (21). We found that when female undergraduates were stressed by being asked to solve problems that were actually unsolvable, they subsequently drank more beer than did control subjects who had been given solvable problems. Interestingly, both groups of women drank similar amounts of ginger ale, implying that their alcohol consumption had been aversively, not appetitively, motivated. That is, mood measures showed that working on unsolvable problems made the subjects hostile, not simply undifferentially thirsty.

In a related vein, Cappell (22) had earlier criticized alcohol and stress experiments for confounding appetitively and aversively motivated drinking. That is, experiments on alcohol and stress were not distinguishing between the influence of negative affect or stress versus general arousal. Therefore, we (23) did another study, comparing the effect of watching slides of repugnant/fearful scenes with that of viewing sexually arousing scenes and neutral scenes. Our male subjects drank more only after viewing the sexually arousing scenes, despite the fact that only repugnant/fearful scenes generated significant autonomic arousal, as measured by changes in skin conductance.

Clearly, the results of this latter study are inconsistent with the vast bulk of published reports demonstrating that laboratory-induced stress will increase alcohol consumption. On the contrary, it shows that increased alcohol consumption does not always follow stress and, furthermore, implies that even when it does, it may sometimes be due simply to effects related to general arousal. This study also suggests that, although physiological criteria are often a major component in the definition of stress, physiological arousal need not take precedence over cognitive variables as antecedents or accompaniments to drinking.

B. *Administration of Alcohol ("Preloading")*

The other major laboratory strategy is to preload subjects in order to assess the impact of specific dosages or blood levels of alcohol on stress. This way of assessing the first corollary of the TRH is illustrated in our (24) study of the effect of different dosages of alcohol on socially anxious, shy males and normally dating, nonanxious males. The crucial performance measures centered around each subject's recorded interaction with a female confederate.

On the basis of an array of observational, physiological, and self-report measures, we concluded that, compared to placebo, alcohol effected a marked impairment of social-interactional performance. Furthermore, this effect was replicated in two parts of the study, and, for the nonanxious males, appeared to be linearly dose-dependent. Finally, our subjects reported experiencing more irrational self-statements during the intoxicated social interaction than they did after consuming placebo. This suggests that cognitive changes may mediate the alcohol-induced exacerbation of stress in shy males.

Compelling as our results appeared to us, they conflict with those of Wilson and Abrams (25). In a similar experiment, they found that simply believing one had received alcohol was sufficient to diminish social anxiety; alcohol did not, however, affect their subjects' responding. And more recently, Sher and Levenson (26) found that the effectiveness of alcohol in altering stress responses depended on particular subject characteristics. That is, alcohol diminished stress responses only for subjects judged to be at risk for alcoholism, based on their scores on the MacAndrew Scale of the Minnesota Multiphasic Personality Inventory (MMPI) (27).

Given these and numerous other reports conflicting with our findings, we felt compelled to once again examine alcohol's anxiolytic properties. Therefore, in our next large (N = 130) study (28, 29), we investigated the effect of two different dosage levels of alcohol, administered immediately before or after stress, on the performance of both male and female college students. Our stressor was uncontrollable aversive noise, administered via learned helplessness procedures (30) that typically create measurable affective change and impairment in subsequent learning.

Earlier work by Tucker, Vuchinich, Sobell and Maisto (31) had shown that when given the choice, subjects will drink following a stressor rather than before. This suggested our experimental hypothesis, to wit, that alcohol consumed following the uncontrollable noise will be the more effective stress reducer. In our paradigm, that would mean that alcohol would thus minimize or prevent problems in subsequent escape learning. Surprisingly, our results were just the opposite, and there were no differences between the performances of men and women. Thus, only the subjects given a moderate dose of alcohol *before* the uncontrollable noise subsequently performed as well as the control groups. It was as if alcohol before stress "prevented" later impairments in learning. In contrast, alcohol *after* stress increased the probability of later task failure, and did so in dose-related fashion.

In trying to explain these counterintuitive results and the apparent contradiction of our earlier data with shy males, we have discussed problems due to differing definitions of stress, procedural distinctions, attributional differences among subjects, and even the effects of alcohol on memory (see 29 for a fuller discussion). Yet none of these provide any systematic solutions, and many questions remain unanswered.

CONCLUSIONS AND RECENT DIRECTIONS

It thus appears that, although people typically assert that alcohol reduces stress, they are often wrong. In short, we may safely conclude only that such effects depend on characteristics of the subjects (e.g., risk for alcoholism, beliefs, and expectancies), particulars of the setting and dosage, time of consumption relative to stress, and definitions of stress or tension. Consideration of these and other methodological issues are superbly detailed in other recent reports (e.g., 32, 33, 34). However, this is not an obligatory, naive call for more studies, each controlling or manipulating the variables just listed, in the hope of finally coming up with "the truth" about alcohol and stress. Unsatisfactory though it may appear, "the truth" is, as just stated above, marked by numerous qualifiers, contingencies, and operational definitions, akin to "the truth" about whether psychotherapy works.

Even at this moment, more studies of the TRH of drinking continue to appear, further elucidating various relevant parameters, in hope of contributing some innovative theoretical perspective. Recent reviews (29, 35, 36, 37) describe and critique many of these theoretical perspectives on alcohol and stress, showing that none can possibly encompass the array of negative and conflicting data. On a more encouraging note, although no theory may currently prevail, several have yet to be more adequately tested and developed.

In our laboratory, this state of affairs has led us to ask questions which differ in kind from those we have entertained to date. For example, we were struck by the report noted above (15) that, despite conflicting scientific evidence, nondrinking adolescents will assert that alcohol reduces stress. When and from which sources do they learn that? Besides making the usual attributions to cultural, familial, and peer influences, we found ourselves examining the widely suspected influence of television (38).

First we conducted a brief observational study of television programming during prime time. We found few portrayals of negative consequences following alcohol consumption, even though alcohol was depicted or alluded to approximately 7.5 times per hour of prime-time viewing (39). Indeed, perhaps we have been underestimating the potential influence of television on children's development of alcohol-related expectancies.

Therefore, we undertook an experiment to discover how children's social problem-solving might be affected by viewing drinking in various contexts on television (40). To this end, we showed third- and fourth-grade children videotaped scenes from M.A.S.H., a very popular prime-time show. The videotapes varied in the type of beverage portrayed (alcoholic or nonalcoholic) and the circumstances under which the beverage was used (tension or enjoyment). After viewing the scenes, the children were presented with five short situations describing various adult social problems of daily living. Each child was asked to rate the appropriateness of different solutions to these problems. Half of the solutions presented involved drinking alcohol.

As we had predicted, those children who had viewed scenes of alcohol consumption judged alcohol-related solutions as more appropriate than did children who saw only the consumption of nonalcoholic drinks. This seems a striking and generalized effect, given that the children viewed our television scenes only for 10–12 minutes in a laboratory setting. Of course, we can only begin to speculate about the meaning and strength of this effect in the possible contexts of viewing a program in its entirety, viewing many programs over many months, and viewing in the child's own home under a variety of other conditions.

An interesting related question is whether this effect would be even more pronounced among the children of alcoholics. That is, given their family environment, might such children be more readily influenced by television portrayals of drinking? And, independent of viewing habits, might not such children be more inclined to construe alcohol as a means to reduce stress or solve problems? This latter consideration has led us to adapt the problem-solving measure for use in an ongoing project with the children of alcoholics.

Finally, we have also begun to examine how alcohol might affect the reaction of an adult listener to a child's cry, a widely documented stressful and aversive event (41). It is our hope that, by utilizing knowledge we have gained from work on alcohol, stress, and aggression, we may soon be able to investigate in a controlled-analogue setting some of the alleged, but untested, links between alcohol and child abuse (42).

Let me conclude by returning to my initial point about the strategy of disconfirmation. Obviously, in this review I chose to highlight studies that appear clearly to refute the TRH. Indeed, a complete box score in this matter has been compiled by Pihl and Smith (43). Yet, contemporary philosophy of science does not equate negative evidence with clear disconfirmation of a theory or hypothesis (44). Often, it is simply a matter of making a good theory more malleable by means of specific adjustments. I submit that, as it now stands, the TRH has become so highly qualified that, in contrast to malleability, it sometimes borders on vacuousness, posing more obstacles than solutions. New theories and new questions are needed. Perhaps this review will stimulate some.

REFERENCES

1. Platt JR: Strong inference. Science 146:347–352, 1964
2. Cappell H, Herman CP: Alcohol and tension reduction: A review. Q J Stud Alc 33:33–64, 1972
3. Horton DJ: The function of alcohol in primitive societies: A cross-cultural study. Q J Stud Alcohol 4:199–320, 1943
4. Field PB: A new cross-cultural study of drunkenness, in Society, Culture, and Drinking Patterns. Edited by Pittman DJ, Snyder CR. New York, Wiley, 1962
5. Conway TL, Vickers RR, Jr, Ward HW, et al: Occupational stress and variation in cigarette, coffee, and alcohol consumption. J Health Soc Behav 22:155–165, 1981
6. Rohsenow DJ: Social anxiety, daily moods, and alcohol use over time among heavy social drinking men. Addict Behav 7:311–315, 1982
7. Mulford HA: Stress, alcohol intake and problem drinking in Iowa, in Stress and Alcohol Use. Edited by Pohorecky LA, Brick J. New York, Elsevier Biomedical, 1983
8. Gleser GC, Green BL, Winget C: Prolonged Psychosocial Effects of Disaster: A Study of Buffalo Creek. New York, Academic Press, 1981.
9. Adams PR, Adams GR: Mount Saint Helens' ashfall: Evidence for a disaster stress reaction. Am Psychol 39:252–260, 1984
10. Rohsenow DJ: Drinking habits and expectancies about alcohol's effects for self versus others. J Consult Clin Psychol 51:752–756, 1983
11. McHugh M, Beckman LJ, Frieze IH: Analyzing alcoholism, in New Approaches to Social Problems. Edited by Frieze IH, Bar-Tal D, Carroll JS. San Francisco, Jossey-Bass, 1979
12. Segal B, Huba GJ, Singer JL: Drugs, Daydreaming, and Personality: A Study of College Youth. Hillsdale, NJ, Lawrence Erlbaum Associates, 1979
13. Brown SA, Goldman MS, Inn A, et al: Expectations of reinforcement from alcohol: Their domain and relation to drinking patterns. J Consult Clin Psychol 48:419–426, 1980
14. Beckman LJ: Perceived antecedents and effects of alcohol consumption in women. J Stud Alcohol 41:518–530, 1980

15. Christiansen BA, Goldman MS, Inn A: Development of alcohol-related expectancies in adolescents: Separating pharmacological from social-learning influences. J Consult Clin Psychol 50:336–344, 1982
16. Berkowitz L, Donnerstein E: External validity is more than skin deep: Some answers to criticisms of laboratory experiments. Am Psychol 37:245–257, 1982
17. Levis DJ: The case for performing research on nonpatient populations with fears of small animals: A reply to Cooper, Furst, and Bridges. J Abnorm Psychol 76:36–38, 1970
18. Marlatt GA: Behavioral assessment of social drinking and alcoholism, in Behavioral Approaches to Alcoholism. Edited by Marlatt GA, Nathan PE. New Brunswick, NJ, Rutgers Center of Alcohol Studies, 1978
19. Miller PM, Hersen M, Eisler RM: Relative effectiveness of instructions, agreements, and reinforcement in behavioral contracts with alcoholics. J. Abnorm Psychol 83:548–553, 1974
20. Nathan PE, Goldman MS, Lisman SA, et al: Alcohol and alcoholics: A behavioral approach. Trans NY Acad Sci 34:602–627, 1972
21. Noel NE, Lisman SA: Alcohol consumption in college females following exposure to unsolvable problems: Learned helplessness or stress-induced drinking? Behav Res Ther 18:429–440, 1980
22. Cappell H: An evaluation of tension models of alcohol consumption, in Research Advances in Alcohol and Drug Problems, Vol 2. Edited by Gibbins RJ, et al. New York, Wiley, 1975
23. Gabel PC, Noel NE, Keane TM, et al: Effects of sexual versus fear arousal on alcohol consumption in college males. Behav Res Ther 18:519–526, 1980
24. Keane TM, Lisman SA: Alcohol and social anxiety in males: Behavioral, cognitive, and physiological effects. J Abnorm Psychol 89:213–223, 1980
25. Wilson GT, Abrams DB: Effects of alcohol on social anxiety and physiological arousal: Cognitive versus pharmacological processes. Cognitive Therapy and Research 1:195–210, 1977
26. Sher KJ, Levenson RW: Risk for alcoholism and individual differences in the stress-response-dampening effect of alcohol. J Abnorm Psychol 91:350–367, 1982
27. MacAndrew C: The differentiation of male alcoholic outpatients from non-alcoholic psychiatric outpatients by means of the MMPI. Q J Stud Alcohol 26:238–246, 1965
28. Noel NE: Effects of Alcohol Before or After Unsolvable Problems: Prevention or Alleviation of Stress Reactions? Doctoral dissertation, State University of New York at Binghamton, 1984
29. Lisman SA, Keane TM, Noel NE: Feeling depressed, angry, shy, sexually aroused?—Why not have a drink? in Stress and Alcohol Use. Edited by Pohorecky LA, Brick J. New York, Elsevier Biomedical, 1983
30. Seligman MEP: Helplessness: On Depression, Development, and Death. San Francisco, Freeman, 1975
31. Tucker J, Vuchinich R, Sobell M, et al: Normal drinkers' alcohol consumption as a function of conflicting motives induced by intellectual performance stress. Addict Behav 5:171–178, 1980
32. Nathan PE, Lansky D: Common methodological problems in research on the addictions. J Consult Clin Psychol 46:713–726, 1978
33. Abrams DB: Psycho-social assessment of alcohol and stress interactions: Bridging the gap between laboratory and treatment outcome research, in Stress and Alcohol Use. Edited by Pohorecky LA, Brick J. New York, Elsevier Biomedical, 1983
34. Connors GJ, Maisto SA: Methodological issues in alcohol and stress research with human participants, in Stress and Alcohol Use. Edited by Pohorecky LA, Brick J. New York, Elsevier Biomedical, 1983
35. Wilson GT: Alcohol and anxiety: Recent research on the tension reduction theory of drinking, in Advances in the Study of Communication and Affect, Vol. 7. Edited by Polivy J, Blankstein K. New York, Plenum, 1982
36. Collins LR, Marlatt GA: Psychological correlates and explanations of alcohol use and

abuse, in Medical and Social Aspects of Alcohol Abuse. Edited by Tabakoff B, Sutker PB, Randall CL. New York, Plenum, 1983

37. George WH, Marlatt GA: Alcoholism: The evolution of a behavioral perspective, in Recent Developments in Alcoholism, Vol. 1. Edited by Galanter M. New York, Plenum, 1983

38. Lisman SA, Futch EJ, Geller MI: Alcohol and television: What children see and how it affects them. Presented at the National Council on Alcoholism Forum, Detroit, April 1984.

39. Futch EJ, Lisman SA, Geller MI: An analysis of alcohol portrayal on prime-time television. Int J Addict 19:403–410, 1984

40. Futch EJ: The Influence of Televised Alcohol Consumption on Children's Social Problem Solving. Doctoral dissertation, State University of New York at Binghamton, 1984

41. Murray AD: Infant crying as an elicitor of parental behavior: An examination of two models. Psychol Bull 86:191–215, 1979

42. Orme TC, Rimmer J: Alcoholism and child abuse: A review. J Stud Alcohol 42:273–287, 1981

43. Pihl RO, Smith S: Of affect and alcohol, in Stress and Alcohol Use. Edited by Pohorecky LA, Brick J. New York, Elsevier Biomedical, 1983

44. Weimer WB: Notes on the Methodology of Scientific Research. Hillsdale, NJ, Lawrence Erlbaum Associates, 1979

SECTION II

Ethanol-Induced Changes in the Stress Response

6

Characteristics of the Interaction of Ethanol and Stress

LARISSA A. POHORECKY and JOHN BRICK

We have determined the interaction of ethanol and stress in rats, using two biochemical measures (levels of corticosterone and nonesterified free fatty acids [NEFA] in plasma). Stressed rats injected with a low dose of ethanol (0.5 g/kg IP) had smaller elevations of plasma corticosterone and NEFA, compared to saline-injected control rats. This effect of ethanol was observed in rats stressed by various physical and psychological stressors, but was not seen in swim-stressed rats. Conversely, a 2.0 g/kg dose of ethanol potentiated the effects of a stressor. The low dose protective effect of ethanol was also noted in chronically stressed rats. In chronically ethanol-treated rats the effect was significant with NEFA but not with corticosterone.

INTRODUCTION

In recent years, there has been an increasing awareness of the general negative health effects of stress. As a result of both popular and scientific concern about the medical consequences of stress, new areas in both

Supported by NIAAA grants AA00045, 04241, and 04238.
We thank E. Rassi, M. Michalak, and E. Kasziba for excellent technical assistance and P. LaSasso for typing expertise.

medicine and psychology have emerged which deal exclusively with the prevention and/or consequences of stress-related behaviors and health problems.

A large body of epidemiological and clinical evidence indicates that stressors have a variety of medical consequences. In fact, some of the most salient medical problems of our society in this century have stress as an important contributing factor (1, 2, 3, 4). Other medical problems, such as duodenal ulcers and alcoholism, may also be linked to stress exposure (5, 6, 7). Susceptibility to stress is generally influenced by individual differences. That is, the genetic constitution, previous experience, and general health of the individual will determine to a large extent the "stressfulness" and thus the stress response to a given stressor (8, 9).

Interest in the interaction of stress and alcohol stems from the pioneering research of Masserman and Yum (10) and subsequently Conger (11). Their studies suggested that ethanol improves the behavior of stressed animals. It was thus postulated that stress was a possible contributing factor to alcohol abuse by humans (11). This research focused attention on the interrelationship of stress and alcohol and provided impetus to this line of research.

An interaction of ethanol and stress has also been demonstrated in Rhesus monkeys (12, 13). In these studies, the stressor was peer separation, which induced marked behavioral despair in the stressed animals (12). Ethanol was found to have a dose-dependent biphasic effect in peer-separated monkeys. A low dose of ethanol had a beneficial effect on the behavior of stressed monkeys (12). Furthermore, this beneficial effect of ethanol was related to ethanol's ability to increase norepinephrine levels in cerebrospinal fluid of the stressed monkeys (13).

The most publicized interaction of stress with alcohol in man has been in reference to the risk of coronary heart disease. Although some epidemiological studies found no statistically significant association between the risk of heart disease and drinking, more recent studies report a strong negative association between moderate alcohol consumption (up to 60 g/d) and the risk of nonfatal myocardial infarction and death from coronary heart disease (14–20). The mechanism of the protective effect of moderate alcohol ingestion against heart disease is unclear. It may be related to changes in blood lipid composition.

Although basic research in this area is scarce, there are indications that a beneficial effect of ethanol on the heart can also be demonstrated in experimental animals (21–24).

It is generally accepted that stress-induced myocardial damage is mediated by catecholamines (25–28). Therefore, it is interesting to note that small doses of ethanol may indeed produce its protective effect by this mechanism. Evidence in both man (29) and experimental animals (30–33) indicates that low doses of ethanol can lower stress-induced release of peripheral catecholamines as well as other classical indices of stress, such as blood levels of corticosterone and nonesterified fatty acids (NEFA).

Our research is aimed at demonstrating the biological basis for an interaction of ethanol and stress. The research presented here describes our findings on the generality of the ethanol-stress interaction, using several different stressors (physical and psychological), as well as the effect of chronicity (stress, ethanol, or both) on this interaction. To delineate the specificity and characteristics of the ethanol-stress interaction, we used two standard biochemical indices of stress, namely changes in plasma levels of corticosterone and NEFA.

METHODS

Subjects

The subjects in our studies were male Sprague-Dawley rats (Charles River, Wilmington, Massachusetts) which, at the time of testing, weighed 250–300 g. Subjects were individually housed in our temperature- ($22.0°C \pm 0.2°$) and light- (12:12 light:dark cycle, lights on 0700) controlled vivarium. Three days prior to testing (2 weeks after arrival), subjects were handled 2–3 minutes per day to minimize the stress of contact with the experimenter during the actual experiment.

Stress Procedures

Footshock stress. Footshock was delivered from a custom-built, high-voltage AC shocker to the steel grid floor of a Plexiglas cage. The cages were enclosed within individual ventilated, sound-attenuating boxes. Shock intensity was 0.50mA, and shock duration was 2 seconds. Shock sessions consisted of 30–180 trials, with an intertrial interval of 1 minute. Saline- and ethanol-treated subjects were run concurrently, and drug treatments were alternated between shock chambers. Ethanol 0.5 g/kg or saline was injected 30 minutes before the stress session. Nonshock control animals were injected with saline but remained in their home cages. In each experiment, animals were randomly assigned to one of the experimental conditions.

Tail pinch stress. The rat's tail was pinched with a plastic clamp approximately 1 cm from the tip of the tail for a predetermined period of time, as previously described (34).

Immobilization stress. Rats were placed into wire mesh restrainers, which prevented significant movement of the animals (31). The restrainers consisted of a 7 cm diameter tube, made of 7.5 mm wire mesh, which was closed off at one end with a perforated metal cap. Rats were placed in the tube headfirst, and two Chinese chopsticks placed at the base of their tails prevented backing out. The chopsticks were adjusted to provide a snug fit without pinching the rat or forcing it into a contorted position.

Cognitive stress. Two rats were placed in a chamber used for the delivery of footshocks. The chamber was divided in half with a partition made of Plexiglas, with a number of holes to facilitate the exchange of auditory and olfactory stimuli. The floor of one side was covered with a sheet of Plexiglas so that the rat on that side of the partition did not receive footshocks. The stress session consisted of 30 trials with shock parameters identical to those used in the footshock stress experiment. The walls and floor of the chamber were washed between pairs of subjects, and the side in which subjects received shock or drug was alternated between pairs of subjects. A subject from either the saline-cognitive or ethanol-cognitive group was tested in pair with a saline-shock subject.

Novel environment stress. A rat was removed from its home cage, placed in a novel plastic cage, and transported in this cage from the animal vivarium to the general biochemistry laboratory. The cage was placed on a laboratory bench for a fixed period of time after which the animals were decapitated.

Swim stress. The swim test was carried out using the apparatus and procedure originally described by Bass and Lester (35). Briefly, rats were placed at one end of a stainless-steel tank (3.05m long, 0.31m wide, and 0.61m high) filled with ambient temperature water (22°C). The time taken by the rat to swim to the opposite end of the tank, where an escape ladder was located, was recorded in seconds. Each test consisted of five trials spaced 5 minutes apart.

Chronic Experiments

Chronic stress. Rats were randomly assigned to a stress or nonstress group. The stress group was immobilized daily for a period of 90 minutes, while the control nonstressed rats remained in their home cages. On the 12th day *all* the subjects were immobilized. In addition, half of the animals in the chronically stressed and control groups were injected with saline and the other half with ethanol 30 minutes before the end of the stress session.

Chronic ethanol treatment. Half of the rats for this experiment were randomly assigned to the chronic ethanol-treatment group and the other half to the chronic control group. The latter group received an equicaloric amount of sucrose rather than ethanol. Since we found that repeated intraperitoneal (IP) injections of ethanol tend to be stressful, all animals were implanted with gastric cannulas 1 week before treatment was initiated. The cannulas were made of PE-100 polyethelyne tubing. After insertion into the stomach, the cannula is secured to the peritoneal wall and funnelled subcutaneously to the back of the neck, where it is exteriorized. Between treatments, the cannula is closed with a metal stylet. The daily dose of ethanol was 3 g/kg (15% solution). On the 12th day, half of the animals in each group were immobilized for 90 minutes, while the other half were not stressed and remained in their home cages. *All* of the subjects were injected with ethanol (0.5 g/kg IP). The stressed animals were injected 60 minutes into the stress session, that is, 30 minutes before sacrifice. Nonstressed animals received the ethanol injection 30 minutes before decapitation.

Chronic stress and ethanol treatment. For this study, a group of animals received chronic ethanol treatment, as well as chronic stress. These subjects were given 3 g/kg/day of ethanol intragastrically. Half of them were also immobilized daily for 90 minutes. The other half stayed in their home cages. This treatment continued for 10 days. On Day 11, all animals were injected with 0.5 g/kg of ethanol or saline before immobilization.

Assays

Corticosterone was measured using a spectrophotofluorometric procedure (36). Nonesterified free fatty acids were measured using a spectrophotometric assay (37). Blood ethanol levels were determined using a sensitive gas chromatographic procedure (38). Concentration of Na+ and K+ in urine was determined using a Digital Flame photometer.

Statistical Analyses

All data were analyzed using analysis of variance or independent paired t-tests. Differences between groups were considered significant when $p \leq .05$.

RESULTS

The first series of experiments examined the generality of the effect of ethanol in stressed animals. We examined first purely physical stressors and then proceeded to investigate psychological stressors.

Footshock Stress

The first experiment examined whether ethanol had an effect in rats stressed by footshock. Focusing on the NEFA results first, it is apparent that footshock produced a significant increase in NEFA levels, while the 0.5 g/kg dose of ethanol had no significant effect on NEFA levels (see Table 1). Furthermore, ethanol-treated stressed animals had significantly lower levels of NEFA compared to the saline-treated shocked group.

A similar pattern of response was seen with plasma corticosterone levels, i.e., ethanol treatment did not alter corticosterone levels, while footshock elevated levels sevenfold. Similarly, corticosterone levels in ethanol-pretreated stressed rats were significantly lower, compared to saline-treated shock animals. These differences between shocked and nonshocked ethanol-treated animals could not be explained by differences in blood ethanol levels, since these were not significantly different (see Table 1).

The results of this first experiment indicated that a low dose of ethanol did indeed modify the stress response. Next, we examined the time course of this interaction in order to determine the time when the effect of ethanol was maximal. Footshock conditions in this study were the same as in the first experiment except that animals were stressed for different periods of time—either 60, 120, or 180 minutes. All animals, except for the two zero time groups, were stressed and randomly assigned to either the ethanol or the saline-control conditions. Ethanol or saline was injected 30 minutes before the stress session.

TABLE 1
Effect of Ethanol Treatment on NEFA and
Corticosterone Levels in Plasma of
Footshock-Stressed and Nonstressed Rats

Treatment	NEFA(uEq/ml)	CS(ug/ml)	BEL(mg/ml)
Saline—no shock	$0.238 \pm .040$	$0.063 \pm .008$	—
Saline—shock	$0.478 \pm .027*$	$0.520 \pm .028$	—
Ethanol—no shock	$0.238 \pm .038$	$0.080 \pm .006$	0.120 ± 0.015
Ethanol—shock	$0.381 \pm .011**$	$0.422 \pm .016**$	0.125 ± 0.014

$*p < .005$, compared to saline-treated nonshocked group.
$**p < .05$, compared to saline-treated shocked group; $p < .02$, compared to ethanol-treated nonshocked group ($N = 8$-12).

Footshock stress resulted in a significant increase in NEFA and corti-costerone levels within 60 minutes (see Figure 1). NEFA levels remained significantly elevated for the duration of the experiment. In fact, NEFA levels were highest at the 180 minute period. By contrast, corticosterone levels gradually declined from its peak increase at 60 minutes. It is apparent from Figure 1 that, for both stress-induced NEFA and corticos-terone levels data, the peak interaction of stress and ethanol occurred at both 60 and 120 minutes. Analysis of variance of these data indicated a significant time x treatment interaction for both corticosterone ($F = 10.89$, $df = 3,32$; $p < .001$) and NEFA ($F = 2.93$, $df = 3,32$; $p < .05$).

In the first two studies, ethanol was injected prior to exposure to stress. The next study examined the interaction of ethanol and footshock with respect to the time of treatment with ethanol. We compared the effect of administering ethanol before (prestress group), during, or after (poststress) the stress session.

In the prestress condition, ethanol (0.5 g/kg) was injected 30 minutes prior to exposure to stress, which was 90 minutes long, as in the first experiment described earlier. In the during-stress conditions, ethanol (0.5 g/kg) was injected 60 minutes into the stress session; that is, 30 minutes before sacrifice. In the poststress condition, animals stressed for 30 minutes were then injected with ethanol (0.5 g/kg) at the termination of the stress session. Those animals were killed 30 minutes after injection of ethanol.

From the results in Table 2 it is apparent that the protective effect of ethanol was similar when it was injected prior to or during the stress session. This is quite interesting considering the differences in time of

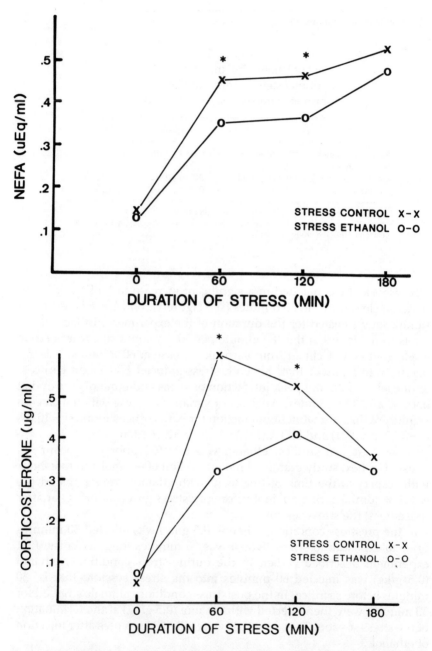

Figure 1. Response to ethanol treatment (0.5 g/kg IP) or saline treatment on plasma corticosterone and NEFA levels in rats stressed by different durations of footshock (n = 6/group). Statistically significant (p = .05 or less) differences between ethanol and saline stressed group are indicated[*].

TABLE 2
Effectiveness of Ethanol Treatment in
Stressed Rats—Dependency on
Time of Administration

Ethanol Injection	Treatment Group	Percent change from saline no-stress group	
		CS	NEFA
Poststress	Saline-stress	+ 97.6	− 13.8
	Ethanol-stress	+ 182.3	+ 58.5
During stress	Saline-stress	+ 546.9	+ 111.1
	Ethanol-stress	+ 374.0	+ 37.8
Prestress	Saline-stress	+ 725.4	+ 100.6
	Ethanol-stress	+ 569.8	+ 60.1

Note. Rats were stressed during a 90-minute footshock session. Ethanol treatment, 0.5 g/kg IP, was administered 30 minutes before, during, or right after the stress session. The results are calculated as percent change from the no stress saline-injected control group.

testing after ethanol. However, ethanol had no protective effect when it was administered after the stress session. In the later group, corticosterone levels were still significantly elevated, while NEFA levels were not. In marked contrast to the prestress and during-stress conditions, both corticosterone and NEFA levels were significantly higher in the ethanol-stress conditions compared to the saline-stress conditions.

Tail Pinch Stress

Another purely physical stressor is tail pinch. Tail pinch was originally described as a model for studying stress-induced behaviors (34).

First, we examined several time parameters to determine optimal conditions needed to obtain maximal elevations in plasma levels of both corticosterone and NEFA. Table 3 shows these results. Using a plastic clamp, tail pinch was applied intermittently for a total duration of 5 or 10 minutes. Animals were then killed either 5 or 10 minutes after discontinuation of the stressor.

Five minutes of tail pinch produced maximal response in corticosterone in rats killed 5 minutes poststress (Table 3). Furthermore, with

TABLE 3
Time Course for Tail-Pinch Induced Changes
in Plasma Corticosterone and NEFA Levels

Treatment	CS(ug/ml)	NEFA(uEq/ml)
Home cage control	0.121 ± 0.015	0.256 ± 0.080
Tail-pinch 5 min +5 min recovery	$0.278 \pm 0.040*$	$0.588 \pm 0.120*$
Tail-pinch 10 min +5 min recovery	$0.191 \pm 0.003*$	$0.592 \pm 0.002*$
Tail-pinch 5 min +10 min recovery	$0.301 + 0.030*$	$0.354 \pm 0.005*$
Tail-pinch 10 min +10 min recovery	$0.336 \pm 0.020*$	$0.340 \pm 0.081*$

Note. Groups of 5 rats were subjected to tail-pinch stress for a total of 5 or 10 minutes. Subjects were decapitated at 5 or 10 minutes after termination of the stressor. Control animals remained in their home cages ($N = 6$-12).
*Significantly different at $p < .05$ level.

either 5 or 10 minutes of tail pinch, corticosterone levels were higher in rats killed at 10 minutes poststress versus 5 minutes poststress. Plasma NEFA levels were highest in the stressed rats irrespective of whether they were stressed for 5 or 10 minutes. NEFA levels of the stressed rats allowed 10 minutes of recovery were lower, compared to those of rats recovering for 5 minutes. On the basis of these results, we selected 5 minutes of tail pinch with 5 minutes of recovery for the studies on the interaction with ethanol.

Figure 2 illustrates the effect of ethanol in animals which were stressed by tail pinch. A 0.5 g/kg dose of ethanol lowered the tail pinch-induced rise in plasma corticosterone levels by 23% and decreased plasma NEFA levels by 34%. By contrast, a 2.0 g/kg dose of ethanol did not modify the corticosterone response of stressed rats, while NEFA levels increased by 150% compared to saline-injected stressed animals.

The results of this experiment were analyzed using an ANOVA test for unweighted means to compensate for unequal number of animals in the different treatment conditions. Focusing on corticosterone results first, stress significantly elevated corticosterone levels ($F = 77.99$, $df = 1,58$; $p < .0001$). Ethanol also had a significant effect on plasma corticosterone levels ($F = 68.382$, $df = 2,58$; $p \leq .0001$), and there was a significant interaction between ethanol and stress ($F = 31.520$, $df = 2,58$; $p < .001$) in the stress condition; the effect of ethanol was significant compared to the

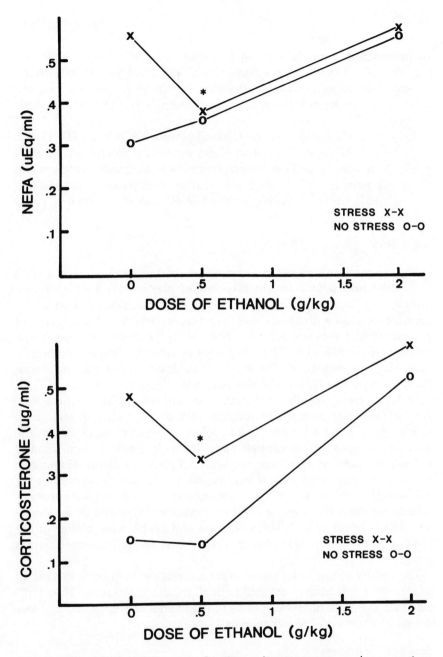

Figure 2. Effect of ethanol (0.5–2.0 g/kg IP) or saline treatment on plasma corticosterone and NEFA levels in rats stressed by tail pinch ($n = 6$/group)(*). Statistically
significant ($p < .001$) differences between saline-treated stressed group and ethanol-
(0.5 g/kg) treated stressed groups.

saline-injected animals for the 0.5 g/kg dose ($F = 12.662$, $df = 1,53$; $p < .001$) as well as the 2.0 g/kg dose ($F = 53.437$, $df = 1,53$; $p < .001$). In the nonstress condition, only the effects of the 2.0 g/kg dose were significantly different from the saline-injected animals ($F = 150.887$, $df = 1,53$; $p < .0001$).

Stress and ethanol significantly altered plasma NEFA levels ($F = 13.487$, $df = 1,58$; $p < .001$, and $F = 8.494$, $df = 2,58$; $p < .001$, respectively). Furthermore, there was a significant interaction between ethanol treatment and stress exposure ($F = 8.529$, $df = 2,58$; $p < .001$). The greatest interaction of ethanol with stress on NEFA occurred at 60 and 90 minutes of stress exposure.

Swim Stress

The last purely physical stressor we examined was swim stress. Table 4 shows the time course for the response of plasma NEFA and corticosterone in swim-stressed animals. Plasma corticosterone showed a progressive increase with duration of the stressor. However, the response of plasma NEFA levels was variable. Thus, with 5 minutes of swim, NEFA levels were decreased by 22%; they were elevated by 13% at 10 minutes, and were unchanged by 30 minutes. Basically, there was no major changes in plasma NEFA with this particular stressor.

Table 5 presents results for the interaction of ethanol and swim stress. Animals were stressed for 15 minutes. Half of them were injected with saline, the other half with 0.5 g/kg of ethanol 30 minutes before the stressor. Animals were decapitated after the swim stress session. Control animals in this case were injected with 0.5 g/kg of ethanol 45 minutes before decapitation. Swim stress increased plasma corticosterone by 117% and NEFA levels by 178%. Pretreatment with ethanol did not attenuate either the corticosterone or NEFA elevations produced by the stressor. In fact, levels of both corticosterone and NEFA were higher in the ethanol-pretreated stress group versus the saline-pretreated stress group.

The results of the swim stress experiment were surprising in view of the similar interaction of ethanol with all the other stressors. They indicate that there might be exceptions to the overall beneficial effect of low doses of ethanol in stressed animals.

Immobilization Stress

Footshock is mostly a physical stressor. The next stressor we examined was restraint or immobilization stress. This stressor is considered to have both physical and psychological components. Figure 3 illustrates the

TABLE 4

Response in Plasma Levels of Corticosterone, NEFA,
Na+ and K+ Ions in Swim-Stressed Rats

Treatment	Corticosterone (ug/ml)	NEFA (uEq/ml)	Na+	K+
			uEq/hr	
Home cage	0.096 ± 0.002	0.356 ± 0.017	145.2 ± 0.63	7.88 ± 0.20
Swim— 5 min	0.156 ± 0.006*	0.278 ± 0.023*	141.9 ± 1.01*	7.16 ± 0.23*
—10 min	0.337 ± 0.004*	0.401 ± 0.092*	138.9 ± 1.34*	7.02 ± 0.14*
—30 min	0.459 ± 0.003*	0.350 ± 0.033	130.9 ± 3.40*	7.22 ± 0.11*

Note. Groups of 5 rats swam for 5, 10, or 30 minutes in ambient temperature water. Animals were sacrificed at the termination of the stress session. Control animals remained in their home cages (N = 6).
*Significantly different at $p < .05$ level.

effect of immobilization stress on plasma levels of corticosterone and NEFA. Fifteen minutes of restraint produced a 450% increase in corticosterone. Peak increase in corticosterone was seen within 30 minutes of stress exposure, and in rats immobilized for 150 minutes corticosterone was less elevated compared to the 30 or 90 minute stressed groups. NEFA levels, on the other hand, showed an initial 110% peak at 15 minutes. This was followed by a decline in levels in the 30 minute

TABLE 5

Lack of Effect of Ethanol Pretreatment on
Plasma Levels of Corticosterone and
NEFA in Swim-Stressed Rats

Treatment	Corticosterone (ug/ml)	NEFA (uEq/ml)
Ethanol (0.5 g/kg)	0.190 ± 0.005	0.210 ± 0.003
Swim	0.413 ± 0.012*	0.584 ± 0.006*
Ethanol (0.5 g/kg) + swim	0.568 ± 0.027*	0.619 ± 0.006*

Note. Groups of rats were swim-stressed for 15 minutes. Half of the animals were randomly assigned to receive ethanol (0.5 g/kg,IP) pretreatment 30 minutes before the stress session. The other half of the animals received an injection of saline. The nonstress control group was injected with 0.5 g/kg ethanol (N = 6).
*Significantly different at $p < .05$ level.

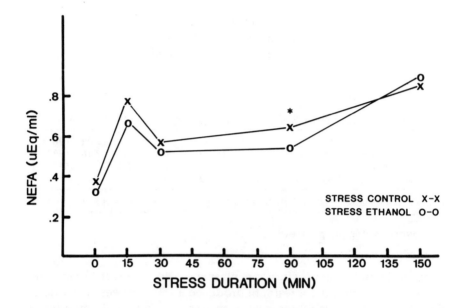

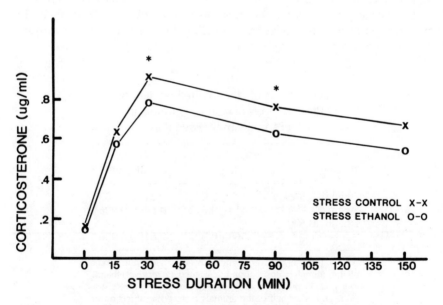

Figure 3. Time course of the effect of ethanol (0.5 g/kg IP) or saline treatments on plasma corticosterone and NEFA levels in rats stressed by immobilization ($n = 8$/group). Statistically significant ($p < .05$).

stressed group, followed by a gradual increase in NEFA levels all the way to 150 minutes. Analysis of variance of these data indicate a significant interaction of ethanol and time for both corticosterone ($F = 2.97$, $df = 4,70$; $p < .05$) and NEFA ($F = 2.90$, $df = 4,80$; $p < .05$).

Cognitive Stress

The next two experiments examined the interaction of ethanol and stress using purely psychological stressors. The first study examined the effect of ethanol on animals which are only exposed to the sound, smell, and possible visual observation of a rat which is being stressed.

The results of this study are presented in Table 6. It is apparent that a purely psychological stressor significantly elevated both plasma corticosterone and NEFA. In fact, levels of NEFA, and less so of corticosterone in the plasma of the rats receiving cognitive stress, were very close to those of the animals which received footshock. Plasma corticosterone levels of the cognitive-stress animals treated with a low dose of ethanol were significantly lower than those of the saline-treated cognitive rats. However, this was not the case with plasma NEFA levels. That is, NEFA levels of the cognitive-stress ethanol-treated group, although lower, did not reach conventional levels of statistical significance.

TABLE 6
Effect of Ethanol, Footshock, and
Cognitive Stress on Plasma Levels of
Corticosterone and Free Fatty Acids

Treatment group	Corticosterone ug/ml	NEFA uEq/ml
Saline-shock	0.560 ± 0.061	0.506 ± 0.014
Saline-cognitive	0.506 ± 0.062	0.485 ± 0.025
Ethanol-cognitive	0.318 ± 0.054[a]	0.442 ± 0.044

Note. Values are expressed as mean levels of corticosterone or free fatty acids $\pm$ S.E.M. ($N = 6$/group).
[a]Significantly different at $p < .05$ level.
Reprinted by permission of the publisher from Neuroendocrine responses to stress and the effect of ethanol, in Stress and Alcohol Use: Proceedings of the First International Symposium on Stress and Alcohol Use. Edited by Pohorecky, LA, Brick, J. New York, Elsevier, 1983, pp. 389–402. Copyright 1983 Elsevier.

Novel Environment Stress

The second study, with a purely psychological stressor, involved what is called a "novel environment" stress. In order to evaluate the "stress-fulness" of this procedure, we measured plasma corticosterone and NEFA levels after 10 or 30 minutes of exposure to a novel (laboratory) environment. It can be seen that exposure to the laboratory environment for 10 minutes raised corticosterone and NEFA levels significantly (see Table 7). If exposure was longer, i.e., 30 minutes, the elevation in corticosterone levels was less (84% versus 102%), while that in NEFA was slightly higher (42% versus 14%).

For the study on the interaction with ethanol, rats were injected with a 0.5 g/kg dose of ethanol or saline and then, 30 minutes later, brought to the laboratory for a period of 15 minutes. Control animals remained in their home cages. Stressed animals were decapitated at the end of the stress period. As can be seen in Table 8, in the ethanol-pretreated animals, corticosterone levels were 23% lower than in the saline-pretreated animals.

We concluded from the last two experiments that pretreatment with a small dose of ethanol also had a protective effect in animals exposed to purely psychological stressors.

There is evidence that catecholamines may regulate plasma potassium concentration (39, 40). Since stress elevates plasma catecholamines (33), we also examined plasma levels of sodium and potassium in this particular experiment. Ten minutes of stress resulted in a downward shift in both ions; however, only the decline in potassium was significant (Table 7). There was some recovery in the levels of potassium ions in the 30

TABLE 7
Novel Environment Stress on Plasma Levels of
NEFA and Corticosterone

Treatment	CS ug/ml	NEFA (uEq/ml)	Na+	K+
			uEq/hr	
Control	0.120 ± 0.01	0.281 ± 0.009	140.5 ± 0.74	7.80 ± 0.15
Stress—10 min	$0.242 \pm 0.02*$	$0.321 \pm 0.012*$	138.3 ± 0.93	$7.22 \pm 0.11*$
—30 min	$0.221 \pm 0.04*$	$0.399 \pm 0.008*$	140.3 ± 0.79	7.61 ± 0.09

Note. Rats were exposed to a "novel environment" for 10–30 minutes. Control animals re-mained in their home cages in the animal vivarium. The stress control group received an injection of saline ($N = 6$).
*Significantly different at $p < .05$ level.

TABLE 8
Changes in Plasma Levels of
Corticosterone/NEFA in Ethanol or
Saline-Treated Rats Exposed to
a Novel Environment

Treatment	Corticosterone (ug/ml)
Control	0.137 ± 0.029
Stress (15 min)	0.430 ± 0.040*
Ethanol (0.5 g/kg)—stress	0.330 ± 0.030

Note. Rats were exposed to a "novel environment" for 15 minutes. Control animals remained
in their home cages in the animal vivarium. The
stress control group received an injection of saline. The ethanol-treated group was injected with
0.5 g/kg 30 minutes before exposure to the "novel environment" (N = 6).
*Significantly different at p < .05 level.

minute group. With this stressor there were time-dependent declines in
both measures. The peak 9.8% decline in sodium ion occurred at 30
minutes, while the peak 10.9% decline in potassium ions was at the 10
minute period.

Chronic Studies

The next question we addressed was what would be the interaction of
ethanol and stress if either stress exposure or ethanol treatment was
chronic. It is conceivable that chronic stress modifies the response to
ethanol. For example, in chronically stressed animals, a small dose of
ethanol may no longer have an effect. Similarly, in rats chronically
treated with ethanol, the protective effect of a small dose of ethanol may
disappear. To examine these issues we have carried out three experiments.

The first of these studies examined the effectiveness of a small dose of
ethanol in rats that had been stressed chronically. Table 9 presents these
data; analysis of variance revealed a significant interaction between
chronic stress treatment and acute ethanol ($F = 9.81$, $df = 1,36$; $p < .001$).

An acute session of immobilization elevated plasma corticosterone levels, with highest levels present in the chronic control group treated with
saline. The saline-treated chronic stress group was lower, compared to

TABLE 9
Effect of Acute Ethanol Treatment on
Stress-Induced Changes in Plasma Levels of
NEFA and Corticosterone in Chronically Stressed Rats

Treatment	Corticosterone (ug/ml)	NEFA (uEq/ml)	BEL (mg/ml)
Chronic stress acute ethanol	0.432 ± 0.010	0.324 ± 0.019	0.094 ± 0.010
Chronic stress acute saline	0.320 ± 0.026*	0.419 ± 0.042*	—
Chronic control acute ethanol	0.418 ± 0.030**	0.340 ± 0.036	0.120 ± 0.011
Chronic control acute saline	0.506 ± 0.028	0.346 ± 0.038	—

Note. A total of 28 rats were randomly assigned to one of four treatments. Half of the animals were stressed daily (immobilization for 90 minutes) for 12 days. The other half of the animals were nonstressed controls. On Day 12 all animals were restrained. Half of the chronically stressed and nonstressed groups were injected with 0.5 g/kg of ethanol and the other half with an equivalent volume of saline.
*Significantly different from chronic stress-acute ethanol group, $p < .05$.
**Significantly different from chronic control-acute saline group, $p < .05$.

the chronic control group, indicating that significant tolerance had developed to the stressor by the last day of testing. On the other hand, there was no statistically significant difference between the two ethanol-treated groups. That is, corticosterone levels were similar in rats injected with ethanol, irrespective of whether they had been previously stressed or not.

However, since the corticosterone levels of the chronically stressed, saline-treated animals were 35% lower than those of the corresponding chronic-control group, the ethanol treatment increased corticosterone levels slightly in the chronic stress group while decreasing corticosterone levels in the chronic control group. Therefore, this dose of ethanol had no protective effect as far as plasma corticosterone levels in subjects that were stressed chronically.

Turning to the plasma NEFA data, we see a difference in response to this measure for the saline-injected animals. Plasma NEFA levels were significantly higher in the chronically stressed group, as indicated by a significant main effect of chronic stress ($F = 5.66$, $df = 1,20$; $p < .05$). That is, no tolerance developed in the response to stress to this particular measure.

However, the two ethanol-treated groups again were almost identical. Therefore, in contrast to the results with corticosterone, the protective effect of ethanol was not significant in the chronic control group, while it was statistically significant in the chronically stressed group. We have no explanation for the lack of the protective effect of ethanol in the acutely stressed group.

We also examined blood ethanol levels in this study. Chronic stress did not significantly alter blood ethanol level.

The second chronic study examined the effectiveness of a small dose of ethanol in rats chronically treated with ethanol. Focusing on corticosterone first, analysis of variance of the data indicated a significant main effect of chronic treatment with ethanol ($F = 22.03$, $df = 1,20$; $p < .001$) and for acute stress ($F = 326.67$, $df = 1,20$; $p < .001$). More important was the significant interaction of chronic treatment with ethanol and the acute stressor ($F = 12.194$, $df = 1,20$; $p < .001$). As before, in previous experiments, immobilization stress elevated plasma corticosterone levels (Table 10). On the other hand, chronic ethanol treatment did not modify plasma corticosterone levels in nonstressed rats.

The elevation in plasma corticosterone produced by acute immobilization stress was similar in both the chronic ethanol group and the chronic control group. However, the corticosterone levels in the acutely stressed animals were lower in those animals that were chronically treated with ethanol. Thus, chronic ethanol treatment did not eliminate the "protec-

TABLE 10
Effect of Acute Ethanol Treatment on Plasma
Levels of Corticosterone and NEFA in
Acutely Stressed, Chronically Ethanol-Treated Rats

Treatment	Corticosterone (ug/ml)	NEFA (uEq/ml)	BEL (mg/ml)
Chronic ethanol acute stress	0.328 ± 0.020*,**	$0.487 \pm .077$*	0.111 ± 0.012
Chronic ethanol no stress	0.166 ± 0.004	$0.128 \pm .034$	0.135 ± 0.009
Control acute stress	0.406 ± 0.003***	$0.436 \pm .090$***	0.144 ± 0.021
Control no stress	0.194 ± 0.017	$0.220 \pm .069$	0.138 ± 0.012

Note. Twenty-eight rats were randomly assigned to one of four groups: half the rats received daily treatment with ethanol (3 g/kg, intragastrically) for 11 days, the other half served as controls. On the 12th day, half of each group was stressed by immobilization for 90 minutes. *All* the animals received 0.5 g/kg ethanol.
  *Significantly different from chronic ethanol—no stress group, $p < .05$.
  **Significantly different from control acutely stressed group, $p < .05$.
  ***Significantly different from control—no stress group, $p < .05$.

tive" effect of the low dose of ethanol. It is conceivable that cross-tolerance could develop between ethanol and stress with respect to elevation
of corticosterone. Therefore, an acute stressor would be less effective in
elevating corticosterone levels in animals given chronic ethanol treatment.

The protective effect of a low dose of ethanol is no longer evident in
chronically ethanol-treated rats, if one examines plasma NEFA values. In
fact, the only significant effect is that of the acute stressor ($F=43.42$,
$df=1,20$; $p<.001$). Blood ethanol levels did not differ statistically in any
one of the four experimental groups.

The last study involved animals receiving chronic ethanol treatment as
well as chronic stress. In this experiment, we wanted to see if chronic
stress and chronic ethanol altered the effect of stress on plasma corticosterone and NEFA levels.

All chronic treatments (ethanol, stress, ethanol plus stress) decreased
the corticosterone response to stress on the last day of the study (see
Table 11). We see again that chronic stress treatment produced tolerance
to the acute stressor. Chronic ethanol treatment did not alter the protective effect of the 0.5 g/kg of ethanol in acutely stressed animals (i.e., the

TABLE 11
Acute Ethanol Treatment on Plasma Levels of
Corticosterone and NEFA Levels in Chronically
Stressed and Chronically Ethanol-Treated Rats

Treatment	Corticosterone (ug/ml)	NEFA (uEq/ml)	BEL (mg/ml)
Chronic ethanol no stress	0.534 ± 0.048*	0.274 ± 0.039*	0.125 ± 0.012
Chronic control no stress	0.754 ± 0.051	0.333 ± 0.090	0.112 ± 0.010
Chronic ethanol chronic restraint	0.539 ± 0.079	0.570 ± 0.073**	0.117 ± 0.012
Chronic control chronic restraint	0.505 ± 0.084*	0.463 ± 0.064*	0.135 ± 0.016

Note. Animals were stressed for 90 minutes daily for a total of 10 days. Control nonstress
animals remained in their home cages. Half of the animals in each group received daily 3
g/kg of ethanol intragastrically. The other half received equicaloric volume of maltose.
The chronic restraint group were restrained daily for 90 minutes. The chronic restrained
control animals were left in home cages. On the last day of the experiment (Day 11), all
animals were restrained for 90 minutes and all animals were injected with 0.5 g/kg of
ethanol.
*Significantly different from chronic control—no stress group, $p<.05$.
**Significantly different from chronic ethanol—no stress group, $p<.05$.

two nonstressed groups). However, this dose of ethanol did not have a protective effect in the chronically stressed animals. Finally, there is no potentiation between the chronic ethanol treatment and stress, since there was no significant difference between the chronically stressed animals treated with or without ethanol or the group of rats chronically treated with ethanol but not chronically stressed. A possible explanation of these results is that ethanol and stress elevate corticosterone by similar mechanism(s).

DISCUSSION

Using a variety of stressors, we have determined that in rats, a low dose of ethanol alters part of the neuroendocrine and sympathetic nervous systems' response to stress. The stressors we evaluated ranged from the physical to purely psychological ones. Some stressors, e.g., immobilization, included both physical and psychological components.

We found that, except for swim stress, a low dose of ethanol was able to modify the elevation of corticosterone and NEFA produced by a variety of different stressors. A most striking finding was the difference in response to the two doses of ethanol we tested. In the study reported here, as well as in others, we found that in contrast to the beneficial action of a low dose of ethanol, a moderately high dose had the opposite effect in stressed animals. That is, a 2.0 g/kg dose of ethanol potentiated the stress response in rats.

This dose-dependence is interesting, but is not unique. Ethanol is known to have other biphasic effects in both experimental animals and in man (41). For example, in rodents a low dose of ethanol can be excitatory and increase general motor activity, while larger doses of ethanol markedly depress motor activity (42, 43).

On the other hand, the effect of ethanol on corticosterone is not biphasic (44, 45). Although the 0.5 g/kg dose of ethanol had no significant effect on plasma corticosterone or NEFA levels, ethanol has a dose-dependent effect on plasma corticosterone.

With respect to the chronic studies, it is interesting to note that rats which received chronic ethanol treatment responded to stress with smaller increases in plasma corticosterone than rats in the chronic control/stress group. This suggests that there may be some cross-tolerance between the effect of ethanol and stress on corticosterone. This was not the case for NEFA. Actually, chronic ethanol caused a slight potentiation of stress-induced elevation in plasma NEFA levels. Further studies are underway to determine the effect of chronic ethanol on subsequent acute ethanol administration.

Several possible explanations can be advanced as mechanism(s) for the interaction of ethanol with stress. With some of the stressors, especially those involving physical pain, such as footshock or tail pinch, it could be argued that ethanol may have an analgesic effect. That is, by decreasing the pain ethanol-treated animals were experiencing, the elevation in corticosterone and NEFA would be smaller. This explanation is unlikely for two reasons. First, although our own work and that of others do indicate that ethanol has an analgesic action, this effect generally requires larger doses of ethanol (46). Secondly, the effect of ethanol on analgesia is dose-dependent; the relationship is monotonic and not biphasic. Therefore, we would expect the protective effect of a 2.0 g/kg dose of ethanol to be greater than that with a 0.5 g/kg dose. This, however, was not the case.

Ethanol could act by partially *preventing* the stress-induced release of plasma corticosterone and NEFA. Alternatively, ethanol could *lower* the stress-induced elevations of both corticosterone and NEFA. In the first case, ethanol would block the stress-induced release of NEFA and corticosterone. In the second case, ethanol would act by accelerating the disappearance from blood of both corticosterone and NEFA. For example, ethanol could accelerate the uptake and metabolism or utilization of NEFA and corticosterone by the liver or by other organs.

We found that ethanol altered the stress response of animals when it was injected before or during the stress session, but not when injected after the stress session. Therefore, ethanol must be present during exposure to the stressor in order to have a protective effect. In fact, when injected after the stress session, ethanol potentiated the stress response.

Our research indicates that ethanol probably acts by the first of the proposed mechanisms, i.e., by preventing the release of NEFA and corticosterone into blood. We can only speculate, at this point, how ethanol may be accomplishing this. One possibility is that ethanol is affecting the release of neurotransmitters mediating the release of corticosterone or the regulation of sympathetic activity. We have additional evidence to indicate that the site of ethanol's action is most likely central and not peripheral. For example, ethanol still has a protective effect on plasma NEFA levels in stressed, adrenalectomized animals (32; also see Brick & Pohorecky, this volume).

Our results also indicate that, although the interaction of a low dose of ethanol occurs with a variety of stressors, there might be exceptions. For example, the 0.5 g/kg dose of ethanol had no effect in rats stressed by swimming. Interestingly, the effect of swim stress on plasma NEFA levels differed from that of all the other stressors. Also there was a marked decline in plasma concentrations of sodium and potassium. This indicates that the metabolic consequences of this particular stressor were different from those of the other stressors evaluated.

There is precedence indicating that the effect of ethanol is dependent on other metabolic factors. For example, the effect of ethanol on blood glucose is highly dependent on the metabolic state of the subject. When metabolic fuels are low, e.g., in partially food-deprived subjects, ethanol produces hypoglycemia (47, 48). On the other hand, hyperglycemia is produced by ethanol in fully satiated subjects (47, 48).

Both NEFA and glucose serve as energy sources for various tissues and organs. It is possible that a stressor that is more physically demanding, such as prolonged swimming, results in greater demands for energy substrates. Under these conditions, it is of greater benefit to the animal that both NEFA levels as well as corticosterone, because of its permissive effects on general metabolism, remain elevated. Therefore, in swim-stressed animals, the potentiation of both plasma levels of NEFA and of corticosterone by ethanol is actually beneficial. This suggests that the protective effect of a low dose of ethanol adjusts to the particular metabolic demands produced by a stressor.

Interestingly, we observed a significant decrease in the plasma concentrations of both potassium and sodium in stressed animals. It has been proposed by Phillis and Wu (49) that skeletal muscles play a major role in the control of plasma potassium levels under normal physiological conditions. A hypokalemic effect of peripheral catecholamines has been described previously (50–51). Therefore, the decline in plasma potassium we observed is consistent with the stress-induced increase in plasma catecholamines.

The results from our studies may be relevant to some of the known effects of ethanol in man. For example, the decline in NEFA produced by low doses of ethanol may partially explain the reported cardioprotective effects of ethanol in man (14–20).

Plasma NEFA contribute significantly to the energy supply of the myocardium (52). Our results indicate that one mechanism by which low doses of ethanol may have a cardioprotective effect in stressed animals is because it decreases NEFA levels in plasma and thus decreases the likelihood for the accumulation of excess lipid deposits in the heart.

Secondly, the physiological changes produced by low doses of ethanol in stressed individuals may result in subtle differences in somatic sensations. These could be perceived as "less stressful" by the subjects and, therefore, more desirable in a tense individual. This mechanism could be one of the mechanisms by which ethanol reinforces its own ingestion. Whether the latter in any way influences ethanol preference is obviously a whole different issue, which needs to be evaluated by future studies.

Thirdly, the decrease in stress-induced corticosterone may have a protective effect in individuals susceptible to ulcer formation. Stress-induced elevations in glucocorticoid levels may play a role in ulcer development (53).

Our data indicate that ethanol has a modifying effect on the stress response in rats. The direction of the interaction will vary with the particular stressor, the dose of ethanol, and the chronicity of the stressor and ethanol treatment. Additional studies are needed to explore these interactions further and to establish their potential usefulness to stressed subjects.

REFERENCES

1. Cebelin MS, Hirsch CS: Myocardial lesions in victims of homocidal assaults with internal injuries. Human Path 11:123–132, 1970
2. Henry FP, Stephens PM (eds): Stress Health and the Social Environment. New York, Springer Verlag, 1977
3. Riley V: Cancer and stress: Overview and critique. Cancer Detection and Prevention 2:163–195, 1979
4. Lown B, DeSilva RA, Lenson R: Roles of psychologic stress and autonomic nervous system changes in provocation of ventricular premature complexes. Amer J Cardiology 41:979–985, 1978
5. Ader R: Experimentally induced gastric lesions. Adv Psychosom Med 6:1–39, 1971
6. Marlatt GA: Stress as a determinant of excessive drinking and relapse, in Stress and Alcohol Use. Edited by Pohorecky LA, Brick J. New York, Elsevier, 1983
7. Mulford HA: Stress, alcohol intake and problem drinking in Iowa, in Stress and Alcohol Use. Edited by Pohorecky LA, Brick J. New York, Elsevier, 1983
8. Hastrup JL, Light KC, Obrist PA: Parental hypertension and cardiovascular response to stress in healthy young adults. Psychophysiology 19:615, 1982
9. Friedman R, Iwai J: Genetic predisposition and stress-induced hypertension. Science 193:161–162, 1976
10. Masserman JH, Yum KS: An analysis of the influence of alcohol on experimental neuroses in cats. Psychosom Med 8:36–52, 1946
11. Conger JJ: Reinforcement theory and the dynamics of alcoholism. Q J Stud Alc 17:296–305, 1956
12. Kraemer GW, Lin DH, Moran EC, et al: Effects of alcohol on the despair response to peer separation in rhesus monkeys. Psychopharmacology 73:307–310, 1981
13. Kraemer GW, Ebert MH, Lake R, et al: Neurobiological measures in rhesus monkeys: Correlation of the behavioral response to social separation and alcohol, in Stress and Alcohol Use. Edited by Pohorecky LA, Brick J. New York, Elsevier, 1983
14. Barboriak JJ, Rimm AA, Anderson AJ: Coronary artery occlusion and alcohol intake. Br Heart J, 39:289–293, 1977
15. Dyer AJ, Stamler J, Paul O: Alcohol, cardiovascular risk factors, and mortality in two Chicago epidemiological studies. CVD Epidemiol Newslett 20:34–39, 1976
16. Klatsky AL, Friedman GD, Siegelaub AB: Alcohol consumption and non-fatal myocar-

dial infarction: Results from the Kaiser-Permanente epidemiologic study of myocardial infarction. Ann Intern Med 81:294–301, 1974

17. Paul O, Lepper MH, Phelan WH: A longitudinal study of coronary heart disease. Circulation 28:20–31, 1963

18. Stason WB, Neff RK, Miettinen OS: Alcohol consumption and non-fatal myocardial infarction. Am J Epidemiol 104:603–608, 1976

19. Yano K, Rhoads GG, Kagan A: Coffee, alcohol, and risk of coronary heart disease among Japanese men living in Hawaii. New Engl J Med 297:405–409, 1977

20. Young LD, Barboriak JJ, Anderson AJ: Coronary prone behavior, stress and alcohol consumption: The relationship to coronary artery disease, in Stress and Alcohol Use. Edited by Pohorecky LA, Brick J. New York, Elsevier, 1983

21. Gerber WF, Anderson TA, vanDyne B: Influence of ethanol on the response of the albino rat to audiovisual and swim stress. Exp Med Surg 24: 25–35, 1966

22. Gerber WF, Anderson TA: Ethanol inhibition of audiogenic stress-induced cardiac hypertrophy. Experientia 23:734–736, 1967

23. Mallov S, Gilmour RF: Inhibition of epinephrine-induced myocardial necrosis in rats by administration of single doses of ethanol. Drug & Alc Depend 2:297–408, 1977

24. Mallov S: Catecholamine-induced myocardial necrosis and the protective effect of alcohol, in Stress and Alcohol Use. Edited by Pohorecky LA, Brick J. New York, Elsevier, 1983

25. Haggendal J, Johansson G, Jonsson L, et al: Effect of propranolol on myocardial cell necroses and blood levels of catecholamines in pigs subjected to stress. Acta Pharmacol et Toxicol 50:58–66, 1982

26. Lombardi F, Verrier RL, Lown B: Relationship between sympathetic neural activity, coronary dynamics, and vulnerability to ventricular fibrillation during myocardial ischemia and perfusion. Am Heart J 105:958–964, 1983

27. Bristow MR, Ginsburg R, Minobe W, et al: Decreased catecholamine sensitivity and β-adrenergic-receptor density in failing human hearts. New Engl J Med 307:205–211, 1982

28. Karlsberg RP, Cryer PE, Roberts R: Serial plasma catecholamine response early in the course of clinical acute myocardial infarction: Relationship to infarct extent and mortality. Am Heart J 102:24–28, 1981

29. Goddard PJ: Effects of alcohol on excretion of catecholamines in conditions giving rise to anxiety. J Appl Physiol 13:118–120, 1958

30. Pohorecky LA, Rassi E, Weiss JM, et al: Biochemical evidence for an interaction of ethanol and stress: Preliminary studies. Alcoholism Clin Exp Res 4:423–426, 1980

31. Brick J, Pohorecky LA: Ethanol-stress interaction: Biochemical findings. Psychopharmacol 77:81–84, 1982

32. Brick J, Pohorecky LA: The neuroendocrine response to stress and the effect of ethanol, in Stress and Alcohol Use. Edited by Pohorecky LA, Brick J. New York, Elsevier, 1983

33. DeTurck KH, Vogel WH: Effect of acute ethanol on plasma and brain catecholamine levels in stressed and unstressed rats: Evidence for an ethanol-stress interaction. J Pharmacol Exp Ther 223:348–354, 1982

34. Antelman SM, Caggiula AR: Tails of stress-related behavior: A neuropharmacological model, in Animal Models in Psychiatry and Neurology. Edited by Hanin I, Usdin E. New York, Pergamon, 1977

35. Bass M, Lester D: Swimming as a measure of motor impairment after ethanol and pentobarbital in rats. J Stud Alcohol 39:1618–1622, 1978

36. Glick D, Von Redlich D, Levine S: Fluorometric determination of corticosterone and cortisol in 0.02–0.05 milliliters of plasma or submilligram samples of adrenal tissue. Endocrinology 74:653–655, 1964

37. Smith SW: A simple salting out procedure in the colorimetric assay of free fatty acids. Anal Biochem 67:531–539, 1975

38. Pohorecky LA: Effects of ethanol on central and peripheral noradrengenic neurons. J Pharmacol Exp Ther 189:380–391, 1974

39. Akaike N: Sodium pump in skeletal muscle: Central nervous system-induced suppression by β-adrenoreceptors. Science 213:1252–1254, 1981
40. Silva P, Spokes K: Sympathetic system in potassium homeostasis. Am J Physiol 241:F151–F155, 1981
41. Pohorecky LA: Biphasic action of ethanol. Bio Behav Rev 1:231–240, 1978
42. Frye GD, Breese GR: An evaluation of the locomotor stimulating action of ethanol in rats and mice. Psychopharmacol 75:372–379, 1981
43. Matchett JA, Erickson CK: Alteration of ethanol-induced changes in locomotor activity by adrenergic blockers in mice. Psychopharmacol 52:201–206, 1977
44. Ellis FW: Effect of ethanol on plasma corticosterone levels. J Pharmacol Exp Therap 153:121–128, 1966
45. Pohorecky LA, Jaffe LS: Noradrenergic involvement in the acute effects of ethanol. Res Commun Chem Pathol Pharmacol 12:433–448, 1975
46. Brick J, Sun JY, Davis L, et al: Ethanol and the response to electric shock in rats. Life Sci 18:1293–1298, 1976
47. Bleicher SF, Freinkel N, Byrne JJ, et al: Effect of ethanol on plasma glucose and insulin in the fasted dog. Proc Soc Exper Biol Medic 115:369–373, 1964
48. Tramill JL, Turner PE, Harwell G, et al: Alcoholic hypoglycemia as a result of acute challenges of ethanol. Physiolog Psychol 9:114–116, 1981
49. Lassers BW, Carlson LA, Kayser L, et al: The nature and control of myocardial substrate metabolism in healthy man, in Effect of Acute Ischaemia on Myocardial Function. Edited by Oliver MF, Julian DG, Donald KW. Edinburgh, Churchill Livingstone 200–212, 1972
50. Ellis S: Metabolic effects of epinephrine and related amines. Pharmacol Rev 8:485–562, 1956
51. Lockwood RH, Lum BKB: Effects of adrenergic agonists and antagonists on potassium metabolism. J Pharmacol Exp Ther 189:119–129, 1974
52. Phillis JW, Wu PH: The role of muscle and glial cells in potassium homeostasis. J Pharmacol 33:340, 1981
53. Weiss JM: Effect of coping in different warning signal conditions on stress pathology in rats. J Comp Physiol Psy 77:1–13, 1971

7

The Limbic System and Ethanol-Induced Changes in Plasma Corticosterone and Nonesterified Fatty Acids

JOHN BRICK and LARISSA A. POHORECKY

The effects of a moderate dose of ethanol (2.0–3.0 g/kg) on corticosterone and nonesterified fatty acid levels were measured in rats with amygdala, hippocampal, septal, or hypothalamic lesions. The elevating effect of ethanol on nonesterified fatty acids was, compared to sham-lesioned rats, potentiated following amygdala and hippocampal lesions but unchanged following septal lesions. The increase in corticosterone following ethanol was potentiated following hippocampal lesions but unchanged in rats with amygdala or septal lesions. In rats with ventromedial hypothalamic lesions, the effect of ethanol depended upon the stress state of the animal. The role of the limbic system in the regulation of, and ethanol's action on, corticosterone and nonesterified fatty acids is discussed.

INTRODUCTION

In the last few years, we have carried out a number of studies demonstrating that ethanol and stress interact at the neuroendocrine level and

We thank Jeffrey Feinberg, Sophia Ahmad, Maryna Adams, and Mark Schackman for excellent technical assistance. We especially thank Halina Szyposzynski for her work on the VMH study. This research was supported by USPHS grants AA00045, 04241, and 94238.

101

within the sympathetic nervous system. So far, our work has focused on three aspects of this interaction.

First, we noted the generality and limitations of ethanol's protective effect. For example, low doses of ethanol protect experimental animals from psychological stressors as well as several, but not all, types of physical stressors.

Second, we have been interested in the effects of chronicity (of either ethanol administration or exposure to a stressor) on the protective effects of ethanol and subsequent responses to a stressor. Our results on the generality of the interaction between ethanol and stress, as well as our initial studies on chronicity, are described in Chapter 6 of this volume and elsewhere (1, 2, 3).

Our third area of interest is in elucidating the possible neural substrates involved in ethanol's action on corticosterone and nonesterified fatty acids (NEFA). This paper will describe our progress so far in searching for the neural mechanisms mediating ethanol's interaction with the neuroendocrine and sympathetic nervous systems.

Up until now, the basic effect we have been reporting is that low doses of ethanol attenuate stress-induced increases in corticosterone and NEFA levels. In the absence of stress, low doses (0.5 g/kg) of ethanol produce small, nonsignificant increases in plasma levels of corticosterone and NEFA. The mechanisms for the interaction of stress and ethanol are invariably quite complex and not easily partitioned out at the physiological level.

The precise mechanisms by which ethanol alters corticosterone and NEFA are not fully understood. It appears that ethanol's action on corticosterone involves changes in the pituitary release of ACTH (4–8), rather than a direct effect on the adrenal cortex.

Ethanol may alter NEFA by one or more of several ways. For example, ethanol may alter liver metabolism (9, 10) or change the release of catecholamines from sympathetic nerve endings directly innervating adipose tissue. Lastly, ethanol may affect brain regions associated with sympathetic nervous system induced changes in NEFA (11–14). Research from several sources implicate monoamines in the effect of ethanol on NEFA (2, 15–17). A recent study (18) showed that ethanol did not alter the release of fatty acids from liver. Research in our laboratory (2) has shown that ethanol and stress probably do not alter NEFA through adrenal catecholamines since in adrenalectomized rats, changes in NEFA in response to stress and moderate doses of ethanol are still present.

In attempting to define the neural substrates of the interaction between ethanol and stress-induced changes in corticosterone and NEFA, we have focused on the possible mechanisms by which ethanol, in the absence of stress, elevates these substances. We have found that, compared to sham-operated controls, rats with locus coeruleus lesions had a significantly attenuated elevation of plasma NEFA in response to a moderate dose (2.0 g/kg) of ethanol (19). In this study, no changes in response to saline injection were observed between lesioned and control subjects. We confirmed these lesion results using a pharmacological manipulation, as well. When rats were pretreated with N-(2-chloroethyl) (N-ethyl-2 bromobenzylamine) (DSP-4), a selective noradrenergic neurotoxin, the elevating effects of a moderate dose of ethanol were again significantly attenuated (19). In both experiments, no changes in the effect of ethanol on corticosterone were observed. Since the locus coeruleus supplies the majority of brain norepinephrine, these results suggested to us that the elevating action of ethanol on NEFA, but not corticosterone, involved noradrenergic neurons.

The above-mentioned experiments gave little indication as to how ethanol altered corticosterone, except that norepinephrine was not involved. We recently reported that treatment of rats with para-chlorophenylalanine (PCPA), a serotonin depletor, significantly elevated plasma corticosterone and NEFA (2). We also noted that a low dose of ethanol attenuated the PCPA-induced increase in corticosterone. Doses of ethanol that elevated corticosterone did not interact with PCPA to alter plasma levels of corticosterone (2). This suggested to us that ethanol may be altering plasma corticosterone via a mechanism involving serotonergic neurons. Several previous studies also support a serotonin x corticosteroid interaction (20–22).

In the brain, the majority of serotonin-containing cells are found in the raphe nucleus of the pons and upper brainstem. To further test the role of serotonergic neurons in ethanol's action, we compared the effect of ethanol on corticosterone and NEFA in rats with dorsal raphe lesions and sham-operated controls. As in our pharmacological studies, raphe lesions increased plasma levels of NEFA in saline-treated rats. Interestingly, dorsal raphe lesions also attenuated the elevating effects of ethanol on NEFA and, to a smaller extent, corticosterone (23).

In a similar study, we also examined the effect of median raphe lesions on the elevating action of ethanol. Median raphe lesions elevated NEFA levels, compared to sham-operated controls, but did not significantly alter the response to ethanol. Similarly, corticosterone levels were also elevated in subjects with median raphe lesions, but the response to ethanol was not impaired (23).

These results support our hypothesis that serotonergic neurons are involved in ethanol's action on corticosterone. Since lesions of the dorsal raphe elevated basal (saline-treated) levels of corticosterone, but attenuated ethanol's elevating action, a simple explanation of these results is not likely. The elevated corticosterone levels in response to saline might suggest that in the intact rat, the raphe has an inhibitory influence on corticosterone regulation. It is not known why ethanol's action would be attenuated by raphe lesions. This may suggest the involvement of other anatomical substrates and that other neurotransmitter interactions participate in this effect.

Very little is known about neuroanatomical substrates involved in ethanol's action on NEFA or corticosterone. Our studies involving locus coeruleus lesions and DSP4 suggested to us that the locus coeruleus or brain structures innervated by the locus coeruleus may be involved in ethanol's action on NEFA. Since the raphe nucleus sends and receives axons to and from the locus coeruleus and both raphe and locus coeruleus neurons contribute to the medial forebrain bundle, the possibility existed that areas innervated by these structures, such as the limbic system, may be involved in ethanol's neuroendocrine and sympathetic nervous system actions. A large portion of brain monoamines come from the raphe and locus coeruleus, and ethanol alters monoamines. Therefore, this is an attractive notion.

The limbic system was a likely candidate for several reasons. First, it received adrenergic and serotonergic input from the raphe and locus coeruelus via the dorsal adrenergic and medial forebrain bundles. In addition, the limbic system includes the hippocampus, septum, and amygdala, structures believed to be important anatomical substrates of emotional behavior (24, 25) as well as for the responses to stress (26–29).

The experiments we performed next were aimed at determining the possible contributions of the limbic system to ethanol's action on corticosterone and NEFA.

GENERAL METHODS/PROCEDURE

Subjects

In all experiments, we used male Sprague-Dawley rats obtained from Charles River (Wilmington, Massachusetts). At the time of testing, the rats weighted 300–350 grams. Subjects were housed singly in our temperature- (22°C ± .2) and light-controlled (lights off 0930, on 2130 hours) vivarium. Tap water and Purina rat chow were available *ad libitum*.

Handling

Subjects were allowed 7-10 days to recover from shipment and adapt to our vivarium. Approximately 3 days prior to each experiment, subjects were handled daily for 2-3 minutes and weighed the night before testing. We found this to be helpful in minimizing confounds caused by experimenter-handling stress during actual experiments.

Surgery

Prior to surgery, subjects were pretreated with atropine sulfate (25 mg), then anesthetized using 50 mg/kg of sodium pentobarbital (Nembutal sodium). Every effort was made to minimize discomfort during surgery. After each operation, subjects were treated with a broad spectrum antibiotic (300,000 units Flo-Cillin).

Lesions

Brain lesions were made electrolytically using a Grass S44 stimulator, with currents ranging from 0.5–1.5 mA and of varying durations. Stainless steel 00 pins, insulated except for the tip, were used as electrodes. Sham operations were identical to lesion treatment except that current was not passed through the electrode. Lesion coordinates were determined using the stereotaxic atlas of Pellegrino and Cushman (30).

Time of Testing

All testing was done between 0930 and 1230 hours. This corresponded to the first quarter of the subject's dark period.

Drugs

Ethanol was injected intraperitoneally. Ethanol was a 20% (w/v) solution for all doses equal to or greater than 1.0 g/kg or a 10% (w/v) solution for all doses below 1.0 g/kg. The use of slightly different doses of ethanol in these studies was based upon pilot studies and/or our expectation as to whether the effects of ethanol would be greater or lesser following each experimental manipulation.

Corticosterone and NEFA Assays

Plasma corticosterone levels were assayed using the fluorometric method of Glick, von Redlich, and Levine (31).

Plasma nonesterified fatty acids were assayed using the spectrophotometric method of Smith (32).

Histology

At the end of each experiment, lesion locations were determined. Brains were removed and placed in a rapid-hardening solution and stained one week later using a metachromic method (33).

Blood Ethanol Levels

Blood ethanol levels were determined using a gas chromatographic technique (34). Duplicate samples were collected at the time of testing, 30 minutes after ethanol administration.

Statistical Analysis

All results were analyzed using a 2 (lesion, control) x 2 (ethanol, saline) analysis of variance, unless otherwise indicated. Post hoc comparisons were made using the method outlined by Keppel (35). In some cases, as indicated, parametric analyses were performed using a two-tailed *t*-test. Differences between groups were considered statistically significant when $p < .05$.

We began our investigations of the possible neural substrates of ethanol action on corticosterone and NEFA using a lesion approach. The rationale was that changes in ethanol-induced elevation of these substances, after lesioning a particular area of the brain, would indicate some association between that neural system and the mechanisms of ethanol's action.

EXPERIMENT 1

To test the possible involvement of the limbic system in ethanol's action on corticosterone and NEFA, subjects were randomly assigned to receive bilateral basolateral and basomedial amygdala lesions or sham operations. One week later, subjects were randomly assigned to receive ethanol (3.0 g/kg) or an equivalent volume of saline (n = 6/group). Thirty minutes later, subjects were removed to a separate room and decapitated, and blood was collected for determination of plasma corticosterone, NEFA, and ethanol levels.

RESULTS

Histological analysis of each brain showed relatively large lesions, which included the basolateral and mediobasal nuclei of the amygdala. In some cases, the lateral amygdala was lesioned. There was no systematic relationship between subjects with basolateral and mediobasal lesions and subjects showing basolateral, mediobasal, and lateral amygdala lesions, with respect to the biochemical responses measured.

The effects of bilateral amygdala lesions on plasma NEFA are shown in Figure 1. An analysis of variance of these data indicated a significant drug × lesion interaction, $F = 8.59$, $df = 1,20$; $p < .01$. Lesions resulted in a decrease in plasma NEFA levels in response to saline. This decrease did not, however, reach conventional levels of statistical significance. In response to ethanol, subjects with amygdala lesions showed a significant ($p < .05$) increase in NEFA levels, compared to sham-operated controls.

In our hands, saline injections do not usually increase either plasma corticosterone or NEFA (30 minutes postinjection), compared to subjects that are left undisturbed. It is therefore tempting to speculate that the levels of either NEFA or corticosterone that we measure after saline injections are at least reasonable approximations of basal levels. In this experiment, it would almost appear as though amygdala lesions decreased sympathetic nervous system induced mobilization of NEFA in saline-treated subjects. We know from previous studies that moderate doses of ethanol elevate catecholamines (34, 36) and NEFA (10). Possibly, amygdalectomy alters sympathetic nervous system activity in such a way so that it sensitizes the subject to ethanol. In the presence of ethanol there is an increase in sympathetic response, which results in a greater than normal mobilization of NEFA. Admittedly, this is speculative, but it would be interesting to measure circulating levels of catecholamines following amygdala lesions.

Amygdala lesions had no effect on the elevating action of ethanol on corticosterone, nor did such lesions alter the response to saline. Present was a significant main effect of drug ($F = 94.1$, $df = 1,20$; $p < .001$), which can be seen in Figure 2 as an increase in response to ethanol.

No significant differences in blood ethanol levels were observed be-

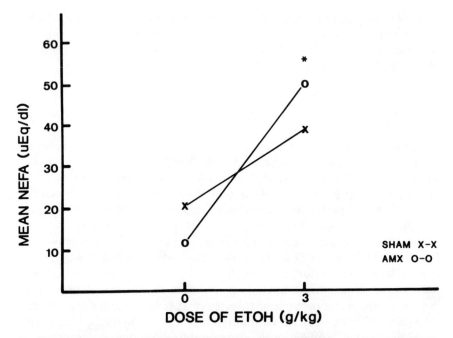

Figure 1. Changes in mean levels of plasma nonesterified fatty acids (NEFA) 30 minutes after ethanol (3.0 g/kg) or saline in rats with bilateral amygdala lesions or or sham-operated controls (N = 6/group). Statistically significant (p < .05) differences between surgical groups are indicated by an [*].

tween sham-operated controls (279.3 ± 17.6 mg/dl) and subjects with bilateral amygdala lesions (265.2 ± 11.8 mg/dl).

EXPERIMENT 2

The hippocampus is a prominent limbic system structure that has been shown to be particularly sensitive to morphological changes following ethanol. In addition, some but not all studies have suggested that hippocampal lesions alter basal and stress-induced changes in plasma corticosterone (37–41). To test the possible involvement of the hippocampus in ethanol's action in corticosterone and NEFA, subjects were randomly assigned to receive bilateral hippocampal lesions, cortical lesions, or sham operations. In this study, lesions were made using the aspiration technique described by Isaacson and Woodruff (42). With this method, the overlying cortical tissue is also removed with the hippocampus. Therefore, a separate cortical control group was included. Ten days after surgery, subjects were randomly assigned to receive ethanol (2.0 g/kg) or an equivalent volume of saline ($n=7$/group). Thirty minutes later, subjects were removed to another room and decapitated, and blood was collected.

RESULTS

By the 3rd day after surgery almost 20% of the subjects died, bringing the total number of subjects per group down to 6. Although most fatalities were in the hippocampal lesion group, several cortical controls also died. (Replications of this study showed a slightly lower [15%] but none-

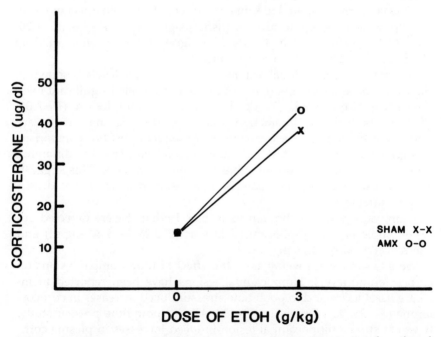

Figure 2. Changes in mean levels of plasma corticosterone 30 minutes after ethanol (3.0 g/kg) or saline in rats with bilateral amygdala lesions or sham-operated controls ($N=6$/group). Statistically significant ($p < .05$) differences between surgical groups are indicated by an [*].

theless high mortality rate, compared to other lesion studies where the rate is usually zero.)

Histological analysis revealed that large portions of hippocampus had been aspirated away. In all subjects, the areas designated CA3 and CA2 were removed and in most cases at least half of the inferior region (CA1) was also removed. Since CA1 receives all its inputs from the superior regions, it can be assumed that there was significant degeneration in any remaining tissue. The lesions did not extend into the thalamus. Where possible, histological analyses were also made of brains from subjects that died shortly after surgery. There did not seem to be any relationship between lesion size or location and postsurgery survival, suggesting that excessive blood loss during surgery may have been a significant contributing factor.

There were no differences between cortical controls or sham-operated subjects following saline or ethanol treatment, so the results from these groups were combined.

In subjects with hippocampal lesions, ethanol caused a small elevation of plasma NEFA compared to saline treatment. This main effect of lesion was not robust enough to reach statistical significance, $F = 3.6$, $df = 1,20$; $p < .08$. As can be seen in Figure 3, a significant main effect of drug ($F = 8.33$, $df = 1,20$; $p < .01$) was present.

The effect of hippocampal lesions on corticosterone levels is shown in Figure 4. The analysis of variance of these data revealed significant main effects for drug ($F = 35.47$, $df = 1,20$; $p < .001$) and lesion ($F = 7.01$, $df = 1,20$; $p < .025$). No interaction was detected using analysis of variance, possibly due to heterogeneity. A subsequent post hoc comparison using an independent t-test did show a significant ($p < .01$) difference between lesioned and control subjects receiving ethanol. This suggests that the use of additional subjects may result in a significant drug x surgery interaction.

Again, no significant differences in blood ethanol were detected between subjects with hippocampal lesions (202.28 ± 3.80 mg/dl) and controls (179.06 ± 14.76 mg/dl).

There is some controversy as to the effect of hippocampal lesions on corticosterone levels. Hippocampal lesions have been reported to increase basal levels and to potentiate stress-induced increases in corticosterone (37, 38, 43). Other studies (39, 40), including the present study, have not shown hippocampal lesion-induced increases in plasma corticosterone.

These results suggest that the hippocampus may have an inhibitory role on ethanol's action on NEFA and corticosterone release. In the

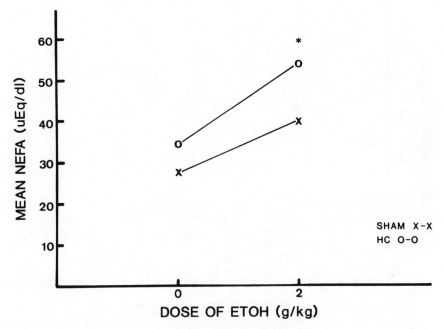

Figure 3. Changes in mean levels of plasma nonesterified fatty acids (NEFA) 30 minutes after ethanol (2.0 g/kg) or saline in rats with bilateral hippocampal lesions or cortical/sham-operated controls ($N = 6$/group). Statistically significant ($p < .05$) differences between surgical groups are indicated by an [*].

present study, the interaction between lesion and drug effect was only hinted at, and certainly more work will need to be done to further implicate the hippocampus in ethanol's action on NEFA and corticosterone.

EXPERIMENT 3

Among the various limbic system structures (excluding the hypothalamus), the one most frequently associated with changes in emotion and neuroendocrine responses to stress is the septum. It has been known for some time that septal lesions result in a rage response (44) and exaggerated physiological changes in response to stress (26). We therefore examined the effects of septal lesions on ethanol's action on NEFA and corticosterone.

Subjects were randomly assigned to receive bilateral lesions of the

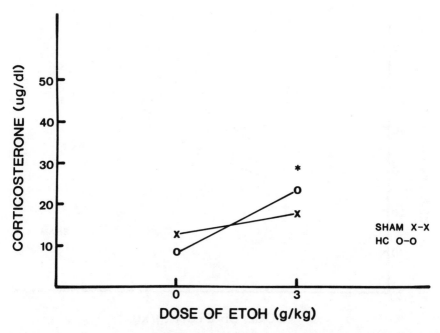

Figure 4. Changes in mean levels of plasma corticosterone 30 minutes after ethanol (2.0 g/kg) or saline in rats with bilateral hippocampal lesions or cortical/sham-operated controls ($N = 6$/group). Statistically significant ($p < .05$) differences between surgical groups are indicated by an [*].

medial septal nuclei. One week later, subjects were assigned to receive ethanol (2.0 g/kg) or an equivalent volume of saline ($n = 6$/group).

RESULTS

In all subjects, large lesions of the medial septum were observed. In all cases, the lesion or necrosis extended into portions of the lateral nuclei but never as far as the walls of the lateral ventricles. Typically, lesions were restricted to the area ventral to the corpus callosum and usually dorsal to the anterior commissure.

Septal lesions did not alter the elevating action of ethanol on NEFA (Figure 5). Analysis of these data revealed only a significant main effect of drug, $F = 7.2$, $df = 1,20$; $p < .01$. Similarly, septal lesions did not alter corticosterone levels (Figure 6) as only a significant main effect of drug was again observed, $F = 29.2$, $df = 1,20$; $p < .001$. There were no significant differences in blood ethanol levels between rats with septal lesions (201.0 ±2.0 mg/dl) and sham-operated controls (194.82 ± 2.7 mg/dl).

These results were very surprising to us, since previous studies have shown rats with septal lesions to have exaggerated corticosterone elevation in response to various stressors, including brief handling (45). It should also be noted that we have repeated this study several times with identical results. Possibly our handling procedure altered the rats' response to ethanol. Postsurgical handling has been shown to greatly reduce many of the behavioral deficits associated with septal lesions.

Although we did not see any indication of an effect of septal lesions on ethanol's action on corticosterone or NEFA, these results do point out that lesions, per se, do not always produce changes in the response to ethanol. Thus, our finding of no effect with septal lesions would suggest that the changes in ethanol's effect following raphe, amygdala, and hippocampal lesions were not the result of some nonspecific effect of the electrolytic lesion technique.

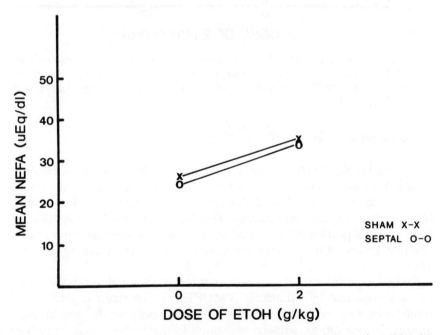

Figure 5. Changes in mean levels of plasma nonesterified fatty acids (NEFA) 30 minutes after ethanol (2.0 g/kg) or saline in rats with bilateral septal lesions or sham-operated controls (N = 6/group). Statistically significant (p < .05) differences between surgical groups are indicated by an [*].

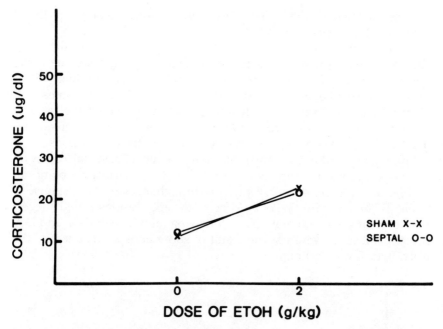

Figure 6. Changes in mean levels of plasma corticosterone 30 minutes after ethanol (2.0 g/kg) or saline in rats with bilateral septal lesions or sham-operated controls ($N = 6$/group). Statistically significant ($p < .05$) differences between surgical groups are indicated by an [*].

EXPERIMENT 4

The last limbic structure we examined was the hypothalamus. Several studies have demonstrated that different nuclear groups of the hypothalamus are involved in the regulation of corticosterone (via feedback inhibition or in release of corticotropin-releasing hormone). More specifically, the ventral portion of the hypothalamus contains neurosecretory cells and may be one of several sites involved in endocrine regulation (see 46, 47).

For this experiment, subjects were randomly assigned to receive bilateral ventromedial hypothalamic (VMH) lesions or sham lesions. One week after surgery, subjects were randomly assigned to one of two groups. In one group, subjects remained in their home cage, as in the previous three experiments. In the other group, subjects were stressed by placing them for 90 minutes in wire restrainers previously described

(1). Subjects were then randomly assigned to receive ethanol (0.5 or 1.5 g/kg) or saline ($n=8$/group). In the home cage group, subjects were sacrificed 30 minutes later. In the stress group, ethanol or saline injections were made 60 minutes into the stress session, and subjects were sacrificed 30 minutes later.

RESULTS

Histological analysis showed discrete lesions of the ventromedial hypothalamic nuclei. Lesions generally did not impinge upon the wall of the III ventricle, although in some subjects the lesion included part of the arcuate nucleus. During the period between surgery and the day before sacrifice (1 week), all subjects showed weight gains, but there were, at this point, no significant differences in weight between subjects with ventromedial hypothalamic lesions and control subjects. These results of stressed and nonstressed groups were analyzed separately. As in the previous studies, there were no significant differences in blood ethanol levels between surgical groups.

Ethanol caused a significant increase in corticosterone, $F=10.65$, $df=2,30$; $p<.01$. We can see from Figure 7 that in sham-operated controls, the low 0.5 g/kg dose of ethanol had no effect on corticosterone levels, but the 1.5 g/kg dose resulted in a significant elevation. Interestingly, VMH lesions increased levels of corticosterone in saline-treated subjects by about 88%, but this lesion-induced increase in levels was attenuated by a 0.5 g/kg dose of ethanol. The larger 1.5 g/kg dose of ethanol did not raise corticosterone significantly above the levels found in saline-treated VMH-lesioned rats. If one compared, within lesion group, the effect of 1.5 g ethanol to saline, it appears that VMH lesions blocked the elevating action of ethanol on corticosterone. Such a comparison must be interpreted cautiously, however, since VMH lesions significantly elevated corticosterone levels in saline-treated subjects.

The response of subjects with VMH lesions to restraint stress and ethanol is shown in Figure 8. The analysis of variance of these data revealed a significant drug x lesion interaction, $F=6.10$, $df=2,30$; $p<.025$. First, we can see (Figure 8) that all subjects had significantly elevated levels of corticosterone. In sham-operated subjects, ethanol (0.5 g/kg) decreased plasma levels of corticosterone, compared to saline treatment. This attenuating effect of ethanol on stress-induced elevation of corticosterone is similar to that which we have previously reported (1, 2,

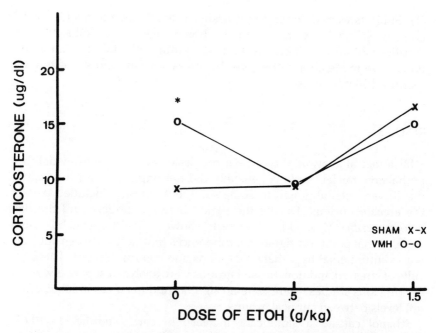

Figure 7. Changes in mean levels of plasma corticosterone 30 minutes after ethanol (0.5, 1.5 g/kg) or saline in rats with bilateral ventromedial hypothalamic lesions or sham-operated controls (N = 8/group). Statistically significant (p < .05) differences between surgical groups are indicated by an [*].

3). In stressed, sham-operated subjects, the 1.5 g/kg dose of ethanol did not significantly elevate corticosterone levels. This may have been because the stress-induced increase in corticosterone was greater than that which would have been produced by ethanol alone. Subjects with VMH lesions and treated with saline or 0.5 g/kg had significantly (p < .01) higher levels of corticosterone than similarly treated sham-operated controls. Lesioned subjects treated with 1.5 g/kg ethanol actually showed a decrease in corticosterone elevation and were not significantly different from similarly treated sham-operated controls.

From these results, it appears that the VMH may play a role in ethanol's action on corticosterone. The precise route of this interaction is not known at this time. Whereas lesion-induced elevations of corticosterone are attenuated by 0.5 g/kg ethanol (and not by the 1.5 g/kg dose), stress-induced corticosterone elevation in lesioned animals is significantly attenuated only by the 1.5 g/kg dose.

DISCUSSION

These experiments were performed in an attempt to determine what possible neural substrates were involved in the elevating action of ethanol on plasma NEFA and corticosterone levels.

Destruction of specific limbic system structures or fibers of passage through them, altered the action of ethanol on corticosterone and/or NEFA. Our results suggest that the amygdala is involved in ethanol's action on NEFA, whereas the hippocampus and hypothalamus may, in part, mediate ethanol's action on corticosterone.

Amygdala lesions potentiated ethanol's action on NEFA. Unfortunately, very little work has been done, to our knowledge, concerning the role of brain structures other than the hypothalamus on NEFA mobilization. Rats with amygdala lesions showed a slight decrease in NEFA levels

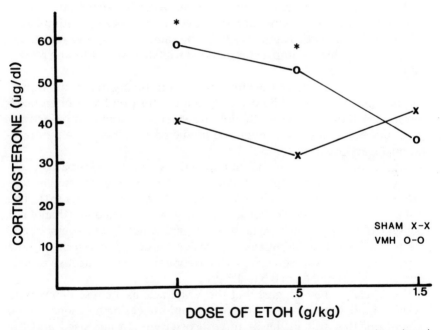

Figure 8. Changes in mean levels of plasma corticosterone 30 minutes after ethanol (0.5, 1.5 g/kg) or saline in restraint-stressed rats with bilateral ventromedial hypothalamic lesions or sham operations ($N = 8$/group). Statistically significant ($p < .05$) differences between surgical groups are indicated by an [*].

following saline treatment which might suggest a facilitory role of the amygdala in the intact animal. The amygdala receives inputs from both the locus coeruleus and the raphe nuclei, so destruction of the amygdala may have altered part of the system involved in ethanol-induced changes of NEFA regulation. It is not known where in the corticotropin-releasing pathway the amygdala is functioning. Perhaps future studies, employing infusion of centrally acting serotonergic drugs, would answer the question.

The effect of hippocampal lesions on ethanol's action on NEFA and corticosterone were only mildly suggested in the present study. No significant changes between lesioned and sham-operated controls were observed. This finding tends to support other studies showing that hippocampal lesions do not alter basal levels of corticosterone (39, 40). Rats with hippocampal lesions tended to show a greater increase in corticosterone in response to ethanol than did sham-operated controls. The effects of ethanol are sometimes referred to as "stress-like" (48). If moderate doses of ethanol are stressful, then these data agree with the results of previous studies showing that during stress, hippocampal stimulation inhibits levels of corticosterone (49). In the same study, under nonstressful conditions, hippocampal stimulation facilitated corticosterone release (49).

Thus, depending upon the stress placed on the organism, the hippocampus may have an inhibitory or facilitory effect on levels of corticosterone (25). If the stressor is ethanol, the absence of hippocampal activity (e.g. hippocampal lesions) might be predicted to increase the pituitary-adrenal response, which it did.

Lesions of the ventromedial hypothalamus elevated plasma corticosterone in nonstressed saline-treated rats. These results are similar to a previous report (50) as well as a study of "lean" VMH rats (51). The lesion-induced elevation of corticosterone was attenuated by ethanol but depended upon whether the rat was stressed or not. In nonstressed rats, a low 0.5 g/kg dose attenuated the lesion-induced increase in plasma corticosterone. In stressed rats, VMH lesions shifted the effective protective dose of ethanol from 0.5 to 1.5 g/kg.

These results may suggest that the VMH acts as a stress-dampening system, inhibiting the release of corticotropin-releasing hormone. In the absence of this system, levels of corticosterone are increased and the effective dose of ethanol required to attenuate the stress-induced release of corticosterone is altered.

Not all limbic system lesions resulted in a change in NEFA or corticosterone levels following saline or ethanol treatment. Septal nuclei lesions had no effect on basal levels of NEFA or corticosterone, nor did they alter the effect of ethanol. This indicates that the changes we observed in other limbic regions were not simply due to a nonspecific effect of brain lesions. In addition, none of our studies revealed any change in blood ethanol levels as a function of brain lesions, suggesting that the results obtained were not due to changes in absorption, distribution, or metabolism of ethanol.

The results from these experiments, along with our previous work, suggest that limbic system monoamines may be involved in ethanol-induced changes in plasma levels of NEFA and corticosterone. Additional work will be needed to further specify the nature of this system in nonstressed and stressed animals.

REFERENCES

1. Brick J, Pohorecky LA: Ethanol-stress interaction: Biochemical findings. Psychopharmacology 77:81–84, 1982
2. Brick J, Pohorecky LA: Neuroendocrine response to stress and the effect of ethanol, in Stress and Alcohol Use. Edited by Pohorecky LA, Brick J. New York, Elsevier, 1983
3. Pohorecky LA, Rossi E, Weiss JM, et al: Biochemical evidence for an interaction of ethanol and stress: Preliminary studies. Alcohol: Clinical Experimental Research 4:423–426, 1980
4. Smith J: The effect of alcohol on the adrenal ascorbic acid and cholesterol of the rat. J Clin Endocrinology 11:792, 1951
5. Forbes JC, Duncan GM: The effect of acute alchol intoxication on the adrenal glands of rats and guinea pigs. Quart J Stud Alcohol 12:355–359, 1951
6. Ellis F: Effect of ethanol on plasma corticosterone levels. J Pharmacol Exp Ther 153:121–127, 1966
7. Noble E, Kakihana R, Butte J: Corticosterone metabolism in alcohol-adapted mice, in Biological Aspects of Alcohol. Edited by Roach M, McIsaac W, Creaven P. Austin, Texas, Faculty for Advanced Studies of the Texas Research Institute of Mental Sciences by the University of Texas, 1971
8. Kakihana R, Butte J: Ethanol and Endrocrine Function in Biochemistry and Pharmacology of Alcohol, vol. 2. Edited by Majchrowicz E, Noble E. New York, Plenum Press, 1979
9. Elko E, Wooles W, Diluzio N: Alterations and mobilization of lipids in acute ethanol treated rats. Am J Physiol 201:923–926, 1961
10. Mallov S: Effect of ethanol intoxication on plasma free fatty acids in the rat. Quart J Stud Alcohol 22:250–253, 1961
11. Bray G, Nishizawa Y: Ventromedial hypothalamus modulates fat mobilization during fasting. Nature 274:900–902, 1978
12. Shimazu T, Takahashi A: Stimulation of hypothalamic nuclei has different effects on lipid synthesis in brown and white adipose tissue. Nature 248:62–63, 1980
13. Steffens AB, Morgenson GJ, Stevenson JAF: Blood glucose, insulin and free fatty acids after stimulation and lesions of the hypothalamus. Am J Physiol 222:1446–1452, 1972
14. Parker R, Hall R, Marr H, et al: Vascular responses in canine subcutaneous adipose tissue to hypothalamic stimulation. Am J Physiol 237:H386–H391, 1979
15. Scheig R: Ethanol, lipids and adipose tissue metabolism, in Biochemistry and Pharma-

cology of Ethanol, vol. 1. Edited by Majchrowicz E, Noble E. New York, Plenum Press, 1979

16. Mallov S, Bloch J: Role of hypophysis and adrenals in fatty infiltration of liver resulting from acute ethanol intoxication. Am J Physiol 184:29–34, 1956

17. Estler CJ, Ammon H: The influence of B-adrenergic blockade on the ethanol induced derangement of lipid transport. Arch Int Pharmacodyn Ther 166:333–340, 1967

18. Topping DL, Clark DG, Illman RJ, et al: Inhibitor by insulin of ethanol-induced hyperglycaemia in perfused livers. Horm Metab Res 14:361–364, 1982

19. Brick J, Pohorecky L: Role of noradrenergic neurons in ethanol-induced elevation of plasma corticosterone and non-esterified fatty acids. Life Sci 35:207–212, 1984

20. Vernikos-Danellis J, Kellar K, Kent D, et al: Serotonin involvement in pituitary-adrenal function. Ann NY Acad Sci 297–318, 1977

21. McElroy JF, Miller JM, Meyer JS: Fenfluramine, p-chloroamphetamine and p-fluoroamphetamine stimluation of pituitary-adrenocortical activity in rats: Evidence of differences in site and mechanism of action. J Pharmacol Exp Ther 228:593–599, 1984

22. DiRenzo, GL, Schettini G, Quattrone A, et al: Monoaminergic control of hypothalamic-hypophyseal-adrenal axis activity, in Catecholamines and Stress. Edited by Usdin E, Kvetnansky R, Kopin I. New York, Elsevier Holland-North, 1980

23. Brick J, Pohorecky L: Monoamines and the effect of ethanol on corticosterone and non-esterified fatty acids. Alcohol 2(2): 261–265, 1985

24. MacLean P: Some psychiatric implications of physiological studies of the frontotemporal portion of the limbic system (visceral brain). Electroencephalogy Clin Neurophysiol 4:407–418, 1952

25. Isaacson RL: The Limbic System. New York, Plenum Press, 1974

26. Brick J, Burright R, Donovick P: Stress responses in rats with septal lesions. Pharmacol Biochem Behav 11:695–700, 1979

27. Kvetnansky R, Kopin I, Saavedra J: Changes in epinephrine in individual hypothalamic nuclei after immobilization stress. Brain Res 155:387–390, 1978

28. Nauta W: Hippocampal projections and related neural pathways to the midbrain in the cat. Brain 81:319–340, 1958

29. Saavedra J, Kvetnansky R, Kopin I: Adrenaline, noradrenaline and dopamine levels in specific brain stem areas of acutely immobilized rats. Brain Res 160:271–280, 1979

30. Pellegrino LJ, Cushman AJ: A Stereotaxic Atlas of the Rat Brain. New York, Appleton-Century-Crofts Meredith Publishing Co, 1967

31. Glick D, von Redlich D, Levine S: Fluorometric determination of corticosterone and cortisol in 0.02–0.05 milliliters of plasma or submilligram samples of adrenal tissue. Endocrinology 74:653–655, 1964

32. Smith SW: A simple salting out procedure in the colorimetric assay of free fatty acids. Anal Biochem 67:521–539, 1975

33. Donovick PJ: A metachromic stain for neural tissue. Stain Technol 49:49–51, 1974

34. Pohorecky LA: Effects of ethanol on central and peripheral noradrenergic neurons. J Pharmacol Exp Ther 189:380–391, 1974

35. Keppel J: Design and Analysis: A Researchers Handbook. Englewood Cliffs, NJ, Prentice-Hall, 1973

36. Myrsten AL, Post B, Frankenhaeuser M: Catecholamine output during and after acute alcohol intoxication. Percept Mot Skills 33:652–654, 1971

37. Knigge K: Adrenocortical response to stress in rats with lesions in the hippocampus and amygdala. Proc Soc Exp Biol Med 108:18–21, 1961

38. Knigge K, Hays M: Evidence of inhibitive role of hippocampus in neural regulation of ACTH release. Proc Soc Exp Biol Med 4:67–69, 1963

39. Lanier L, Van Hartesvel C, Weis B, et al: Effects of differential hippocampal damage upon rhythmic and stress-induced corticosterone secretion in the rat. Neuroendocrinology 18:154–160, 1975

40. Murphy HM, Wideman CH, Brown TS: Plasma corticosterone levels and ulcer formation in rats with hippocampal lesions. Neuroendocrinology 28:123–130, 1979

41. Usher D, Kasper P, Birmingham M: Comparison of pituitary adrenal function in rats lesioned in different areas of the limbic system and hypothalamus. Neuroendocrinology 2:157–178, 1967
42. Isaacson RL, Woodruff M: Spontaneous alternation and passive avoidance behavior in rats after hippocampal lesions, in Experimental Psychobiology: A Laboratory Manual. Edited by Hart BL. San Francisco, Freeman & Co, 1975
43. Fendler K, Karmos G, Telegdy G: The effect of hippocampal lesions on pituitary adrenal function. Acta Physiol Hung 20:293–297, 1961
44. Brady J, Nauta W: Subcortical mechanisms in emotional behavior: Affective changes following septal forebrain lesions in the albino rat. J Comp Physiol Psychol 46:339–346, 1978
45. Seggie J, Brown G: The effects of ablation of the septal nuclei in the rat on circadian variation and stress response pattern of corticosterone, growth hormone and prolactin, in The Septal Nuclei: Advances in Behavioral Biology, vol 20. Edited by DeFrance JF. New York, Plenum Press, 1976
46. Rose J, Ganong W: Neurotransmitter control of pituitary function, in Perspectives in Clinical Endocrinology. New York, Spectrum, 1980
47. Ganong WF: Brain mechanisms regulating the secretion of the pituitary gland, in The Neurosciences, Third Study Program. Edited by Schmidt FO, Worden FG. Cambridge, MIT Press, 1974
48. Van Thiel D: Adrenal response to ethanol: A stress response? in Stress and Alcohol Use. Edited by Pohorecky LA, Brick J. New York, Elsevier, 1983
49. Kawakami M, Setu K, Terasawa E, et al: Influence of electrical stimulation and lesion in limbic structure upon biosynthesis of adrenocorticoid in the rabbit. Neuroendocrinology 3:337–348, 1968
50. Coover G, Welle S, Hart R: Effects of eating, meal cues and ventromedial hypothalamic lesions on serum corticosterone, glucose and free fatty acid concentration. Physiol Behav 25:641–651, 1980
51. King B, Levine S, Grossman S: Pituitary-adrenocortical response to shock-induced stress in normal and hypothalamic hyperphagic rats. Physiol Behav 22:753–757, 1979

8

Effects of Ethanol on Plasma Catecholamines and Heart Rate in Unstressed and Stressed Rats

WOLFGANG H. VOGEL, JOANNE MILLER, and
HEDWIG ROGGENDORF

A high, almost hypnotic, dose of alcohol increased norepinephrine (NE) and epinephrine (E) levels in unstressed rats not initially but after 1 hour. However, a second dose of alcohol on the next day caused marked increases in both catecholamines indicative of sensitization. Immobilization stress-induced increases in NE and E levels were initially antagonized by alcohol but later levels of both catecholamines were increased even further. Heart rate increased in unstressed rats after alcohol, and alcohol did not affect the stress-induced tachycardia. There was, at best, a poor correlation between plasma catecholamine levels and heart rate. The results, obtained with a high dose of alcohol, only partially support the Tension Reduction Hypothesis.

Recently, we observed that a small dose of ethanol (0.5 g/kg) had no effect on plasma catecholamine levels in unstressed rats but significantly reduced stress-induced increases of these plasma catecholamines during and after immobilization stress (1). Similar reductions in stress-induced

The financial support of this study by a grant from the Distilled Spirits Council of the U.S. and by grant AA06017 from the Department of Health and Human Services is gratefully acknowledged.

increases in corticosterone levels by alcohol have been reported (2), although levels of this steroid were elevated significantly by alcohol in unstressed rats (3). To extend our findings, we studied the effect of a high dose of alcohol (4 g/kg) on plasma norepinephrine (NE) and epinephrine (E) levels in stressed and unstressed rats. In addition, we studied the heart rate and ECG in these animals to obtain a physiological correlate of our biochemical findings.

METHODS

Male Sprague-Dawley rats weighing about 300 g were used in these experiments. Animals were housed in groups (12 hr light/12 hr dark) and received food and water *ad libitum*.

For the biochemical studies, rats received an indwelling jugular catheter under Ketamine/pentobarbital anesthesia (1). The catheter was shielded by a steel spring and supported by a swivel pulley above the cage. The catheter was filled with heparinized (100 U/ml) saline. Blood samples were centrifuged, the plasma frozen, and assayed by the radioenzymatic procedure (Cat-A-Kit, Upjohn Diagnostics, Kalamazoo, Michigan).

For the physiological studies two gold-plated disk electrodes (Grass Instruments Company) were attached under the skin to the thoracic muscles. The leads were exteriorized through a small incision in the back of the animal, and were then supported by a swivel pulley above the cage. Heart rate and ECG (lead II) were recorded on a Grass Model 7 polygraph equipped with a cardiotachometer.

For the unstressed animals, saline or alcohol was given and measurements were made before and after the IP injection. For the stressed rats, measurements were made before saline or alcohol injection, and 15 minutes following the injection. Immediately after this measurement, animals were immobilized for 30 minutes and then released. Subsequent measurements were taken in the home cage.

Statistical analyses of the results involved an analysis of variance with Dunnett's Ad Hoc test or Student's *t*-test.

RESULTS

The effects of a high, almost hypnotic, dose of alcohol on plasma catecholamine levels in unstressed rats are shown in Table 1. Animals were unable to move, were completely relaxed, and were unresponsive

TABLE 1
Effect of Ethanol (4 g/kg) on Plasma Norepinephrine and
Epinephrine Levels in Unstressed Rats

Condition	Time (minutes)				
	0	15/20	30	45	60
Norepinephrine (pg/ml)					
Saline	160 ± 25	235 ± 25	288 ± 31	214 ± 12	188 ± 11
Ethanol (Day 1)	240 ± 21	364 ± 40	403 ± 69	359 ± 60	$511 \pm 75^{a,b}$
Ethanol (Day 2)	302 ± 20	$966 \pm 112^{a,b,c}$	$1197 \pm 199^{a,b,c}$	$2513 \pm 610^{a,b,c}$	$1747 \pm 172^{a,b,c}$
Epinephrine (pg/ml)					
Saline	95 ± 4	99 ± 19	117 ± 15	73 ± 8	86 ± 12
Ethanol (Day 1)	106 ± 18	269 ± 40	268 ± 35	$427 \pm 209^{a,b}$	$643 \pm 100^{a,b}$
Ethanol (Day 2)	141 ± 25	$1585 \pm 316^{a,b,c}$	$2941 \pm 385^{a,b,c}$	$5818 \pm 971^{a,b,c}$	$5555 \pm 922^{a,b,c}$

Note. Values represent means ± SEM of 4–5 animals. Saline or ethanol was given after a blood drawing at 0 minutes. Blood was then drawn at specified times. Experimental animals received 4 g/kg of ethanol on two consecutive days.
[a]$p < .05$ (comparison with 0 minutes).
[b]$p < .05$ (comparison with saline value).
[c]$p < .05$ (comparison with Day 1).

10 minutes after the injection. This dose produced no major effects on plasma catecholamine levels except at later times when NE and E levels started to rise. E levels were more affected than those of NE. Of particular interest is that a second administration of alcohol to these animals on the following day produced extremely elevated levels of both catecholamines. In addition, almost all of the animals died shortly after the last sample was drawn on the second day, while only an occasional animal died after the first exposure of 4 g/kg.

Table 2 shows the effects of ethanol on plasma catecholamine levels in immobilized rats. No force had to be used to restrain the alcohol-treated animals, since they lay immobile on the laboratory bench; nevertheless, they were tied to the bench in the same way the saline-treated animals were restrained. The latter fought and vocalized a great deal during restraint and appeared exhausted upon release. As expected, both NE and E levels increased markedly during immobilization in the saline-treated animals but returned to normal after the animals had been released for 30 minutes. Alcohol reduced the stress-response of NE and E at the beginning of immobilization (5 min) but increased the stress-response of E at the end of restraint (30 min). After release, the levels of

NE and E did not return to normal but remained highly elevated in the alcohol-treated animals.

Table 3 shows some of the individual differences which were encountered during stress alone as well as after injection of alcohol.

Table 4 shows the effects of ethanol on heart rate in the conscious, unstressed or stressed rat. Heart rate remained relatively constant over a period of 120 minutes after saline injection in unstressed rats. Injection of ethanol at two doses increased heart rate significantly at most times. In the stressed animals, immobilization increased heart rate markedly. Injection of alcohol had no effect on the stress-induced increases in heart rate.

DISCUSSION

As reported previously (1), administration of a small dose of alcohol (0.5 g/kg) showed no major effects on gross behavior and did not change plasma catecholamine levels in unstressed rats. During immobilization, these rats fought and vocalized as much as did the saline-treated controls. However, it reduced significantly immobilization stress-induced increases in plasma NE and E levels. Although this decrease was statisti-

TABLE 2

Effect of Ethanol (4 g/kg) on Plasma Norepinephrine and
Epinephrine Levels in Stressed Rats

Condition	Time (minutes)				
	0	5	15	30	60
Norepinephrine (pg/ml)					
Saline	147 ± 22	1254 ± 219^a	754 ± 82^a	554 ± 65^a	255 ± 35
Ethanol	119 ± 22	$960 \pm 370^{a,b}$	518 ± 114^a	698 ± 119^a	$688 \pm 184^{a,b}$
Epinephrine (pg/ml)					
Saline	49 ± 8	1182 ± 301^a	792 ± 81^a	563 ± 64^a	84 ± 15
Ethanol	56 ± 16	$419 \pm 88^{a,b}$	577 ± 162^a	$1645 \pm 850^{a,b}$	$869 \pm 416^{a,b}$

Note. Values represent means $\pm$ SEM of 6–10 animals. Saline or ethanol were given after a blood drawing at 0 minutes and the animals were restrained 15 minutes later. Blood was drawn at 5, 15, and 30 minutes of immobilization. The animals were then released, returned to the home cage, and blood was again obtained after 30 minutes (Time 60).
[a]$p < .05$ (comparison with 0 minutes).
[b]$p < .05$ (comparison with saline value).

TABLE 3
Effects of Saline and Alcohol (4 g/kg) on Norepinephrine/
Epinephrine (pg/ml) in Individual Rats

Condition	Time (minutes)				
	0	5	15	30	60
Saline					
Rat 26	235/60	758/400	936/652	667/554	275/134
Rat 41	105/55	2331/1459	1092/477	1101/464	345/90
Alcohol					
Rat 38	186/51	348/276	204/243	285/198	273/51
Rat 29	182/100	984/164	614/140	6240/4730	1070/814

Note. Values represent individual values for norepinephrine/epinephrine. Animals received saline or alcohol and samples were obtained before (0 minutes), during (5, 15, and 30 minutes) and after (60 minutes) immobilization.

cally significant, large individual differences were observed. These differences appeared during stress as well as during alcohol exposure.

In this study, a much larger dose of alcohol was used. This dose produced a flaccid, immobile, and unresponsive animal about 10 minutes after injection. In spite of this large dose, NE and E levels in these unstressed rats were unaffected at first but became elevated after about 1 hour. Levels of both NE and E were normal at the next day or after about 24 hours. However, a second dose in these animals produced dramatic increases in NE and E levels already after 15 minutes. Most animals died within the next 12 hours. Thus, alcohol seems to sensitize the catecholamine-releasing tissues to a second administration of alcohol. It is perhaps this sensitization process which makes rats, in general, avoid alcohol ingestion.

During the immobilization or stress experiments, saline-treated rats had to be forcefully restrained, and they fought, struggled, and vocalized during the 30-minute restraint period. Alcohol-treated animals were motionless, offered no resistance or struggle, and seemed to be "unaware of the restraint." In spite of this behavior, catecholamine levels rose. Initially, alcohol reduced stress-induced increases but later on increased these increases even further and prevented the return of NE and E levels to normal. As seen in earlier experiments with smaller doses, drastic differences in the response of different animals to stress and alcohol were seen.

Although catecholamine levels were not significantly elevated after alcohol in unstressed rats until about 60 minutes, heart rate increased immediately after alcohol administration. No difference between the two doses were noted. No reduction on stress-induced increases in heart rate were noted although NE and E levels were reduced, and increased later on. Thus, no correlation between catecholamine levels and heart rate was apparent.

It has been hypothesized that alcohol reduces anxiety and that some alcoholics drink to relieve this tension; this has been referred to as the "Tension Reduction Hypothesis" (4). Available data in the literature both support and refute this hypothesis, and it has even been shown that alcohol can induce anxiety (5). Our studies show that alcohol can indeed have different effects depending on a number of variables.

First, the state of the animal is important. In unstressed animals, a small dose produced certain changes in central catecholamines which were also seen during stress when the animal is presumably anxious (1). A high dose of alcohol raises plasma catecholamine levels, which are often assumed to be biochemical indicators of stress. This rise could be interpreted as anxiety. Furthermore, the heart rate increases, which can also be interpreted as a sign of anxiety in the animal. Different data are obtained during stress. A small dose of alcohol reduces stress-induced increases in plasma catecholamines and conceivably reduces anxiety (1).

TABLE 4

Effect of Ethanol (4 ml/kg) on Heart Rate (Beats Per Minute)
in Unstressed and Stressed Rats

Condition	Time (minutes)					
	0	5	15	30	60	120
Unstressed Rats						
Saline	330 ± 14	360 ± 19	358 ± 13	344 ± 15	335 ± 16	374 ± 14
Ethanol (1 ml/kg)	334 ± 8	399 ± 24^a	$426 \pm 12^{a,b}$	$453 \pm 18^{a,b}$	$413 \pm 22^{a,b}$	$363 \pm 7^{a,b}$
Ethanol (4 ml/kg)	319 ± 14	415 ± 22^a	417 ± 25^a	$412 \pm 24^{a,b}$	370 ± 31	$410 \pm 19^{a,b}$
Stressed Rats						
Saline	328 ± 12	475 ± 1^a	495 ± 11^a	506 ± 8^a	430 ± 7^a	430 ± 16^a
Ethanol (1 ml/kg)	342 ± 13	499 ± 12^a	490 ± 8^a	485 ± 9^a	458 ± 17^a	444 ± 22^a
Ethanol (4 ml/kg)	323 ± 12	496 ± 7^a	494 ± 5^a	491 ± 9^a	437 ± 6^a	463 ± 8^a

Note. Values represent means ± SEM of 5–6 animals. For unstressed rats, heart rate (HR) was measured at 0 time followed by saline or alcohol (IP) injection. Measurements were taken at specified times. For stressed rats, HR was measured at 0 minutes followed immediately by saline or alcohol (IP) injection. Fifteen minutes later, animals were immobilized. Measurements were taken after 5, 15, and 30 minutes. Animals were released and measurements were taken in the home cage after 30 minutes (60) and 90 minutes (120).
[a]$p < .05$ (comparison with 0 minutes).
[b]$p < .05$ (comparison with saline value).

A large dose of alcohol decreases stress-induced plasma catecholamine levels at first, but augments these increases later on. This could mean that anxiety is reduced initially but increased afterwards.

Second, the measure of anxiety in animals is important. A small dose of ethanol causes no obvious signs of tension reduction during immobilization (1), whereas the large dose used here produced an animal which was unresponsive and did not mind at all being restrained. This would support the Tension Reduction Hypothesis; however, this measure is largely based on the interpretation of the observer. Plasma catecholamine level reduction during stress would also partly support the hypothesis; here it has to be kept in mind that a large dose can augment these levels later on. The measure of heart rate shows an increase in unstressed and no effect during stress. In this case, alcohol causes only "anxiety."

Third, the amounts of alcohol given plays a major role in the effects observed as outlined above.

Thus, the effects of alcohol on "anxiety" in rats depend on many factors including the state of the animal, measure of anxiety, and dose of ethanol used. In addition, large individual differences found among our animals will probably never allow a universal hypothesis of the etiology of alcoholism. Nevertheless, evidence is available which indeed shows that alcohol reduces stress and anxiety in some, although not all, rats.

REFERENCES

1. DeTurck KH, Vogel WH: Effects of acute ethanol on plasma and brain catecholamine levels in stressed and unstressed rats: Evidence for an ethanol stress interaction. J Pharm Expt Ther 223:348–354, 1982
2. Pohorecky LA, Rassi E, Weiss JM, et al: Biochemical evidence for an interaction of ethanol and stress: Preliminary studies. Alcohol Clin Exp Res 4:423–426, 1980
3. Ellis FW: Effect of ethanol on plasma corticosterone levels. J Pharmacol Expt Ther 153:121–127, 1966
4. Cappell H, Herman P: Alcohol and tension reduction. Quart. J Stud Alcohol 33:33–64, 1972
5. Pohorecky LA: The interaction of alcohol and stress. A review. Neurosci Biobehav Rev 5:209–238, 1981

9

The Effect of Maternal Handling on Ethanol Sensitivity in Adult Offspring

KATHRYN H. DeTURCK and
LARISSA A. POHORECKY

The authors determined the effects of prenatal maternal handling (5 min/ day x 7 days; Days 14–21 of gestation) of rats on behavioral and biochemical responses to ethanol (2.0 g/kg, ip) in the adult offspring.

Treated (stressed) subjects exhibited significantly less ethanol-induced hypothermia and adrenocortical activation, although their performance in the swim test was more impaired by ethanol, compared to controls. Blood ethanol levels did not differ in both groups of offspring. Thus, the rate of ethanol metabolism was not altered by prenatal handling; rather, the differences seen between groups were the result of stress-induced changes in CNS sensitivity to acute ethanol.

Prenatal stress is a well recognized teratogen in animals. Exposure to stress *in utero* is capable of producing a wide range of effects on the offspring, including growth deficiencies, somatic abnormalities, and biochemical imbalances, which have been noted at a relatively early age (1–7). In addition, other effects have been shown to persist into adulthood and may therefore represent permanent alterations in the off-

Supported by USPHS grants AA-00045, 04238, and 04241.

spring. When tested as adults, prenatally stressed animals exhibit the following differences from control offspring: decreased emotional and sexual behavior (5, 8–14), lower body and gonadal organ weights (15), decreased pituitary-adrenocortical activity (16, 17), thermoregulatory deficits (18), and various neuro-chemical changes (19–22).

The variety of the reported long-term consequences of prenatal stress indicate severe, widespread, and persistent biobehavioral impairments. It is likely that other changes exist, but they have not as yet been investigated. It is conceivable that such exposure may also result in changes in the adult organism's reaction to other types of stimuli, including pharmacological. Specifically, we examined the possibility that prenatal handling may produce long-term alterations in the rat's biobehavioral responses to acute ethanol administration.

Because stress and ethanol consumption are both so prominent in our society, it is highly desirable that more studies be conducted to delineate the interaction of ethanol and stress. Both stimuli activate the pituitary-adrenocortical system in adults when administered separately (23–25). However, treatment of animals with low doses of ethanol (0.5 g/kg) prior to stress has been shown to result in a significant attenuation of the "stress response" (26–28).

Not surprisingly, stress has long been implicated in the development of alcoholism in man. According to the Tension Reduction Hypothesis (29), ethanol consumption relieves anxiety and may serve as an alternate coping response due to its tension-reducing effect. Although this hypothesis may help to explain what motivates an individual to drink, the underlying processes of ethanol tolerance and physical dependence remain to be defined.

Central nervous system (CNS) mechanisms must certainly be involved; in fact, tolerance to ethanol has been postulated to involve alterations in levels and/or turnover of CNS neurotransmitters (30, 31). Since prenatal stress has been shown to affect these substances, resulting in permanent changes in content, rate of synthesis, etc. (20), an individual's potential degree of tolerance may also be permanently altered.

Activation of the hypothalamic-pituitary adrenal axis during early exposure to stress could also alter the predisposition of adult offspring to ethanol. Since stress is known to elevate both corticosteroids and arginine-vasopressin (32, 33), it is conceivable that prenatally stressed animals have altered sensitivities to the neuroendocrine effects of these hormones. One of the proposed effects of both of those hormones is their role in the development of tolerance to ethanol (34). Therefore, it is possible that this particular ethanol-related phenomenon might be altered in adult animals which have been stressed neonatally. Furthermore, since tolerance is believed to be intimately related to physical dependence, it is likely that neonatally stressed animals will differ in their susceptibility to physical dependence on ethanol.

We tested the hypothesis that maternal handling can exert long-lasting influence upon several ethanol-induced responses in adult offspring, i.e., motor depression, hypothermia, and adrenocortical activation. Taylor, Branch, Liu et al. have demonstrated that in utero ethanol exposure renders the offspring more responsive to the hypothermic and adrenal activating effects of an acute challenge dose of ethanol as adults (35, 36). It is conceivable that prenatal handling may also alter ethanol sensitivity in the offspring.

This study provides an animal model in which the developmental and persistent consequences of prenatal stress exposure on ethanol sensitivity can be studied without the interference of socioeconomic and psychological factors which influence ethanol consumption in humans. It should, therefore, enhance our understanding of the possible sensitizing and/or predisposing factors for ethanol use and/or abuse.

METHODS

Male and female Sprague-Dawley rats were obtained from Charles River Breeding Laboratory at approximately 80 days of age. The animals were housed individually in stainless-steel hanging cages within a temperature-controlled vivarium with a reverse light/dark cycle (lights off from 0900-2100) and with water and Purina lab chow available *ad libitum*.

Prenatal Treatment

On Day 14 of gestation, dams were rehoused in plastic cages, with pine shavings, and randomly assigned to one of two treatment groups: (a) Three were handled for 5 minutes per day for 7 days; and (b) Three remained undisturbed in their home cages without gestation.

Postnatal Treatment

The animals were allowed to litter normally and the day of birth was designated postnatal Day 0. On postnatal Day 1, pups were counted, sexed, weighed, and marked by toe clipping within each prenatal treatment group. To control possible postnatal influence of maternal stress and equalize litter size, some offspring of the handled dams were cross-fostered to control mothers. Remaining pups of handled mothers were fostered within the group.

On Day 21 (weaning), all offspring were weighed and segregated by sex. The onset of eye opening, the onset of puberty (vaginal opening), and body weight at this time were recorded to provide an indication of possible growth deficiencies or morphological abnormalities inherent in neonatally stressed rats.

As adults, male and female offspring in the two treatment groups were tested for their behavioral and biological responses to an acute dose of ethanol. Changes in ethanol-induced behavior were evaluated using swim training (37). To determine the subject's physiological sensitivity to ethanol, two biological responses known to be elicted by ethanol were employed, i.e., hypothermia (38) and adrenocortical activation (23–25).

Behavioral Testing

The behavioral characteristics of the two treatment groups were assessed by observing the 35-50 day-old offspring in a swim performance test. Testing was carried out between 0900 and 1300 hours in a 3.05m long, 0.31 wide stainless-steel swim tank. It was filled with 25 °C water to a depth of 0.35 meters.

Animals received 10 training sessions per day for 4 days, followed by three predrug warm-up trials on the day of testing. A predrug baseline was determined for each rat by taking the mean of the second and third predrug swimming times. Thirty, 60, and 90 minutes after ip injection of 2.0 g ethanol/kg or saline, the rats were again placed in the tank and the transit time recorded. Drug effects were measured as changes from predrug performance, such that each rat served as its own control. Ethanol has been shown to produce a dose-dependent impairment of swim test performance, using the above apparatus (37).

Body Temperature Measurement

Body temperature of the rats was recorded before ethanol or saline injection and 30, 60, and 90 minutes after injection. Body temperature was measured with a Yellow Springs Telethermometer and a lubricated rectal thermistorprobe, inserted 5 cm into the rectum of the animal.

Biochemical Determinations

Seventy days postpartum, the rats were decapitated 30 minutes after ethanol or saline injection and trunk blood was collected on ice for the evaluation of ethanol and corticosterone levels. Ethanol was determined by a sensitive gas chromatographic method currently in use in our laboratory (39). Levels of corticosterone were assayed according to the method of Glick, von Redlich, and Levine (40).

Statistics

Student's *t*-test was used throughout.

RESULTS

Gestation time and litter size were both significantly lower for prenatally stressed animals compared to controls ($t = 2.24$, $p \le .05$). In addition, on the day of birth, litters born to handled mothers weighed 20% less than litters of nonstressed dams ($t = 2.56$, $p \le .05$). A single preweaning mortality occurred in the stress group, as did two cases of gross physical abnormalities. The remaining parameters did not differ for stressed and nonstressed rats.

Tested 42 days postpartum, prenatally stressed rats exhibited significantly less ethanol-induced hypothermia (Figure 1) than nonstressed rats ($t = 2.98$, $p \le .01$). Whereas controls demonstrated a $1.21 \pm 0.12\,°C$ drop in body temperature 30 minutes after acute ethanol administration (2g/kg,ip), temperatures among stressed animals were only $0.85 \pm 0.16\,°C$ lower. Decrements did not differ for male and female offspring.

Acute ethanol treatment impaired swimming performance of stressed rats significantly more than that of controls ($t = 3.77$, $p \le .01$). Maximum increases in transit time (Figure 2) were 65% and 38% greater among males and females, respectively, compared to nonstressed values ($t = 4.38$, $p \le .01$; $t + 3.14$, $p \le .01$).

Stressed rats showed a significantly lower adrenocortical response to ethanol at 70 days of age ($t = 2.62$, $p \le .01$). Peak plasma corticosterone levels (Table 1) in handled males were decreased 35% compared to controls ($t = 2.95$, $p \le .01$), while females exhibited a 20%–25% decrease in responsiveness ($t = 2.41$, $p \le .05$).

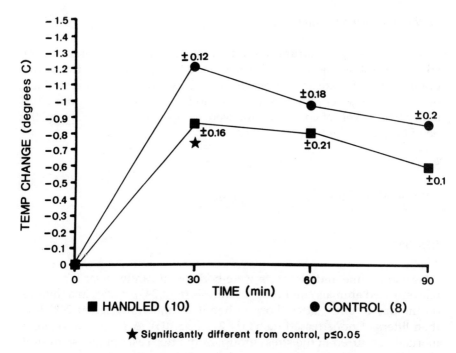

Figure 1. Ethanol (2g/Kg)-induced hypothermia in 40–44 day old rats.

Blood ethanol levels at time of sacrifice were not significantly different for the two groups of offspring (Table 2).

DISCUSSION

Consistent with previous work on prenatal stress influences, maternal handling resulted in a decreased sensitivity of the adult offspring to the hypothermic and adrenocortical activating effects of acute ethanol treatment. Ethanol-induced impairment of swimming performance, however, was more pronounced in the handled rats. Blood ethanol levels did not differ in both groups of offspring. Thus, the rate of ethanol metabolism was probably not altered by prenatal handling; rather, the differences seen between groups were more likely the result of stress-induced changes in CNS sensitivity to acute ethanol.

Earlier investigations of the long-term effects of prenatal maternal handling on the offspring generally demonstrated decreased adult physio-logical and behavioral responsiveness among stressed rats. Upon expo-sure of their animals to handling at 90 days postpartum, Ader and Plaut (16) noted significantly less adrenocortical reactivity, vocalization, and physical resistance in the prenatally handled group, compared to non-stressed animals. However, stressed rats were found to be more suscepti-ble to immobilization-induced gastric ulceration.

Other prenatal handling influences on offspring behavior have includ-ed decreased defecation and increased exploration in the open field, as well as increased exploration in home cage emergence testing (8, 10, 13), indicating a lower level of fear/apprehension, and hence decreased emo-tionality, among stressed animals.

Premating avoidance-conditioning followed by exposure to the condi-tioned stimulus during pregnancy has also been found to result in an increase in exploratory behavior of adult offspring in the cage emergence test (13). In this same study, however, the offspring of females presented

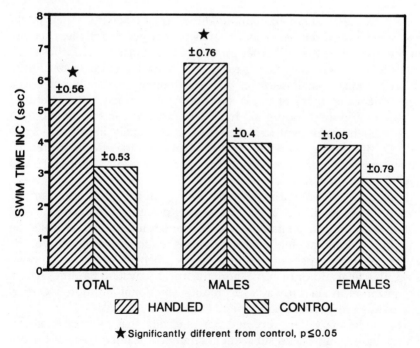

Figure 2. Performance deficits with ethanol in 54–58 day old rats.

TABLE 1
Plasma Corticosterone Responses to Ethanol
(2.0 g/kg) or Saline in Adult Offspring
of Handled and Control Dams

Treatment Group (N)	Corticosterone (ug/100 ml)	
	Handled	Control
Ethanol		
Total	42.42 ± 2.80(12)*	60.60 ± 2.41(7)
Males	26.13 ± 1.95(6)*	39.90 ± 1.54(3)
Females	61.80 ± 3.87(6)*	76.20 ± 2.66(4)
Saline		
Total	12.17 ± 0.61(9)	12.90 ± 0.59(7)
Males	8.70 ± 0.57(5)	7.50 ± 0.60(2)
Females	16.51 ± 1.14(4)	15.06 ± 0.93(5)

$p \le .05$ compared to control.

only with the conditioned stimulus during pregnancy (i.e., their mothers were handled but never shocked) displayed significantly less activity in the open field than all other groups of rats. Furthermore, these animals demonstrated heightened copulatory behavior, in direct contrast to the reductions in male sexual activity and potency generally noted as a consequence of prenatal stress exposure. Interestingly, stress-induced release of arginine-vasopressin has been implicated in the inhibition of testicular androgen synthesis observed in prenatally immobilized rats (41, 42). It appears, therefore, that the biobehavioral effects of prenatal stress depend to some extent on the specific stressor being employed pre- as well as postnatally.

Long-term consequences of prenatal stress in the adult organism are believed to be mediated, at least in part, by pituitary-adrenocortical activation with the concomitant increase in corticosteroid release. Based on the proposition that emotional reactivity is reduced as a function of the degree of stress experienced during development, it has been hypothesized that fetal and/or maternal adrenocortical activation modifies neural organization in such a way as to reduce emotional and adrenocortical reactivity in response to subsequent stimulation (17, 43).

The preliminary data reported here indicate that prenatal maternal handling indeed reduces subsequent adrenocortical reactivity of the offspring to acute ethanol. Handled animals were 30% less responsive to acute ethanol-induced adrenocortical activation compared to controls. As was also the case for acute ethanol-induced impairment of swim performance, male rats demonstrated a greater effect of prenatal treatment on adult ethanol sensitivity than did the females. However, behavioral responsiveness, as measured in the swim test, appears to be increased in prenatally stressed animals.

Interestingly, studies on swim performance conducted by Bass and Lester have shown that differential responsiveness was reversed among rats selectively bred for ethanol-induced behavioral depression (44). The rats bred for insensitivity to ethanol's soporific effects and locomotor depression on a stabilimeter platform were, surprisingly, more impaired by ethanol in the swim test, compared to the sensitive line. Different mechanisms may, therefore, subserve what appear to be similar effects of ethanol.

In conclusion, the pituitary and target organ hormones exert important actions on the CNS to influence biochemistry and behavior both in adult life and during development. Through their actions on neuroendocrine systems, stressful prenatal events may be considered as organizational factors for the developing CNS, with profound consequences for the adult organism. Some of the actions of prenatal stress exposure reflect stress-induced hormonal alterations during development, such as

TABLE 2
Effect of Prenatal Handling
on Blood Ethanol Levels of
Adult Rats 30 Minutes
After IP Ethanol (2.0 g/kg)
Administration

Treatment Group (N)	Ethanol Levels (mg %)
Handled	
Total	$181.60 \pm 17.8(11)$
Males	$174.14 \pm 12.2(6)$
Females	$190.55 \pm 18.4(5)$
Control	
Total	$184.74 \pm 18.2(7)$
Males	$197.53 \pm 15.7(3)$
Females	$175.15 \pm 11.8(4)$

activation of the hypothalamo-pituitary adrenal axis. Such prenatal organizational factors might well produce persistent alterations in adult responses, neuroendocrine or otherwise, to ethanol and/or stress and point to possible hormonal bases for the individual differences in ethanol sensitivity which may influence one's susceptibility to dependence on the drug. It is possible that the effects of early stress exposure interact with genetic factors in determining human predisposition to alcoholism and/or alcohol sensitivity in adulthood (45).

REFERENCES

1. Barlow SM, McElhatton PR, Sullivan FM: Relation between maternal restraint and food deprivation, plasma corticosterone, and induction of cleft palate in the offspring of mice. Teratology 12: 97–104, 1975
2. Smith DJ, Joffe JM, Heseltine GFD: Modification of prenatal stress effects in rats by adrenalectomy, dexamethasone and chlorpromazine. Physiol Behav 15:461–469, 1975
3. Jonson KM, Lyle JC, Edwards MJ, et al: Effect of prenatal heat stress on brain growth and serial discrimination reversal learning in the guinea pig. Brain Res Bull 1:133–150, 1976
4. Milkovic K, Joffe J, Levine S: The effect of maternal and fetal corticosteroids on the development and function of the pituitary-adrenocortical system. Endokrinology 68:60–65, 1976
5. Herrenkohl LR: Prenatal stress reduced fertility and fecundity in female offspring. Science 206:1097–1098, 1979
6. Weisz J, Brown BL, Ward IL: Maternal stress decreases steroid aromatase activity in brains of male and female rat fetuses. Neuroendocrinology 35:374–379, 1982
7. Wilke DL, Tseu SR, Rhees RW, et al: Effects of environmental stress or ACTH treatment during pregnancy on maternal and fetal plasma androstenedione in the rat. Horm Behav 16:293–302, 1982
8. Ader R, Conklin RM: Handling of pregnant rats: Effects on emotionality of their offspring. Science 142: 411–412, 1963
9. Hutchings DF, Gibbon J: Preliminary study of behavioral and teratogenic effects of two "stress" procedures administered during different periods of gestation in the rat. Psychol Rep 26:239–246, 1970
10. Archer JE, Blackman DE: Prenatal psychological stress and offspring behavior in rats and mice. Develop Psychobiol 4:193–248, 1971
11. Ward IL: Prenatal stress feminizes and demasculinizes the behavior of males. Science 143:212–218, 1972
12. Herrenkohl LR, Whitney JB: Effects of prepartal stress on postpartal nursing behavior, litter development and adult sexual behavior. Physiol Behav 17: 1019–1021, 1976
13. Masterpasqua F, Chapman RH, Lore RK: The effects of prematernal and prenatal stress on the sexual behavior and reactivity of male rats. Dev Psychobiol 9: 403–411, 1976
14. Meisel RL, Dohanich GP, Ward IL: Effects of prenatal stress on avoidance acquisition, open-field performance and lordotic behavior in male rats. Physiol Behav 22:527–530, 1979
15. Smith PG, Mills E: Abnormal development of blood pressure and growth in rats exposed to perinatal injection stress. Life Sci 32:2497–2501, 1983
16. Ader R, Plaut SM: Effects of prenatal maternal handling and differential housing on offspring emotionality, plasma corticosterone levels, and susceptibility to gastric erosions. Psychosom Med 30:277–286, 1968

17. Smotherman WP: In utero chemosensory experience alters taste preferences and corticosterone responsiveness. Behav Neural Biol 36:61–68, 1983
18. Dailey JW: Effects of maternally administered reserpine on the development of the cold stress response and its possible ralation to adrenergic nervous system function. Res Comm Chem Pathol Pharmacol 19:389–402, 1978
19. Huttunen MO: Persistent alteration of turnover of brain noradrenaline in the offspring of rats subjected to stress during pregnancy. Nature 230:53–55, 1971
20. Moyer JA, Herrenkohl LR, Jacobowitz DM: Stress during pregnancy: Effect on catecholamines in discrete brain regions of offspring as adults. Brain Res 144:173–178, 1978
21. Peters DAV: Prenatal stress: Effects on brain biogenic amine and plasma corticosterone levels. Pharmacol Biochem Behav 17:721–725, 1982
22. Plaut SM, Graham CW, Leiner KY: Effects of prenatal maternal handling and rearing with aunts on behavior, brain weight, and whole-brain serotonin levels. Develop Psychobiol 5:215–221, 1972
23. Ellis FW: Effect of ethanol on plasma corticosterone levels. J Pharmacol Exp Ther 153:121–127, 1966
24. Mendelson JH, Ogata M, Mello NK: Adrenal function and alcoholism. I. Serum cortisol. Psychosom Med 33:145–157, 1971
25. Pohorecky LA, Jaffe LS: Noradrenergic involvement in the acute effects of ethanol. Res Comm Chem Pathol Pharmacol 12:433–447, 1975
26. Pohorecky LA, Rassi E, Weiss JM, et al: Biochemical evidence for an interaction of ethanol and stress: Preliminary studies. Alc Clin Exp Res 4:423–426, 1980
27. Brick J, Pohorecky LA: Ethanol-stress interaction: Biochemical findings. Psychopharmacology 77: 81–84, 1982
28. DeTurck KH, Vogel WH: Effects of acute ethanol on plasma and brain catecholamine levels in stressed and unstressed rats: Evidence for an ethanol-stress interaction. J Pharmacol Exp Ther 223:348–354, 1982
29. Cappell H, Herman P: Alcohol and tension reduction. Q J Stud Alcohol 33:33–64, 1972
30. Tabakoff B: Neurochemical aspects of ethanol dependence, in Alcohol and Opiates. Edited by Blum K. New York, Academic Press, 1977
31. Tabakoff B, Hoffman PF: Alcohol and neurotransmitters, in Alcohol Tolerance and Dependence. Edited by Righter H, Crabbe J C. New York, Elsevier/North Holland, 1980
32. Konzett H, Hortnagl H, et al: On the urinary output of vasopressin, epinephrine and norepinephrine during different stress situations. Psychopharmacologia (Berlin) 21:247–256, 1971
33. Husain MK, Manger WM, Rock TW, et al: Vasopressin release due to manual restraint in the rat: Role of body compression and comparison with other stressful stimuli. Endocrinology 104:641–644, 1979
34. Sze PY: The permissive role of glucocorticoids in the development of ethanol dependence and tolerance. Drug Alc Depend 2:381–396, 1977
35. Taylor AN, Branch BJ, Liu SH, et al: Fetal exposure to alcohol enhances pituitary-adrenal and temperature responses to ethanol in adult rats. Alcoholism 5:237–246, 1981
36. Taylor AN, Branch BJ, Liu SH, et al: Long-term effect of fetal ethanol exposure on pituitary-adrenal response to stress. Pharmacol Biochem Behav 16:585–589, 1982
37. Bass MB, Lester D: Swimming as a measure of motor impairment after ethanol and pentobarbital in rats. J Stud Alcohol 39:1618–1622, 1978
38. Freund G: Hypothermia after acute ethanol and benzyl alcohol administration. Life Science 13:345–349, 1973
39. Poherecky LA, Brick J: A new method for the determination of blood ethanol levels in rodents. Pharmacol Biochem Behav 16:693–696, 1982
40. Glick D, von Redlich D, Levine S: Fluorometric determination of corticosterone and cortisol in 0.02-0.05 milliliters of plasma or submilligram samples of adrenal tissue. Endocrinology 74:653–655, 1964
41. Adashi TY, Hsueh AJW: Direct inhibition of testicular androgen biosynthesis of argi-

nine-vasopressin: Mediation through pressor-selective testicular recognition sites. Endocrinology 109:1793–1795, 1981
42. Charpenet G., Tache Y, Bernier M, et al: Stress-induced testicular hyposensitivity to gonadotropin in rats. Role of the pituitary gland. Endocrinology 110: 48–55, 1982
43. Ader R, Grota LJ: Adrenocortical mediation of the effects of early life experience, in Progress in Brain Research, vol 39, Drug Effects on Neuroendocrine Regulation. Edited by Gispen WH, Marks BH, deWied D. Amsterdam, Elsevier, 1973
44. Bass MB, Lester D: Rats bred for ethanol sensitivity: Impairment of swimming by ethanol and pentobarbital. Psychopharmacology 63:161–167, 1979
45. Deitrich RA, Collins AC: Pharmacogenetics of alcoholism, in Alcohol and Opiates. Edited by Blum K. New York, Academic Press, 1977

SECTION III

Contributions from Human Studies

10

Autonomic Nervous System Dysfunction in Alcoholism

LEONARD S. RUBIN

In this study, measurement of pupillary diameter during reflex constriction in response to light and during reflex dilation in response to darkness are used as indices of parasympathetic and sympathetic mechanisms. Normal subjects and abstinent alcoholics free of medical and psychiatric problems served as subjects in both resting and stress conditions. Subjects were also tested after receiving a controlled amount of alcohol. Results of the studies suggest that alcoholics are characterized by an autonomic dysfunction when free of stress. They are also incapable of optimal arousal on mobilization as is required for adequate coping when confronted with stress. It is postulated that normals may drink alcohol to reduce tension whereas alcoholics may consume alcohol to provide self-stimulation.

Psychological, social, biological, or chemical variables have not yet been shown uniquely to differentiate alcoholics from nonalcoholics. The "alcoholic personality" has been associated with traits such as hostility, immaturity, depression, and dependency in spite of the lack of experimental confirmation (1).

A study by Goodwin, Schulsinger, and Hermansen (2) has suggested the importance of genetic factors in the development of alcoholism. Danish alcoholics who had been separated from their biological parents soon

143

after birth and raised by nonrelatives without subsequent contact with their biological parents had 4 times the rate of alcoholism than the control group. The control adoptees were equivalent to the alcoholics with alcoholic biological parents with respect to diagnosed depression, anxiety, neurosis, sociopathy, drug addiction, and the incidence of these factors was low in both groups. Furthermore, no significant correlation was found between the drinking patterns of the adoptees and the presence or absence of alcoholism in their foster parents. This study suggests that the biological influence of an alcoholic parent is far more important than exposure to an alcoholic parent in predicting the development of alcoholism in the offspring.

The search for a phenotypic expression of this genetic predisposition in chemical or biological systems has been and continues to be the concern of numerous investigators. A number of studies have contrasted autonomic nervous system function of alcoholics and nonalcoholics. Wenger (3) found no gross autonomic imbalance in alcoholics at rest. Stern, Schwartz, and Gospodinoff (4) reported that salivary output was lower in alcoholics, and Cutshall (5) reported that diastolic blood pressure was relatively higher in alcoholics. Kissin and Hankoff (6) found that alcoholics were characterized by impaired sympathetic nervous system activity and increased parasympathetic nervous system outflow.

In other studies, Kissin, Schenker, and Schenker (7, 8, 9) demonstrated that alcoholics evinced a high frequency of abnormal values in a number of tests of endocrine and autonomic nervous system functions (measures of adrenocortical response, regulation of arterial blood pressure, etc.). Kissin et al. concluded that these abnormalities were primarily constitutional in nature, rather than due to the effects of alcoholism, since they were found in alcoholics who had been abstinent for at least 2 years.

A reanalysis of Wenger's data by Naitoh (10) again demonstrated no significant difference in the autonomic balance of alcoholics and nonalcoholics. However, only 1 of the 13 variables in Naitoh's analysis approached statistical significance—relatively imprecise measurements of static pupillary diameter. Studies by Rubin (11, 12, 13) and other investigators (14) used precise measurements of the dynamic characteristics of pupillary reactivity to elucidate the role of sympathetic and parasympathetic mechanisms in schizophrenia and other behavior disorders. In the studies to be described, measurements of pupillary diameter during reflex constriction in response to light and during reflex dilation in response to darkness were used, respectively, as indices of parasympathetic and sympathetic mechanisms in healthy controls and alcoholics.

An anatomical and physiological survey describing the extensiveness of the nervous network that makes the pupil an ideal indicator of the physiology of the autonomic nervous system is found in Lowenstein and Lowenfeld (15). The cholinergic sphincter muscle, innervated by parasympathetic oculomotor nerve fibers, is the effector organ for pupillary contraction in response to light; the dilator pupillae, innervated by sympathetic fibers, act as antagonist to the sphincter. Bonvallet and Zbrozyna (16, 17) have demonstrated that the reticular activating system reciprocally controls the antagonist innervation of the pupil; its discharge simultaneously intensifies sympathetic tone, as manifested by increased pupillary dilation, and inhibits tonic activity and resultant parasympathetic outflow of the Edinger-Westphal nucleus.

The extent and shape of any pupillary movement depends, then, on the dynamic equilibrium of the following mechanisms: parasympathetic innervation causes active pupillary constriction, and its central nervous inhibition (supranuclear inhibition) causes slow, passive dilation of the pupil; sympathetic excitation dilates the pupil rapidly and completely, while relaxation of sympathetic activity facilitates constriction.

The details of the apparatus and the procedure employed to obtain the pupillometric measurements have been described by Rubin (11, 12, 13).

Briefly, continuous changes in pupillary diameter of the 1-minute dark-adapted eye were recorded by an infrared monocular TV Pupillometer following 10 seconds of light-adaptation. Then, after a 2-minute period of dark-adaptation, pupillary contraction to a high intensity light source was recorded for 10 seconds. These procedures were administered to determine tonic sympathetic and parasympathetic activity. Phasic responsivity of these systems was elicited by a 1½-minute cold pressor test, during which time pupillary dilation and constriction were recorded. Homeostatic recovery of autonomic nervous system activity was monitored for several minutes following termination of the cold pressor test.

All subjects were paid volunteers. The controls were 10 normal, healthy adults screened by means of the Cornell Medical Index Health Questionnaire (18). On the basis of the controls' responses, no follow-up medical examination or psychiatric interview was deemed necessary. Several additional questions were asked in order to exclude as controls anyone receiving medication; questions were also asked about the controls' drinking habits. Uniformly, the controls drank infrequently, usually modest quantities of alcohol on social occasions, and never to the point of inebriation. Six of the controls were men and 4 were women; they ranged in age from 21 to 40, the average age being 28.5.

The 25 alcoholics studied were inpatients at the Alcoholic Treatment and Research Unit of the Coatesville Veterans Administration Hospital, the unit established by Gottheil, Corbett, and Grasberger (19). None of the alcoholics had had access to alcohol during the preceding 6 days. All the alcoholics were male, 17 white and 8 black; the average age was 41.8 years, the range being 24 to 52 years.

Lidsky, Hakerem, and Sutton (14) found no significant differences in the pupillary reactivity of normal adults as a function of age (18 to 45 years) or sex. Lowenstein and Lowenfeld (15) had previously reported similar findings and, in addition, stated that pupillary reactivity was independent of eye color or a subject's being nearsighted or farsighted. These studies provided reasonable assurance that these variables did not confound the results reported here.

The alcoholics' drinking histories were positive with respect to three or more of the following characteristics: previous hospitalization or imprisonment for drinking; "spree" drinking within the last 5 years; interrupted work history due to excessive drinking; family strife due to drinking; and amnesia, blackouts, hallucinations, or delirium.

The results of medical and neurological examinations were carefully reviewed to ensure that the alcoholics did not have a neurological disease, psychotic illness, and hepatic, renal, pulmonary, cardiac, gastrointestinal, genitourinary or serious nutritional or metabolic disorder. The alcoholics received no medication and required no medical treatment.

The first study (20) used pupillometry to measure parasympathetic-cholinergic and sympathetic-noradrenergic mechanisms of alcoholics and nonalcoholics under a no-alcohol condition at rest, during stress, and throughout a period of homeostatic recovery following the cessation of stress.

At rest, the alcoholics were characterized by deficient pupillary contraction in response to light and attenuated dilation during adaptation to the dark. As pupillary contraction is mediated by parasympathetic outflow, and pupillary dilation in darkness is mediated by a rapid initial increase in supranuclear inhibition which is then followed by more sustained and prolonged sympathetic outflow, these results suggest that alcoholics in a no-alcohol state are characterized by reactive deficiencies of both components of the autonomic nervous system.

Alcoholics and nonalcoholics also differed in systematic variation of contraction and dilation under stress and during homeostatic recovery. Evaluation of changes in the diameter of the dark-adapted pupil revealed that the alcoholics' response to stress was significantly attenuated, and their recovery therefore was faster. In the alcoholics, inadequate sympathetic outflow during stress was accompanied by an aberrant decrease in supranuclear inhibition, as shown by the modest increase in pupillary diameter of the light-adapted pupil. In contrast, the nonalcoholics responded with significantly greater sympathetic outflow and greater supranuclear inhibition. On the whole, the alcoholics were characterized by inadequate autonomic mechanisms that would presumably preclude effective optimal adjustment to stress and subsequent homeostatic recovery.

The question arises whether these patterns of sympathetic-parasympathetic activity are specific to alcoholism. In Rubin's (11, 12, 13) experiments using pupillometry in conjunction with the cold pressor test for the differential diagnosis of psychotic and neurotic behavior, neither neurotics nor schizophrenics manifested the patterns of autonomic responsivity found in the alcoholics who participated in the present study. However, neurotic and psychotic processes do not exhaust the list of socially defined aberrant syndromes.

It is conceivable that an unknown number of people share a biological substratum consisting of tonic, low autonomic arousal and attenuated phasic responsiveness to stress which is perceived as uncomfortable and which is not relieved by a socially defined and sanctioned life style. Perhaps the abnormal patterns of sympathetic-parasympathetic activity observed in alcoholics are present in other syndromes that involve dependency and tolerance. These are moot questions, especially when the results of a cross-sectional study cannot establish a clear temporal or causal relation between specific aberrant patterns of autonomic responsivity and alcoholism. It is possible that the autonomic impoverishment is an invariable antecedent to psychological states that predispose an individual to alcoholism rather than an insidious consequence of alcoholism.

The unique structure of the Alcoholic Treatment and Research Unit at the Coatesville Veterans Administration Hospital permitted a comparison of the autonomic nervous system (ANS) responsivity of alcoholics who could voluntarily abstain from drinking when it was available with that of alcoholics who could not abstain (21).

The 25 alcoholics studied were inpatients at the Alcoholic Treatment and Research Unit of the Coatesville Veterans Administration Hospital. The unit conducts 6-week studies during which alcoholics who are voluntarily hospitalized and detoxified are given the choice of drinking or not drinking at frequent fixed intervals. The cycle, which takes place in a closed ward, begins with a 1-week predrinking phase during which no alcohol is available. Every alcoholic in the present study was examined at the end of this period and had had no access to alcohol for at least 9 days. During the next 4 weeks of the cycle, patients can elect to drink no alcohol or 2 ounces of a beverage containing 43% alcohol each hour on the hour from 0900 to 2100, Monday through Friday; during the final week of the cycle, no alcohol is available.

Of the 25 men studied, 17 were white and 8 black; their average age was 41.8 years, the range being 24 to 52 years. Fifteen abstained from drinking during the entire month that alcohol was available ("non-drinker alcoholics") and 10 drank varying quantities when it was available ("drinker alcoholics"). Evaluation of the patients' histories revealed no significant factor, i.e., years of heavy drinking and previous hospitalizations, related to their drinking decisions.

The drinker alcoholics and the nondrinker alcoholics were compared to each other and to nonalcoholics with respect to: tonic sympathetic and parasympathetic activity (at rest); phasic sympathetic and parasympathetic activity (cold pressor test); and homeostatic recovery of sympathetic and parasympathetic activity following termination of the cold pressor test. It was found that, at rest, drinker and nondrinker alcoholics were equally defective with respect to the rate of pupillary contraction in response to light. Since pupillary contraction is mediated by parasympathetic outflow, this finding suggests that alcoholics in a no-alcohol state are characterized by deficient parasympathetic outflow.

The rate and amplitude of pupillary dilation during adaptation to darkness also revealed intergroup differences. Both groups of alcoholics were defective in rate and amplitude of pupillary dilation; however, alcoholics who chose to drink alcohol showed an even slower rate and a more attenuated amplitude of response. It may be concluded that under the no-alcohol condition, and at rest, drinker alcoholics show a more marked sympathetic deficiency than do nondrinker alcoholics.

These findings do not agree with the conclusions of Kissin et al. (7–9), who reported that alcoholics are characterized by impaired (excessive or deficient) central sympathetic activity and increased parasympathetic nervous activity. Nor are the results in agreement with the overall conclusion of Wenger and Naitoh that there is no gross autonomic imbalance in alcoholics. A prospective study of larger samples would be required to substantiate this potentially useful and suggestive finding.

Systematic variation of contraction and dilation under stress and during homeostatic recovery also differed in alcoholics and nonalcoholics, both drinker and nondrinker alcoholics demonstrating significant impairment in the amount of change in contraction occasioned by stress. Since the amount of change is proportional to the extent of supranuclear inhibition, it may be concluded that, on the average, alcoholics were characterized by inadequate, attenuated supranuclear inhibition during stress.

Sympathetic reactivity to stress seems to be the autonomic component concomitant with the subsequent decision to drink or not drink. Alcoholics who refrained from drinking when alcohol was made available at some later date reacted to stress in the same manner as nonalcoholics and manifested similar homeostatic recovery of sympathetic function. On the other hand, alcoholics who drank alcohol when it was available demonstrated a marked attenuation of sympathetic outflow during stress and, as a consequence, rebounded rapidly to the baseline.

The physiologically adaptive response to stress was exemplified by nonalcoholics who simultaneously showed maximum sympathetic outflow and maximum supranuclear inhibition. The reciprocity of these processes was not observed in alcoholics who abstained from drinking for at least 1 month, who were characterized only by impairment of the supranuclear inhibitory mechanism. Alcoholics who did not exercise restraint were characterized by defective, inadequate levels of sympathetic outflow and markedly attenuated supranuclear inhibition.

The third study (22) was conducted to determine whether alcohol differentially affected the autonomic nervous system responsivity of alcoholics and controls.

The nonalcoholics were 10 healthy adults (4 women), screened by means of the Cornell Medical Index Health Questionnaire and interviewed to establish that they drank only modest quantities of alcohol on social occasions, never to the stage of inebriation, and that they were not taking any medication. Their ages ranged from 21 to 40 years (mean = 28.5).

The alcoholics were six white men, aged 25 to 50 years (mean = 40), who were inpatients in the Alcoholic Treatment and Research Unit of the Coatesville Veterans Administration Hospital. As previous experiments have shown no significant differences in pupillary reactivity in adults as a function of age (18 to 45 years), sex, eye color, or whether the subject was myopic or hyperopic, we may assume that these variables did not confound the results reported here. The patients' drinking histories were positive with respect to three or more of the criteria enumerated in our earlier studies. Before a patient participated in the study, his medical and neurological examination results were carefully reviewed to ensure that numerous diseases were not clinically present. None of the patients had received any medication prior to examination, nor did they require any medical treatment.

During the 6 weeks of the study, the hospitalized alcoholics had the choice of drinking or not at frequent fixed intervals. Alcohol was not available during the 1st week, however, and every alcoholic in the study was tested initially during this period, when he had had no access to alcohol for at least 9 days. Over the next 4 weeks, patients could elect to drink either no alcohol or 2 ounces (59 ml) of whiskey (43% alcohol) at any hour on the hour between 0900 and 2100 hr, Monday through Friday. The alcoholics were tested twice: at the end of the nondrinking period and after they had taken their first drink in the drinking-decision phase.

The nonalcoholics were also examined before and after the consumption of 2 ounces of whiskey. All subjects were required to imbibe the alcohol within 5 minutes, and testing began 30 minutes later. All subjects were tested at 1100 hr and had eaten at 0730-0800 hr.

Measurements of pupillary dilatation and constriction were obtained at rest, during stress (cold pressor), and following the termination of stress (homeostatic recovery), before and after the imbibition of alcohol.

The discussion and interpretation of the results are limited by at least two considerations, however. First, subjects were tested after only a single dose of alcohol. In the absence of systematic variation of dose, we cannot assume that a linear relationship exists between dose and the amplitude or direction of the autonomic effects. Second, as alcoholism is in part defined by increased tolerance, we cannot assume that equal doses in nonalcoholics and alcoholics equally modify ANS reactivity.

Unstressed alcoholics without alcohol had significantly less extensive and slower pupillary change in response to both darkness and light when compared with nonalcoholics, suggesting that they may have an autonomic dysfunctional state, characterized by deficient sympathetic and parasympathetic outflow.

After alcohol, parasympathetic outflow was increased in both alcoholics and nonalcoholics at rest, an effect that was significantly more pronounced in the nonalcoholics. Perhaps the smaller response in alcoholics relates to an increased tolerance for the drug. In contrast, sympathetic outflow was unaffected by alcohol in both groups at rest. It is important to note that the increased parasympathetic outflow produced in alcoholics by alcohol was sufficient to establish a level of activity identical to that in the nonalcoholics before alcohol. Thus, a small dose of alcohol appears to normalize parasympathetic outflow in alcoholics at rest.

The groups also reacted differently during stress and homeostatic recovery before alcohol. Nonalcoholics responded to the cold pressor test with a pronounced increase in sympathetic outflow and a marked increase in supranuclear inhibition, as represented by reduced parasympathetic outflow.

The complementarity of these processes provides for optimal mobilization of the ANS, as demonstrated by Lowenstein and Loewenfeld (15) in humans and by Bonvallet and Zbrozyna (16, 17) in cats. They reported that arousal is characterized by simultaneous active sympathetic discharge to the dilator of the pupil and convergence of inhibitory impulses from cerebral centers on the oculomotor nucleus, preventing it from sending impulses that would constrict the pupil.

In sharp contrast, the autonomic reactivity of the stressed alcoholics revealed pronounced deficiencies in both sympathetic outflow and the degree of supranuclear inhibition. Under stress, the alcoholics responded with attenuated sympathetic outflow and inadequate supranuclear inhibition and, consequently, inappropriate excessive parasympathetic outflow. These preliminary findings suggested that alcoholics were characterized by autonomic dysfunction when free of stress and that they were incapable of adequate arousal or mobilization, a prerequisite for effective coping, when confronted with stress.

Alcohol affected the autonomic responses to stress in several ways. It did not significantly affect the degree of supranuclear inhibition of either group; the inhibition remained appropriately high in the nonalcoholics and abnormally low in the alcoholics. There was a slight but insignificant tendency for alcohol to further depress supranuclear inhibition in the alcoholics. This tendency toward even more pronounced parasympathetic outflow during stress represents a deleterious interference in appropriate parasympathetic responsiveness. Alcohol did exert a differential effect on autonomic sympathetic responsivity during stress in both groups, significantly attenuating the sympathetic outflow in the nonalcoholics and augmenting it in alcoholics.

Therefore, there was a tendency toward normalization of sympathetic outflow in the alcoholics given alcohol. If this effect were dose-dependent and linear, perhaps larger doses of alcohol would permit the alcoholics to manifest that degree of sympathetic outflow appropriate to effective mobilization of the ANS under stress. Whether proprioceptive feedback from this partly normalized state under stress may be involved in the acquisition of the propensity to consume large quantities of alcohol merits further investigation.

In any event, the dose of alcohol used in the experiment elevated sympathetic outflow in alcoholics but did not produce the extent of supranuclear inhibition requisite for effective mobilization. These preliminary results are especially noteworthy in view of the elevated tolerance of alcoholics and suggest that, whereas nonalcoholics may drink alcohol in order to reduce tension, alcoholics may drink to provide self-stimulation as an escape from an endogenous autonomic state that may be equivalent to manifest boredom.

REFERENCES

1. Mello NK: Alcoholism and the behavioral pharmacology of alcohol, in Psychopharmacology: A Generation of Progress. Edited by Lipton MA, DiMascio A, Killam KF. New York, Raven Press, 1978, pp 1619–1637
2. Goodwin DW, Schulsinger F, Hermansen L: Alcohol problems in adoptees raised apart from alcoholic biological parents. Archives of General Psychiatry 28:238–243, 1973
3. Wenger MA: Studies of autonomic balance in Army Air Force personnel. Comparative Psychology Monographs No 101, 1948
4. Stern JA, Schwartz L, Gospodinoff ML: Salivary output of the alcoholic: Effect of treatment with amitriptyline. Conditioned Reflex 3:254–262, 1968
5. Cutshall BJ: The Sanders-Sutton syndrome; an analysis of delirium tremens. Quarterly Journal of Studies of Alcohol 26:423–448, 1965
6. Kissin B, Hankoff L: The acute effects of ethyl alcohol on the Funkenstein mecholyl response in male alcoholics. Quarterly Journal of Studies of Alcohol 20:696–703, 1959
7. Kissin B, Schenker V, Schenker A: The acute effects of ethanol ingestion on plasma and urinary 17-hydroxycorticoids in alcoholic subjects. American Journal Medical Science 239:690–705, 1960
8. Kissin B, Schenker V, Schenker A: Adrenal cortical function and liver disease in alcoholics. American Journal Medical Science 238:344–353, 1979b
9. Kissin B, Schenker V, Schenker A: The acute effects of ethyl alcohol and chlorpromazine on certain physiological functions in alcoholics. Quarterly Journal of Studies of Alcohol 20:480–492, 1959a
10. Naitoh P: The effect of alcohol on the autonomic nervous system of humans; psychophysiological approach, in Biology of Alcoholism, vol 2 Physiology and Behavior. Edited by Kissin B, Begleiter H. New York, Plenum Press, 1972
11. Rubin LS: The utilization of pupillometry in the differential diagnosis and treatment of psychotic disorders, in Pupillary Dynamics and Behavior. Edited by Janisse MP. New York, Plenum Press, 1974
12. Rubin LS: Pupillary reactivity as a measure of adrenergic-cholinergic mechanisms in the study of psychotic behavior. Journal of Nervous and Mental Disease 130:386–400, 1960
13. Rubin LS, Barry T: The effect of cold pressor test on pupillary reactivity of schizophrenics in remission. Biological Psychiatry 5:181–197, 1972
14. Lidsky A, Hakerem G, Sutton S: Pupillary reactions to single light pulses in psychiatric patients and normals. Journal of Nervous and Mental Disease 153:286–291, 1971
15. Lowenstein O, Loewenfeld IE: The pupil, in The Eye. Edited by Davson H. New York, Academic Press, 1962
16. Bonvallet M, Zbrozyna A: Les commandes reticulaires du systeme autonome, et en particulier, de l'innervation sympathique et parasympathique de la pupille. Archives Italliene Biology 101:174–207, 1963a
17. Zbrozyna A, Bonvallet M: L'influence tonique inhibitrice de bulbe sur l'activite du noyan d'Edinger-Westphal. Archives Italliene Biology 101:208–222, 1936b
18. Weider A, Brodman K, Mittelman B: The Cornell Index: A method for quickly assaying personality and psychosomatic disturbances, to be used as an adjunct to interview. Psychosomatic Medicine 8:411–413, 1946

19. Gottheil E, Corbett LO, Grasberger JC: Treating the alcoholic in the presence of alcohol. American Journal of Psychiatry 128:475–480, 1971
20. Rubin LS, Gottheil E, Roberts A, et al: Effects of stress on autonomic reactivity in alcoholics. Pupillometric studies: I. Journal of Studies on Alcohol 38:2036–2048, 1977
21. Rubin LS, Gottheil E, Roberts A, et al: Autonomic Nervous System concomitants of short-term abstinence in alcoholics. Pupillometric studies: II. Journal of Studies on Alcohol 39:1895–1907, 1978
22. Rubin LS, Gottheil E, Roberts A, et al: Effects of alcohol on autonomic reactivity in alcoholics. Pupillometric studies: III. Journal of Studies on Alcohol 41:611–622, 1980

11

Individual Differences in Cognitive Impairment from Alcohol: Prevention and Treatment Implications

KENNETH C. MILLS

Data are presented from a series of five laboratory studies that examine the relationship between social and moderate drinking practices and cognitive impairment from alcohol. In addition, recent studies are highlighted which report that certain moderate drinking practices are coincident with greater levels of cognitive impairment and self-reported depression. The field and laboratory methods to gather information about alcohol consumption and its short-term aftereffects are compared. The different data sets indicate that a continuum of effects may be proportional to an individual's level of absolute alcohol intake. An example prevention trial and implications for early intervention are discussed.

INTRODUCTION

Researchers and clinicians who study alcohol abuse often confront the paradox that some of the short-term effects that follow an evening of drinking—cognitive impairment, memory loss, slurred speech, and decreased judgment—do not show up as reliably measurable events until

The author wishes to gratefully acknowledge the work of Eilene Z. Bisgrove in the collection and analysis of data for the studies described in this paper.

late stage alcoholism is evident. Unfortunately, some individuals suffer these effects permanently. This is a paradox because the noticeably obvious cognitive deficits should provide an excellent starting point to experimentally verify the relationship between consumption and its consequences. This research could be used to construct a predictive model for those interested in prevention and early intervention. Because many of the consequences of drinking are aversive and stressful, such as hangover, depression, and family conflict, researchers might begin to understand the long-term relationship between stress and drinking that has been so difficult to document.

Until recently the short- and intermediate-term *cognitive* aftereffects of drinking have not been systematically examined in social or heavy drinkers. Consequently, it has become popular for many to make assertions about the benign nature of drinking practices of nonalcoholics. Recent research with human subjects, however, questions these assertions. These studies strongly suggest that short-term exposure to moderate amounts of alcohol can produce changes in the central nervous system (CNS). Although these changes do not seem to be either severe or permanent, the CNS does not return to normal as soon as the alcohol leaves the blood stream. These findings are consistent with ideas forwarded by Ryback in 1971 (1) when he proposed a continuum of alcohol-related memory impairments that included memory loss from cocktail party drinking, blackouts, and amnesia associated with the Wernicke-Korsakoff syndrome. With the exception of those studies that have examined withdrawal and hangover in alcoholics, our knowledge about the aftereffects of different drinking practices is limited.

The purpose of this paper is to review some of the current research which attempts to define the continuum of cognitive impairment that follows acute and chronic patterns of alcohol consumption. The late stage effects of a lifetime of alcohol intake are fairly well documented. Thus, recent studies will be reviewed that examine the end of the continuum occupied by social, moderate, and heavy drinkers. Because the research is relatively new and the conclusions are still "working hypotheses," research *methods* that have been used to assess cognitive functioning and alcohol-induced impairment will be emphasized.

Among the variety of methods that are currently used to assess cognitive performance, data will be presented from a series of studies that were specifically designed to assess cognitive performance in samples of light and moderate drinkers before and after they achieved different blood alcohol levels. Our laboratory requirements were somewhat different from those who have studied more permanent cognitive effects in large populations, and the studies have given us some unique insights into the nature of impairment from alcohol.

BACKGROUND RESEARCH

Traditionally, researchers and clinicians have dichotomized drinking behavior into two categories: (1) alcoholic consumption which harms the individual, and (2) social drinking which does not. As a result, there has been a disproportionate amount of research which centers on the cognitive functioning of chronic alcoholics. These classic investigations have uncovered a range of neuropsychological deficits associated with prolonged intake, including measurable impairment in visual-motor performance, abstract reasoning, problem solving, and memory (2–4). Sober alcoholics have particular difficulty in rapidly processing new information, especially on those tasks that require visual scanning, problem-solving, or the systematic application of information-processing strategies (5).

New studies suggest an alternative, namely, that we consider alcohol use as a variable on a continuum that ranges from total abstention to very high levels of intake (6). The impetus for this view has derived from the work of Cahalan, Cisin, and Crossley (7) and other survey researchers (8–10) who have extensively documented the relationship between self-reports of alcohol intake and life problems. These studies have taken both cross-sectional and longitudinal samples from the American public to demonstrate, in general, that lifetime problems increase proportionately with the average amount of alcohol consumed daily. The studies typically do not find two subpopulations that can be conveniently labelled alcoholic and nonalcoholic, but rather distribute the drinking and problem variables continuously.

Studies by Parker and Noble (6) and Parker, Birnbaum, Boyd, et al. (11) have recently described the continuum of cognitive impairment that results from moderate drinking. The first study examined 102 men who were classified according to drinking status as heavy drinkers, light and moderate social drinkers, infrequent drinkers, and abstainers. Drinking history questionnaires were initially mailed to 450 males whose names were randomly selected from a suburban California telephone book. The questionnaires asked about quantity and frequency of current drinking practices, periods of heavier and lighter drinking, age that regular use of alcohol began, and sociodemographic variables. After screening, 102 males agreed to participate in the study. The subjects were tested individually on a battery of four cognitive tests that had been shown previously to be sensitive to impairment in sober alcoholic patients. The cognitive test battery included: (1) the Shipley-Hartford Institute of Living Scale, (2) the Halstead Category Test, (3) the Wisconsin Card Sorting Test, and (4) a multi-trial free-recall test. It should be noted that all of the tests measured cognitive status and not cognitive performance.

The results of the study showed that neither lifetime consumption nor current frequency of drinking was significantly related to cognitive status. However, there was a consistent pattern of significant correlations between the average amount of alcohol consumed per drinking occasion and test scores which measured abstraction, adaptive abilities, and conceptualization impairment.

The finding that cognitive performance declined as the quantity of alcohol consumed per occasion increased was confirmed in a second study by Parker et al. (11). An independent replication by MacVane, Butters, Montgomery, et al. (12), with 106 male social drinkers, found that total consumption measures significantly influenced cognitive performance, especially the short-term memory performance of heavy social drinkers. Both investigative teams concluded that social drinking may result in negative consequences that are qualitatively similar to those reported for long-term alcoholics.

In more recent work, Birnbaum, Taylor, and Parker (13) examined the relationship between alcohol consumption and both cognitive functioning and sober mood state in a sample of 93 female social drinkers. The first part of the study did not find a strong relationship between self-reported alcohol consumption and sober cognitive performance, but the women in the sample drank considerably lower amounts and less often than the men who were sampled from the same community 5 years earlier. However, a strong relationship was observed between alcohol consumption and self-reported depression and anger in the sober state.

Thus, a second phase of the study attempted to directly investigate the possible causal effect of alcohol consumption on these variables by asking half of the subjects to eliminate their intake of alcohol as completely as possible during a 6-week interval. Comparison subjects were encouraged to drink as much as they normally would. All subjects kept records of their daily alcohol consumption. In the second session 6 weeks later, women who had reduced their alcohol intake showed decreases in depression, anger, and mental confusion when they were sober relative to the women who maintained or increased their alcohol consumption over the same period. There were no differences or changes in the cognitive performance of the two groups.

SOME HUMAN LABORATORY DATA

Before we introduce new data on cognitive impairment from alcohol that is given in a laboratory setting, it is important to carefully examine the emerging relationship between the two variables that have peaked our interest. The variables are (1) measures of the amount of alcohol consumed over a specified interval, usually 1 hour, 1 week, or 1 month, and (2) measures of cognitive functioning and/or cognitive performance.

Perhaps these social scientists who conduct surveys and who are forced to depend on self-report instruments with great potential bias have taught us more about measuring alcohol intake than the lab scientist who can pour the desired volume into a beaker and cajole the subjects into drinking while they are watched. The surveyors have learned to request the exact number of ounces of beer, wine, fortified wine, and distilled spirits consumed in a specified interval. They are able to calculate the absolute amount of alcohol that an individual has been exposed to relative to his or her body weight. Given, shorter intervals yield more reliable estimates, especially when intervals are as short as 1 day or 1 week. This type of information is important because the quantity-frequency of consumption variable is the common link between survey, field, and laboratory studies.

The time base for evaluating the effect of alcohol in laboratory investigations is shorter than the intervals estimated in interview and survey studies. The acute exposure data offer several advantages over the retrospective, self-report data. Most importantly, when the amount of alcohol is precisely administered and blood alcohol levels are measured on a time scale, the investigators may derive a dose-response relationship between the actual blood alcohol level and the amount of impairment. The nature of this relationship (e.g., the slope, intercept, and degree of linearity) is critical to determine whether the measures of cognitive performance are, in fact, *causally* related to the use of alcohol. However, the measures used in the field studies on cognitive status discussed earlier have been validated by comparing samples of alcoholics and nonalcoholics. These comparisons may reflect a combination of influences including aging, living conditions, and mood state that may not be directly attributable to alcohol use. With the exception of the multi-trial free-recall test, the cognitive status measures have not been validated with controlled trials of alcohol administration.

Ryan and Butters (14) caution that while the correlation between blood alcohol concentration and short-term memory is strong, the dose-response relationship is influenced by variables such as alcohol metabolic rate, elimination rate, age, and the nature of the cognitive task. They assert that blood alcohol levels trigger changes in the information-processing strategies used by both social drinkers and alcoholics. However, the long-term cognitive consequences of alcohol consumption by chronic alcoholics are inconsistent, with findings that vary with demographics, consumption levels, abstinence intervals, and medical complications. They conclude that alcoholic brain damage is not necessarily responsible for all of the cognitive deficits seen in alcohol users, since the performance on all of the tests used currently is influenced by a wide range of psychological variables.

Hill (15) also expressed conservative opinions, stating that few studies exist on alcohol's effects on cognitive functioning in large samples of nonalcoholics and it is difficult to establish a cutoff value for defining impairment. Factors that are especially relevant to the accurate assessment of alcoholic brain damage (head trauma, high fevers, liver disorders, drug use, depression, and family problems) may be important in assessing social drinkers as well. However, we currently do not know whether the cognitive changes reported for social drinkers are relatively permanent or reversible. Hill cautioned that, in view of the problems encountered in the studies of nonalcoholic drinkers, it seems unwarranted to conclude that there are long-term cognitive dangers for social drinkers.

DEVELOPING A TEST OF IMPAIRMENT

In order to specify more precisely the nature of the relationship between drinking and its outcomes, there is a need for laboratory based tasks that can be used to measure cognitive *performance* in investigations where it is possible to administer alcohol to the participants.

Our early literature review indicated that laboratory tasks that have been used to measure impairment varied widely from study to study in the procedures for administration, methods for data analysis, and criteria for impaired performance. More importantly, very few studies had exposed subjects to multiple doses of alcohol and multiple performance evaluations over time.

We therefore decided to design and test an impairment-sensitive task by specifying the criteria for an ideal task. The design criteria were as follows:

1. The task should be a divided-attention task and have at least two *visual* stimulus sources that the subject would monitor simultaneously (16–19).

2. The task should be quickly administered.
3. The task should be simple enough to be administered repeatedly without strong practice or fatigue effects, thus allowing evaluation of rising and falling Blood Alcohol Concentrations (BACs) at different dose levels.
4. The task should also be easy to learn so that subjects could reach asymptotic levels of performance with a minimum number of practice trials.
5. The task should require minimal instructions and be amenable to standardized procedures for administration to a wide variety of subject populations.
6. The apparatus should record response latencies to a precision of 1 msec.
7. The apparatus should have automatic data recording and storage capabilities.
8. The apparatus should be inexpensive to produce and not depend on multichannel video or movie equipment.
9. The apparatus should be portable enough to facilitate use in field studies.
10. The task should be sensitive to disruption by moderate doses of orally administered pharmacological agents.

Many of the requirements for the new task could only be met through application of microelectronics technology. The first SEDI (the acronym for *S*imulated *E*valuation of *D*rinker *I*mpairment) consisted of an AIM-65 microprocessor (Rockwell Corporation) in which we burned the program into an IC chip. The test unit consisted of the microprocessor, a 4-button response panel, and three 2-cm high, 7-segment numeric displays mounted in plastic cases (see Figure 1).

The stimulus displays were arranged on the arc of a circle with a radius of 52 cm and were approximately 86 cm from the subjects' eyes. The four response buttons were 5 cm apart and were operated with both hands. The task required subjects to monitor, in the central field of vision, a display that presented digital information that changed approximately every 1/2 second. In addition, the two peripheral displays were monitored for changes that occurred an average of every 2 seconds. Subjects were required to respond to both central and peripheral changes, thus dividing their attention between central and peripheral displays. A more complete description of the task parameters are presented elsewhere (20).

The first study using the AIM-65 SEDI sought to establish the dose-response relationship with human subjects who consumed alcohol in a controlled setting (20). The study was also concerned with establishing

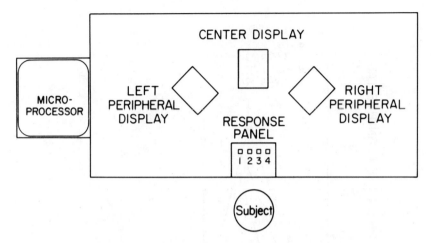

Figure 1. Diagram of the AIM-65 SEDI task displays and response panel.

standardized procedures for administering the task, especially across different doses and different sessions. The protocol enlisted 40 males, half with a mean age of 20 years, half with a mean age of 28.5 years. Half of each age group were light drinkers who reported a mean monthly alcohol intake of 7.3 g/kg. The other half of each group were heavy drinkers who reported a mean alcohol intake of 33.7 g/kg/month. The 10 subjects in each of the four independent groups were given placebo and two doses of alcohol in a random order across sessions. The impairment in their abilities to perform the task was measured as the difference from the baseline score (before drinking) to the scores achieved at 20, 40, 60, and 80 minutes after drinking.

Figure 2 shows the absolute impairment score for all subjects at all dose and time conditions. Both baseline trials are shown to illustrate the initial practice effect that leveled off rapidly upon repeated exposure to the task. A baseline-placebo analysis of variance revealed no significant differences between the four subject groups, indicating that the second baseline scores did not differ significantly from the test scores obtained during the placebo sessions. This demonstrated that once initial practice effects were overcome on the AIM-65 SEDI, performance over nonalcohol sessions showed neither significant improvement (practice effects) nor degradation (fatigue effects).

The analysis of variance on the difference scores between baseline and tests under alcohol showed no significant main effects for age, drinking history, or the interaction of these between-subject variables. Significant

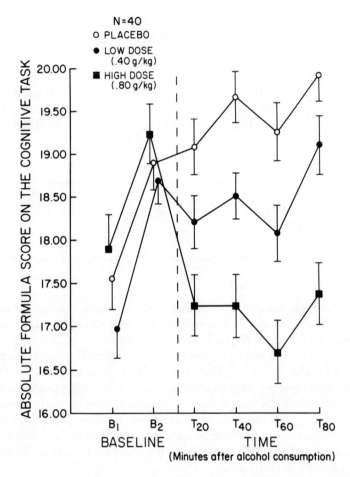

Figure 2. Cognitive impairment for all subjects across placebo, low, and high alcohol doses.

main effects were obtained for dose and time of test. There were no significant second- or third-order interactions of dose and time with age or drinking history. The most important finding was the linearity of the dose-reponse curve for cognitive impairment across all test times and all subject groups. The AIM-65 SEDI test was relatively insensitive to age and drinking-history influences and primarily sensitive to changes in the subjects' BAC.

A subsequent study using the AIM-65 SEDI compared women and men on divided-attention performance, whole-body sway, and subjective impairment (21). Twelve female and 12 male subjects were given placebo, low, and moderate alcohol doses in a random order across sessions. Each subject was tested three times during each session on all measures of impairment. The study controlled for recent drinking history by restricting participation to light drinkers, who were matched on age and education. Alcohol doses were adjusted for body fat and essentially equivalent BAC's were attained in the two gender groups. The results showed that women and men did not differ in their extent of impairment at the placebo and low alcohol doses. However, women showed significantly more cognitive impairment than their male counterparts at the high alcohol dose, even with equivalent BAC's.

Jones and Jones (22) have previously described the relationship between the amount of administered alcohol and cognitive impairment in a sample of women who were social drinkers. The researchers administered a single dose of alcohol to achieve blood alcohol levels that ranged from 60–70 mg/100 ml and examined a number of variables related to the menstrual cycle. The women in the study obtained higher blood alcohol levels than males when bodyweight and the amount of alcohol consumed were held constant. Females that were tested during the premenstrual period (Days 21–28) had higher peak blood alcohol levels and a faster absorption rate than females in the menstrual or intermenstrual period. Their results suggested that females became more intoxicated than males at an equivalent dose of alcohol, particularly if they drank during the premenstrual phase of their cycle. These findings are being replicated in our lab and have important implications for the study of interactions between drinking and premenstrual syndrome (PMS), a disorder often associated with greater levels of self-reported stress.

The SEDI software has also been used by other investigators who were interested in measuring cognitive performance relative to other variables that might predict a liability to alcoholism, e.g., stress history, family history, or history of other drug use. For example, Schuckit (23, 24) has demonstrated that individuals with a family history of alcoholism are less sensitive than controls to the subjective effects of a moderate amount of alcohol. His studies have suggested that these individuals are also less impaired than their counterparts in a natural drinking situation, and he has hypothesized that a lack of impairment feedback might prompt them to consume more alcohol than their peers. If this is the case, the family-history-positive (FHP) individual would be more prone to become tolerant and subsequently dependent upon alcohol. An objective measure of cognitive impairment would be necessary to validate the reported differences in perceived "high" between different risk groups.

Schuckit has adopted a software version of SEDI to test differences between FHP and family-history-negative (FHN) subjects. After running eight matched pairs of FHP and FHN subjects, preliminary data indicate the two groups recover at different rates from the SEDI impairment produced by a relatively high BAC (120 mg/100 ml).[1] Schuckit reports that the SEDI divided-attention task is the most sensitive measure used to date to separate the short-term reactions of his subjects to alcohol.

Two of our most recent pilot investigations have asked the questions: (1) how does performance on SEDI compare with other measures of cognitive performance at different alcohol doses, and (2) are these different measures sensitive to a sustained exposure to alcohol (3–5 hr) instead of the normally administered 20-minute drinking schedule?

Figure 3 compares different laboratory tests of cognitive performance: whole-body sway, recall, and SEDI divided-attention. The tests share the features that they can be administered repeatedly without strong practice effects, they can be administered quickly and automatically, and they yield quantitative estimates of performance. We enlisted 8 male college students as participants in the pilot study to compare performance on the three tasks at blood alcohol levels of 0 (placebo), 44, and 100 mg/100 ml. As Figure 3 illustrates, all three measures showed some dose-response relationship to BAC. The correlation between divided-attention performance and BAC was .55 ($p < .01$). Similarly, the correlation between BAC and recall was .58 ($p < .01$). The correlation between BAC and sway was .40 ($p < .05$), indicating that sway did not show a strong and consistent relationship to BAC in this study. However, the two measures of cognitive performance showed a strong relationship to an individual's BAC.

Figures 4–7 present the results of the second pilot study and compare the performance of 12 male light drinkers who were each given two different types of exposure to alcohol in different test sessions: an acute dose and a maintenance dose. The acute dose exposed each subject to a sufficient quantity of alcohol to bring his BAC to a one-time peak of approximately 100 mg/100 ml. As Figure 4 shows, the blood alcohol level declines thereafter during the course of the 5-hour session. On a different test day, the maintenance dose keeps the subject's blood alcohol level at approximately 100 mg/100 ml for the first 3 hours of the 5-hour session, thus extending the time base for examining cognitive effects.

The figures illustrate that the cognitive deficits induced by alcohol generally persist as long as alcohol is in the bloodstream. Table 1 summa-

---

[1]M. Schuckit (personal communication, March, 1983)

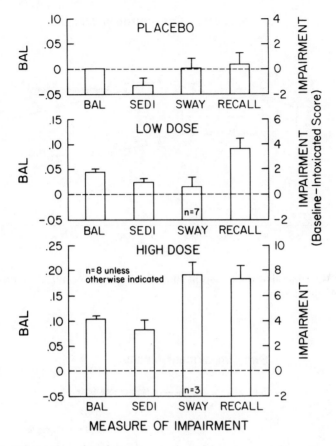

Figure 3. Comparison of performance on three lab measures of impairment across placebo, low, and high alcohol doses.

rizes the repeated measures analyses of variance that execute an orthogonal decomposition of the linear and quadratic components of the data (25, 26). The analyses revealed significant main effects for dose and time on the sway and recall measures. The main effect for time was significant for divided-attention performance, but the dose effect was not. Further, all of the measures showed a significant linear trend when they were examined against time, indicating that the acute and maintenance doses had significantly different effects on performance over the two 5-hour sessions. The data indicate that all of the measures used in this study (sway, recall, and divided-attention performance) were sensitive to the

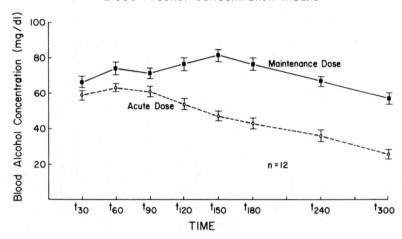

Figure 4. Mean blood alcohol concentrations for acute and maintenance doses during two 5-hour sessions.

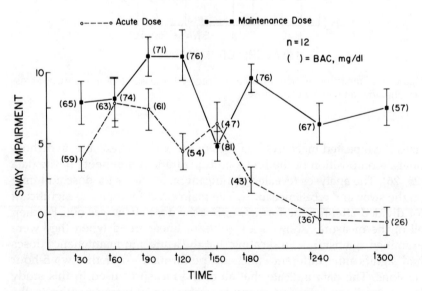

Figure 5. Mean sway performance for acute and maintenance doses during two 5-hour sessions.

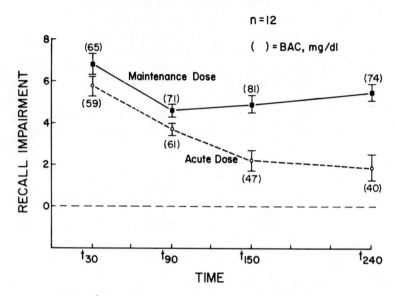

Figure 6. Mean multi-trial recall test scores for acute and maintenance doses during two 5-hour sessions.

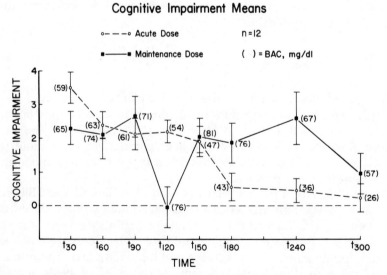

Figure 7. Mean SEDI divided-attention scores for acute and maintenance doses during two 5-hour sessions.

TABLE 1
Summary of Repeated Measures
Orthogonal Decomposition on
ANOVA for Sway, Recall, and
Divided-Attention Measures

Source of Variance	df	F	Probability
Sway			
Dose	1,11	4.98	.05
Time	7,77	3.21	.005
Dose × time	7,77	1.35	.24
Time linear	1,11	11.34	.006
Recall			
Dose	1,11	7.06	.02
Time	3,33	10.29	.0001
Dose × time	3,33	2.12	.12
Time linear	1,11	31.01	.0002
Divided-Attention			
Dose	1,11	0.01	.92
Time	7,77	2.15	.05
Dose × time	7,77	2.24	.04
Time linear	1,11	14.68	.003

prolonged action of alcohol. The subjects in this study did not show cognitive adaptation, or tolerance, to the effects of alcohol when they were given the maintenance dose.

IMPLICATIONS FOR PREVENTION

The second program in which the AIM-65 SEDI became involved was a formally evaluated primary prevention project funded by the National Institute on Alcohol Abuse and Alcoholism (NIAAA) (27–29). The "replication projects" were targeted to college populations throughout the United States, and they varied widely in the types of services and formal evaluations that they provided.

One of the goals of the University of North Carolina-Chapel Hill project was to design effective educational interventions that reduced the prevalence of drinking and driving among high-risk college students (30). High-risk groups for drinking and driving incidents were defined through locally administered surveys and interviews (31). The primary target group on the Chapel Hill campus consisted of 19–22 year-old males who were sophomores, juniors, or seniors *and* who were members of a fraternity.

It should be noted that during the first 2 years of the 3-year project, the students and staff had grown somewhat callous toward conducting alcohol-oriented interventions with the fraternity population. Workshops had been planned and organized for months and attendance would seldom exceed 2 or 3 persons. One spring, an alternative beverage party that demanded 3 weeks of preparation from a group of peer student educators attracted 8 people. To add insult to injury, an adjacently located fraternity house cosponsored a keg party with a local beer distributor and attracted over 1,000 students, who stood patiently in line for one free beer! Besides the lack of project impact on drinking and driving, the fraternity interventions had a devastating effect on student and staff morale.

Meanwhile, back at the lab, we were looking for an environment to test subjects on the AIM-65 SEDI that was less rigidly controlled. We were also interested in impairment that would be produced by a pattern of voluntary alcohol consumption as opposed to scheduled drinking. We approached a fraternity and asked permission to set up a computer test in a room of their fraternity house. The social chairman presented the details to the membership and outlined the conditions for participation. Forms which described the testing protocol and elicited demographic information were then distributed to all participants. The study required each participant to take two baseline tests on the AIM-65 SEDI task during the afternoon before a party. Individuals were informed that they had to return for one test later in the evening when they felt "the first noticeable influences from drinking." The students were encouraged not to drink excessively to fulfill the requirements of the study.

Two findings emerged from the fraternity field study. First, the linear BAC-impairment relationship demonstrated in the laboratory setting held up under less controlled, extremely noisy conditions (22). Second, SEDI was incredibly popular before and during the party. Imagine the surprise of the prevention project personnel when they were told that the fraternity members enthusiastically welcomed the computer experiment as a part of their planned Saturday night Bacchanalia. However, after only one evening of participation and curiosity about SEDI, we remained cautious. We suspected that this was, perhaps, an unusual fraternity group. We replicated the study at another fraternity house within the month. We found similar data and similar enthusiasm.

Since those two formal interventions, the AIM-65 SEDI has been invited to numerous college and community gatherings in North Carolina.

Almost all of the educational demonstrations with SEDI take place in a group setting. Typically, the students are given a brief written description of the nature of the divided-attention task, how to perform well, and what the performance means in terms of the demands placed upon the driver of a motor vehicle.

Detailed instructions on how to play have been prepared on poster boards for group presentation. After a few students demonstrate their performance on SEDI for the audience, all who choose to participate are encouraged to take three or four practice "baseline" trials until their scores level off. The students become very competitive at improving their formula score. Again, performance decrements are explained verbally along with a review of the meaning of blood alcohol levels, the nature of a divided-attention task, and how much impairment could be expected at each BAC. After a number of participants have consumed two or three alcoholic drinks (usually beer), they again perform the task. Performance decrements are charted on a flip chart or a blackboard. It is not unusual for a heavy drinking young male to express surprise at the amount of impairment that follows the drinking, especially when he thought he was invulnerable to the effects of just a few beers.

IMPLICATIONS FOR EARLY INTERVENTION

A small selection of studies currently suggest that specific population subgroups are particularly sensitive to the effects of alcohol on the central nervous system. These studies represent the beginning of research efforts to describe the range of individual differences in response to alcohol. When the data are more complete, one hope is to isolate those subgroups and individuals who may be "insensitive" to the effects of drinking and who may be at increased risk of alcohol-related problems if they drink to feel similar effects as their peers. This data base would be critical to describe the risk factors for alcohol problems and may form the basis for a technology of early intervention.

Unfortunately, we still lack a data base that uses a battery of standardized instruments to assess the effects of alcohol on the central nervous system. Those rather narrowly defined lab measures that show a dose-response relationship to acutely administered doses are not used in the more widely applicable field studies. Similarly, the more comprehensive measures that have been adopted in the field studies have not appealed to the laboratory investigators because of cumbersome methods for test administration.

Ironically, the cognitive impairment produced by an evening of drinking may eventually become a stressor in its own right to the drinker. If we wait until drinking and its effects become a permanent stressor in an individual's life, then we may have waited too long. Clearly, practitioners could benefit from a technology that would be able to accurately assess the subtle effects of alcohol consumption.

REFERENCES

1. Ryback R: The continuum and specificity of the effect of alcohol on memory: A review. Quarterly Journal of Studies on Alcohol 32:995–1016, 1971
2. Tarter R: Psychological deficit in chronic alcoholics: A review. International Journal of the Addictions 10:327–368, 1975
3. Kilsz DK, Parsons OA: Hypothesis testing in younger and older alcoholics. Journal of Studies on Alcohol 38:1718–1729, 1977
4. Ryan C, Butters N: Further evidence for a continuum-of-impairment encompassing male alcoholic Korsakoff patients and chronic alcoholics. Alcoholism: Clinical and Experimental Research 4:190–198, 1980
5. Ryan C: Alcoholism and premature aging: A neuropsychological perspective. Alcoholism: Clinical and Experimental Research 6:22–30, 1982
6. Parker ES, Noble EP: Alcohol consumption and cognitive functioning in social drinkers. Journal of Studies on Alcohol 38:1224–1232, 1977
7. Cahalan D, Cisin IH, Crossley HM: American drinking practices; a national study of drinking behavior and attitudes. Rutgers Center of Alcohol Studies, Monograph No 6, New Brunswick, NJ, 1969
8. Polich MJ, Orvis BR: Alcohol problems: Patterns and prevalence in the U.S. Air Force. R-2308-AF, Santa Monica, CA, RAND Corp, 1979
9. Jessor R, Chase JA, Donovan JE: Psychosocial correlates of marijuana use and problem drinking in a national sample of adolescents. American Journal of Public Health 70:605–613, 1980
10. Clark WB, Cahalan D: Changes in problem drinking over a four-year span. Addictive Behaviors 1:251–259, 1976
11. Parker EL, Birnbaum IM, Boyd RA, et al: Neuropsychological decrements as a function of alcohol intake in male students. Alcoholism: Clinical and Experimental Research 4:330–334, 1980
12. MacVane J, Butters N, Montgomery K, et al: Cognitive functioning in men social drinkers. Journal of Studies on Alcohol 43:81–95, 1982
13. Birnbaum IM, Taylor TH, Parker ES: Alcohol and sober mood state in female social drinkers. Alcoholism: Clinical and Experimental Research, 7:362–368, 1983
14. Ryan C, Butters N: Cognitive deficits in alcoholics, in Biology of Alcoholism. Edited by Kissin B, Begleiter H. New York, Plenum, 1983
15. Hill SY: Alcohol and brain damage: Cause or association? American Journal of Public Health 73:487–489, 1983
16. Moskowitz H, DePry D: Differential effect of alcohol on auditory vigilance and a divided-attention task. Quarterly Journal of Studies on Alcohol 29:54–63, 1968
17. Moskowitz H, Burns M: Effect of alcohol on the psychological refractory period. Quarterly Journal of Studies on Alcohol 32:782–790, 1971
18. Tharp VK Jr, Rundell OH, Lester BK, et al: Alcohol and information processing. Psychopharmacologia 27:131–140, 1972
19. Mills KC, Ewing JA: The effect of low dose intravenous alcohol on human information

processing, in Studies in Alcohol Dependence. Edited by Gross MM. New York, Plenum, 1977
20. Mills KC, Bisgrove EZ: Cognitive impairment and perceived risk from alcohol: Laboratory, self-report and field assessments. Journal of Studies on Alcohol 44:26–46, 1983
21. Mills KC, Bisgrove EZ: Body sway and divided-attention performance under the influence of alcohol: Dose-response differences between males and females. Alcoholism: Clinical and Experimental Research 7:393–397, 1983
22. Jones BM, Jones MK: Alcohol effects in women during the menstrual cycle. Annals of the New York Academy of Sciences 273:576–587, 1976
23. Schuckit MA: Self-rating of alcohol intoxication by young men with and without family histories of alcoholism. Journal of Studies on Alcohol 41:242–249, 1980
24. Schuckit MA: Peak blood alcohol levels in men at high risk for the future development of alcoholism. Alcoholism: Clinical and Experimental Research 5:64–66, 1981
25. Winer BJ: Statistical Principles in Experimental Design. New York, McGraw-Hill, 1962
26. Dixon WJ: BMPD Statistical Software. Berkeley, University of California Press, 1981
27. Staulcup H, Kenward K, Frigo D: A review of federal primary alcoholism prevention projects. Journal of Studies on Alcohol 40:943–968, 1979
28. Mills KC, Pfaffenberger B, McCarty D: Guidelines for alcohol abuse prevention on the college campus: Overcoming the barriers to program success. Journal of Higher Education 52:399–414, 1981
29. Mills KC, McCarty D, Ward J, et al: A residence hall tavern as a collegiate alcohol abuse prevention activity. Addictive Behaviors 8:105–108, 1983
30. McCarty D, Poore M, Mills KC, et al: Direct-mail techniques and the prevention of alcohol-related problems among college students. Journal of Studies on Alcohol 44:162–170, 1983
31. Mills KC, McCarty D: A data-based alcohol abuse prevention program in a university setting. Journal of Alcohol and Drug Education 28:15–27, 1983

12

Alcohol, Affect, and Physiology: Positive Effects in the Early Stages of Drinking

ROBERT W. LEVENSON

This paper reviews the findings of this research group concerning the effects of alcohol on state and reactivity variables drawn from response systems that span the brain, self-disclosing behavior, the autonomic nervous system, and emotional facial expression. This work has focused exclusively on the acute, short-term consequences of alcohol consumption. The bulk of the evidence indicates that for nonalcoholic drinkers these short-term consequences can be viewed as being positive, beneficial, and reinforcing. In addition to studying what alcohol does, the paper reports on individual differences in these effects in relation to risk for subsequent alcoholism.

Over the past five years, our laboratory has been engaged in a program of psychophysiological research that has sought the answer to two ques-

The author would like to acknowledge Linda Grossman, Patricia Meek, David Newlin, Joseph Newman, and Kenneth Sher, all of whom made significant contributions to this research program while they were graduate students at Indiana University. Of particular note are the contributions of Kenneth Sher to the work with high-risk populations and of Patricia Meek to the EEG work.

This research has been supported by National Institute on Alcohol Abuse and Alcoholism grant AA05004.

tions: (a) What are the acute, short-term effects that alcohol has on nonalcoholic individuals? and (b) Do differences among these individuals in the magnitude and nature of alcohol's effects play a significant role in the etiology of alcoholism? In this chapter, I will be primarily focusing on the first question, which could be simply restated as asking: What does alcohol do? In presenting this research, I intend to describe our findings and to offer a careful consideration of which short-term effects of alcohol consumption can be construed most readily by the drinker as being positive, beneficial, and thereby reinforcing.

This seems to be an opportune time for taking such stock, for we have now run close to 400 subjects in four different experiments that have studied the effects of alcohol on a broad range of biological and behavioral variables. The major portion of this work has examined the effects of alcohol on the functioning of the autonomic nervous system (ANS), both in terms of how alcohol affects resting autonomic levels and how it affects the responsivity of the ANS to stressful stimuli. Also in the physiological domain, we have studied the central nervous system effects of alcohol by evaluating how it alters brain reactivity. We have explored the effects alcohol has on processes of self-disclosure by having sober and intoxicated subjects compose and deliver brief speeches about their strengths and weaknesses. Using video recordings obtained in our most recent study, we have begun to examine in a new way the old question of how alcohol affects emotional responding. Instead of relying on self-report data exclusively, we have utilized fine-grained measurement of facial expressive behavior to afford a better understanding of what alcohol does to subjects' internal emotional states. Taken in sum, the breadth of this data set should prove adequate to support a thorough examination of the potentially reinforcing consequences of drinking.

Lest it seem overly strange to be talking about the positive and reinforcing consequences of drinking in a climate of opinion that clearly views alcohol consumption as highly pernicious, some mention should be made of the conceptual thrust of this work. Early in our thinking about this research area, we grappled with the issue of whether to focus on the negative or the positive outcomes associated with alcohol use. We considered studying such negative outcomes as the disruptive effects of alcohol on cognitive performance, motor performance, and the production of socially adaptive behavior. Similarly, we considered focusing on its deleterious long-term effects on physical health, mental health, job performance, economic welfare, and family life.

These negative outcomes are of great consequence, but it seemed that studying them was not the optimal strategy for achieving an understanding of *why* people start drinking and of *why* they keep drinking. Surely people are not initially attracted to alcohol because they want to destroy their health, lose their jobs, and ruin their social and family lives. Rather, it is almost certain that these dire outcomes recede into a very distant corner of awareness during the early stages of drinking.

Of course, one could posit the existence of some intrinsic self-destructive psychopathology that leads people to alcohol abuse, but we decided instead to look for outcomes in the early stages of drinking that could be viewed as being positive, beneficial, and reinforcing. From this viewpoint, people start drinking because they get something valuable, functional, helpful, and even pleasurable from it. Following this reasoning, it seemed that the place to start our study of alcohol and alcoholism was early in the process, when drinking was still pleasant, helpful, and rewarding, and long before the negative outcomes begin to emerge.

Psychophysiologists make lousy hedonists. In thinking about "pleasure," our thoughts usually drift down toward the viscera. In our laboratory, we initially operationalized pleasure and positive outcome in two ways. First, in terms of *state*, we thought that alcohol consumption might transport the drinker into a more enjoyable and pleasurable physiological state. Second, in terms of *reactivity*, we thought that alcohol might serve to buffer the individual from the physiological chaos that results from the hostile insults served up in the typical laboratory experiment. As the work progressed, this focus broadened to include psychological and behavioral effects as well, and these too were considered in terms of the state and reactivity hypotheses.

We will examine each of these hypotheses in turn, but before proceeding, one additional prefatory comment is in order. I will be adopting the strategy of trying to make the strongest statement possible about the positive and reinforcing consequences of alcohol, in hopes of articulating a point of view that has not been well represented in the literature. I will undoubtedly be overstating the case; clearly, alcohol use can be both highly reinforcing *and* extremely harmful.

THE ALCOHOL-INDUCED STATE

The Brain

We know from 40 years of biological research that alcohol has a depressant effect on the central nervous system. A very reliable finding has been that alcohol slows the dominant alpha frequency in the *resting* brain

(4, 6, 8, 15, 20, 25, 31). Some researchers have interpreted this biological effect in terms of a weakening of the inhibitory functions of the neocortex and, by metaphor, to a loosening of behavioral inhibition. To continue with this analysis, being less inhibited and thereby more spontaneous could be considered to be positive outcomes, and thus these first characteristics of the physiological state produced by alcohol are potentially reinforcing ones.

Behavior

From a clinical point of view, behavioral inhibition requires that the person maintain a continuing state of vigilance and self-awareness. Behavior cannot be selectively inhibited unless the person is continually aware of how he or she is behaving or is about to behave. We have obtained experimental evidence that alcohol consumption reduces self-awareness. In four different studies, we have asked subjects to make a 3-minute speech on the topic of what they like and dislike about their bodies and personal appearance. Applying a coding system developed by Exner (9) to these speeches, we have consistently found (16) that alcohol reduces the proportion of speech statements that are coded "self-focused"—that is, those statements that concern only the speaker. Further, alcohol increases the proportion of statements that are coded "external-focused"—that is, those that concern someone other than the speaker.

This finding is well illustrated from data obtained in our most recent study. In this study ($N = 192$), which I will refer to as the "dose-response study," a double-blind balanced placebo design (28) was used to enable separation of effects attributable to alcohol's pharmacologic action from those attributable to expectancies about this action. Subjects were administered one of three doses of vodka in grapefruit juice—O g ethanol/kg body weight, 0.5 g/kg, or 1 g/kg. Appropriate procedures, based upon our previous work (22), were adopted to manipulate subjects' expectations as to whether they were consuming alcohol or not.

In this dose-response study, alcohol had significant effects both in reducing self-focused statements, $F(2,179) = 6.18$, $p = .003$, and in increasing external-focused statements, $F(2,179) = 7.40$, $p = .001$. Examination of Figure 1 will reveal that both effects were incremental at increasing doses. These results indicate that alcohol enabled subjects to divert the focus of critical attention away from themselves and redirect it toward other people; thus alcohol reduced their compliance with the experimenter's explicit request to be self-critical. It is uncertain whether this

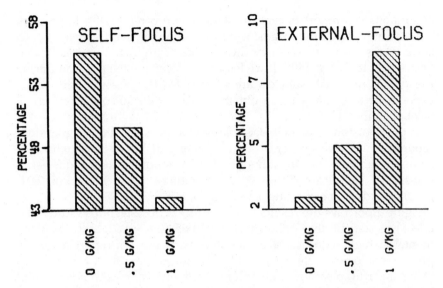

Figure 1. Effects of alcohol dose on self-disclosure. Alcohol reduces percentage of self-focus statements and increases percentage of external-focus statements.

result reflected an empowering effect of alcohol (which would enable the normally compliant laboratory subject to reject the unpleasant request) or a lowering of the level of cognitive functioning (which would cause subjects to drift "off-task"). In either case, the end result is readily construed as being positive and reinforcing for the intoxicated subject, who managed at least a partial escape from the onerous self-disclosure.

Mood

The next piece of this puzzle is the effect of alcohol on mood. The logic of the argument here is straightforward. If the state produced by alcohol is to be construed as being pleasurable and positive, then subjects should report feelings that are congruent with such a pleasurable state. In two studies (22, 29) using different mood questionnaires we found this to be true. Compared to subjects consuming tonic only, subjects consuming the 1 g/kg dose reported feeling more "cheerful" in the first study, $F(1,88) = 12.48$, $p < .001$, and reported feeling more "pleasure" in the second, $F(1,79) = 12.67$, $p < .001$.

There is additional evidence from yet another source. In all of our studies, we have used a device that we call the "anxiety dial" to obtain a continuous self-report of tension. This device consists of a large black plastic knob with a long translucent plastic cursor that traverses a 180° scale. The scale is anchored by the legends "extremely calm" at 0° and "extremely tense" at 180°. If we look at the average dial position during the period in which subjects are waiting for the stressor part of the experiment to begin, we can obtain another indicator of the effects of alcohol on mood.

In the two studies just cited, subjects who consumed the 1 g/kg dose reported lower levels of tension on the rating dial than those who consumed tonic only, but in only one of these studies was the difference statistically significant (Study 1: mean rating 2.0 vs. 2.8, $t(88) = 2.31$, $p < .05$; Study 2: mean rating 3.14 vs. 3.70, $t(78) = 1.33$).

Figure 2 portrays the results from our recent dose-response study; the effect was statistically significant, $F(2,180) = 5.10$, $p = .007$, and was incremental at higher doses. Taken together with the self-report data, the phenomenological state produced by alcohol, which can be described as being cheerful, pleasant, and with reduced tension, is both positive and reinforcing.

Autonomic Nervous System

The final, and probably most complex, component of the state produced by alcohol is the ANS. Historically, the entire issue of the physiological effects of alcohol has lost clarity when different terminologies have been used interchangeably. For example, dimensions such as depressant-stimulant, arousing-relaxing, and tension reducing-tension increasing have had different meanings when used by different investigators. These semantic problems have increased when investigators have attempted to aggregate results across multiple response systems. In the case of the ANS, there has been a historical bias toward viewing it as responding in an "all or none" fashion, but this bias is contradicted by five decades of research showing the capacity of the ANS for specificity and differentiation in response when activated by pharmacological agents, cognitive states, and emotional states.

With due awareness of this historical background, our research rejected the view of the ANS as a monolith, but rather tried to characterize the effects of alcohol separately for each autonomic response system that we were able to study. I will summarize our findings using the arousing-relaxing dimension and then evaluate the complete set of ANS effects in terms of whether they might be viewed as being positive and reinforcing.

In terms of *arousal effects*, we have consistently found that consuming a

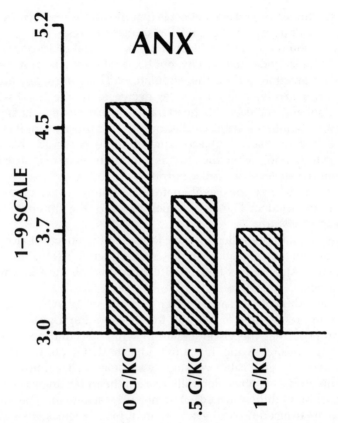

Figure 2. Effects of alcohol dose on self-report of tension. Alcohol reduces self-reported tension (ANX).

1 g/kg dose of alcohol increases both heart rate (by about 6 bpm) and skin conductance (by about 4 umhos). These two changes both indicate higher levels of arousal. In terms of *relaxant effects*, we have consistently found that alcohol increases pulse transmission times by about 11 msec (indicating decreases in cardiac contractile force and/or decreases in mean arterial blood pressure). Other investigators, using more direct measures of cardiac contractile force, have found a similar reduction in myocardial performance (2, 19). We have also found that alcohol produces dilation in the arteries of the finger. A similar dilation in the arteries of other skin areas (32) accounts for the flushing that often accompanies alcohol consumption. Our basis for characterizing vasodila-

tion in the finger as a relaxant effect is that the opposite effect, peripheral vasoconstriction, is part of the ANS response to stress.

Thus, it would appear that alcohol has an arousal effect on the heart's rate and on electrodermal activity, but has a relaxant effect on the heart's force of contraction and on the vasculature. There are many additional complexities involved. For example, decreases in the heart's force of contraction and increases in heart rate are *compensatory* changes that function to maintain a stable cardiac output. For this reason, it is entirely possible that in resting subjects, one of these observed changes is a response to alcohol, while the other is a compensatory response to avoid an inappropriate level of cardiac output.

This complex, but consistent, pattern of autonomic nervous system effects is depicted in Figure 3, which presents the findings from our dose-response study.

Finally, in all four studies we have looked at the effects of alcohol on a global measure of somatic nervous system activity (i.e., gross motor movement). Alcohol has had no effect on this measure in any of the experiments.

It is very difficult to say whether a given set of ANS changes are positive and reinforcing or not. But the thrust of our argument compels us to propose that the visceral state in which we find our intoxicated subjects is a desirable one. It is a hybrid state that could metaphorically be described as being calm, yet slightly stimulated. The intoxicated subject in our studies is physiologically relaxed (heart beating easily, arteries dilated, skin slightly warmed), but not excessively so. The subject is moderately aroused (heart beating more rapidly, increased sweat gland activity), but not overly so.

ALCOHOL AND REACTIVITY

The next group of effects we have studied pertain to *reactivity*—the influence of alcohol on physiological and emotional responses to external stimuli. The question here has been whether alcohol dampens the physiological perturbations caused by stressful environmental events. We have looked at three groups of effects: (1) the brain response to tones; (2) the ANS response to two different stressors (a moderately painful electric shock and having to deliver a self-disclosing speech); and (3) the facial expressive responses to electric shock. I will present each of these in turn, briefly describing the experimental procedures that were utilized.

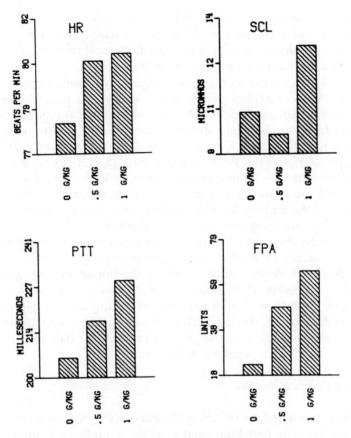

Figure 3. Effects of alcohol dose on prestressor autonomic nervous system levels. Alcohol increases heart rate (HR), increases skin conductance (SCL), increases pulse transmission time (PTT), and increases dilation of blood vessels in finger (FPA).

The Brain

We have studied alcohol's effects on brain reactivity in two experiments. In both, we used standard procedures to obtain cortical evoked potentials, which provide a reasonable index of brain reactivity. For each subject the cortical electroencephalogram (EEG) measured from the vertex (C_z) was recorded during one hundred 1-sec trials. Each 1-sec trial consisted of 300 msec of silence and then an 80 db, 400 Hz tone of 700 msec duration. Trials were separated by a random interval. Eyeblink activity was monitored on-line by a digital computer and trials on which the subject blinked were discarded and replaced. The computer stored the EEG's and averaged the 100 blink-free trials. The averaging technique enables the separation of the specific cortical response to the tone from the background of noncontingent EEG activity.

Figure 4 presents the averaged evoked potentials from subjects at three different doses of alcohol ($N = 64$ at each dose). The progressive reduction of the overall amplitude of the evoked potential at higher doses can be seen. In Figure 5, the significant reductions can be seen in the P1-N1 component, $F(2,138) = 4.77$, $p = .01$, the N1-P2 component, $F(2,176) = 26.88$, $p < .001$, and the P2-N2 component, $F(2,145) = 21.67$, $p < .001$. In an earlier study ($N = 39$) that used only the 1 g/kg and O g/kg doses, we had found the same pattern of results. In both studies, alcohol only diminished the amplitude of the evoked response; the latencies of the various response components were not affected.

We consider diminished cortical reactivity to be a potentially reinforcing consequence of alcohol consumption, especially if the subject is desirous of achieving a state in which the impact of jarring external stimulation is lessened. Although our EEG data do not bear directly on this point, we believe alcohol also reduces the impact of unpleasant and unwanted "internal" stimuli, such as those associated with anxiety, with reliving unpleasant events that occurred during the day, with intrusive thoughts, and with worries about the future.

Autonomic Nervous System

We have examined the effects of alcohol on ANS responses to stress in three studies. The paradigm used in all three studies was quite similar. Subjects consumed their beverages over a 45-minute period and then sat quietly for 30 minutes to allow for absorption. The stressor portion of the experiment lasted for 23 minutes, consisting of a 7-minute baseline, a 6-minute countdown period in which a timer ticked off the seconds remaining until the stressor was administered, the stressor (the electric shock or giving the 3-minute self-disclosing speech), and then 10 more minutes of recording.

Across studies, the most consistent finding was that alcohol reduced the cardiovascular responses to these stressors. In Figure 6, the heart rate response of sober subjects and subjects who had consumed a 1 g/kg dose of alcohol are shown. The dampening of the response is shown at two points—at the beginning of the countdown to the stressor, and at the stressor itself. The same dampening effect was found for both the shock stressor and for the self-disclosing speech. In Figure 7, the pulse trans-

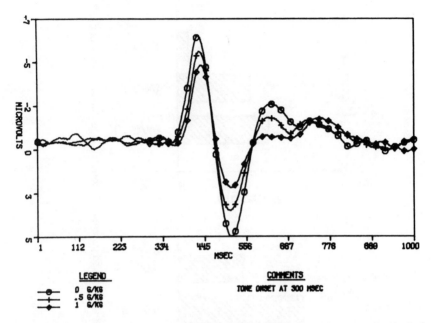

Figure 4. Effects of alcohol dose on the cortical average evoked potential. Alcohol diminishes the amplitude of the evoked potential.

mission time response is shown with similar dampening of the two peaks.

The results from our dose-response study provide additional data on the nature of this stress-response dampening effect of alcohol. Figure 8 portrays the results at several points of maximal reactivity, showing that in the case of the heart rate response to the speech, the heart rate response to the shock, and the pulse transmission time response to the shock, the major stress response dampening effect occurred at the 1 g/kg dose, with relatively little evidence of the effect at the 0.5 g/kg dose. Prior to this study, we had speculated (29) that the higher dose might be necessary before the cardiovascular response was significantly dampened. This dose dependence is supported by a study by Wilson, Abrams and Lipscomb (33), in which dampening of the heart rate response to a stressful social interaction was found at a 1 g/kg dose but was not found at the lower 0.5 g/kg dose.

It is not at all certain whether the stress-response dampening effects of alcohol extend to ANS systems other than the cardiovascular system. Dampening of the cardiovascular response to stimulation at moderately

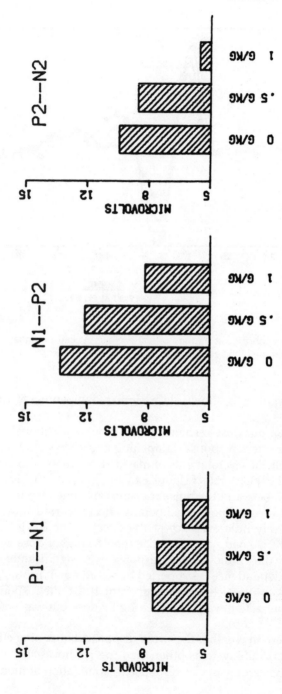

Figure 5. Effects of alcohol dose on the individual components of the average evoked potential. Alcohol reduces the amplitude of the P1-N1, N1-P2, and P2-N2 components.

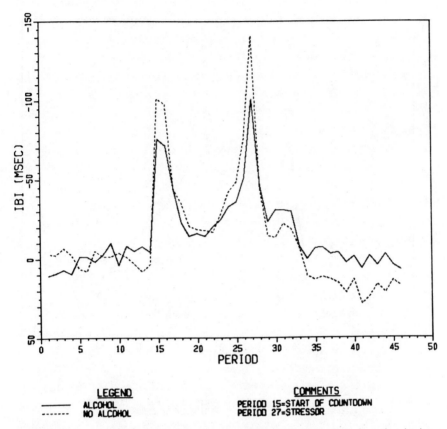

Figure 6. Effects of alcohol on heart rate response. Data are plotted so that higher arousal (i.e., faster heart rate) is in the upward direction.

high dosages of alcohol has been reported in several other laboratories (e.g., loud tones [21]). Results with electrodermal response, on the other hand, are less consistent. Skin conductance responses to simple stimuli, such as tones (1, 13) and words (3, 23), have been found to be dampened by alcohol, but in our laboratory and others, alcohol has not significantly affected skin conductance responses to more complex stressors.

It is likely that the skin conductance responses to simple sensory stimuli have a different psychophysiological meaning than the responses to complex social stimuli. With simple stimuli, we may be seeing the well-documented sweat gland responses that accompany signal detection; these responses may be dampened in much the same way as are cortical responses to sensory stimuli (e.g., our findings with tones). Extending this line of reasoning, the skin conductance responses to complex social

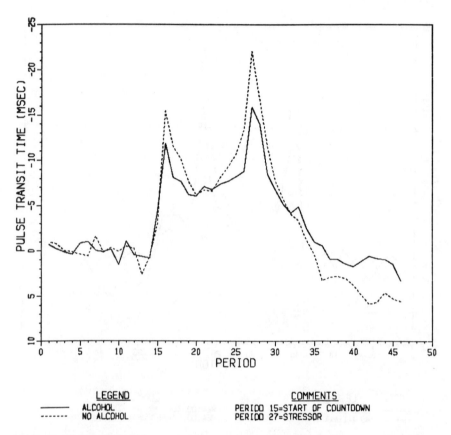

Figure 7. Effects of alcohol on pulse transmission time response. Data are plotted so that higher arousal (i.e., shorter pulse transmission time) is in the upward direction.

stressors could be more indicative of the role of the sweat glands in emotional sweating, and these latter responses may be less susceptible to the stress response dampening effects of alcohol.

Even if the stress response dampening effect of alcohol is limited to the cardiovascular system, this lowering of reactivity in a major ANS system must be viewed as highly positive and reinforcing. It is one of the great ironies of alcohol use that despite the devastating effects of alcoholism on the heart and liver, moderate drinking affords several potentially valuable benefits for cardiovascular health. Since heightened beta-adrenergic reactivity (e.g., heart rate increases and increases in cardiac contractility in response to acute stressors is a component of several etiological models of hypertension (26) and coronary heart disease (12), alcohol's dampening of heart rate and cardiac contractile responses could be quite beneficial. Possibly related to this are the findings from several epidemiological studies (14, 18) that show lower rates of coronary heart disease in moderate drinkers, as compared to abstainers and heavy drinkers.[1]

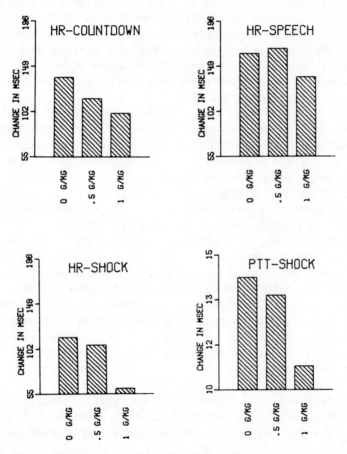

Figure 8. Effects of alcohol dose on cardiovascular responses at points of maximal reactivity. Alcohol reduces heart rate response to the countdown (HR-COUNT-DOWN), heart rate response to the speech (HR-SPEECH), heart rate response to the shock (HR-SHOCK), and pulse transmission time response to the shock (PTT-SHOCK).

---

[1]Another possible mediator of this relationship is the increase in high density lipoprotein (HDL) that is associated with alcohol consumption (30). HDL is thought to be an anti-atherogenic factor. High HDL levels in the blood have been shown to be associated with low levels of coronary heart disease, but the entire issue is controversial (5).

Emotional Responding

In our most recent work, we have started to examine the effects of alcohol on emotional responding in a new way. We undertook this work to try to better understand the basis for our consistent findings of diminished cardiovascular responses to stress. These findings have begged the question of how these effects are mediated. Does alcohol act peripherally to directly dampen the reactivity of the heart and blood vessels? Or does it act centrally to raise hypothalamic thresholds for triggering autonomic activity? Or does it act to change subjects' appraisal processes, making them see the threat inherent in our shock and speech stressors as being much lower than they would if sober?

Given the fact that our subjects were consuming different doses of alcohol, using self-report measures of emotional state to attempt to determine mediating mechanisms would be even more suspect than usual. Thus, we decided to utilize fine-grained measurement of facial expressive behavior using Ekman and Friesen's Facial Action Coding System (FACS). FACS is an anatomically based coding system that utilizes repeated viewing of slow-motion video recordings to decompose each facial expression into its underlying muscle contractions.

Unfortunately, FACS is very time-consuming, taking about one hour to score one minute of facial behavior. For this reason, we decided to focus initially only on the facial responses to the shock stimulus, since these occurred in a brief time period. We have now completed the scoring of 21 female subjects, all with a positive expectancy for alcohol, and distributed equally into our three dosage conditions. With all due caution, owing to the small sample size, the results are extremely interesting. But before presenting these findings, an introduction to the facial reactions to electric shock is in order.

Facial reactions to shock. Based on our viewing of the facial responses of hundreds of subjects to electric shock, there seem to be three "windows" of expression that are distinguishable and theoretically important:

> *Anticipation.* The first window is the final 5 seconds of the countdown to the shock. In this window some subjects show an expression in anticipation of the shock. There is great variability in the nature of this expression. Some subjects show the prototypical expression of fear, some show attempts at emotional control, and some show contempt.

Shock. The second window is the shock itself. Virtually all subjects show some facial reaction to the shock. There is much less variability here, since almost all show some variant of the prototypical expression of fear. Figure 9 shows a full-face prototype of fear. In the 21 subjects scored so far, almost all of the expressions included contraction of the risorius muscle which pulls the lip corners straight back toward the ears. Contraction of this muscle is part of the prototypical expression of fear and may have an evolutionary function in terms of causing the mouth to assume the proper shape for screaming.

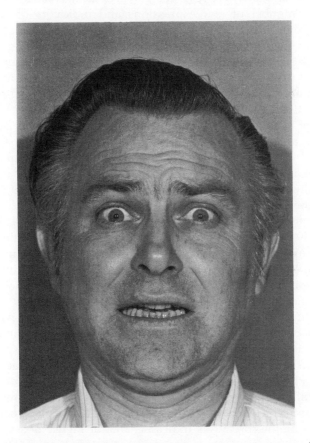

Figure 9. The prototypical facial expression of fear. Note that brows are drawn up and together, upper eyelid is raised, lower eyelid is tensed, lip corners are pulled back horizontally. (Photograph copyright by Paul Ekman)

Reaction. The third window occurs between 3 and 5 seconds after the shock, at which time some subjects show a new expression. This is often a "reaction to their reaction" to the shock. Again, there is much variability. Some subjects smile; some subjects show contempt.

Effects of alcohol on facial responses to shock. The effects of alcohol in each of the three windows will be examined in turn. In the *anticipation* window, alcohol sharply reduced the occurrence of several kinds of preparatory facial behaviors. Figure 10 shows the reduction in overall expressiveness, and in two specific categories of facial behavior: (a) reduction in the number of fear expressions and indicators of attempted emotional control (i.e., lip biting, lip pressing, lip tightening); and (b) reduction in the number of "unfelt" or "false" smiles (citing evidence tracing back to Darwin, Ekman and Friesen [7] describe these as smiles that include the action of zygomatic major, which pulls the lip corners up, but do not include contraction of orbicularis oculi, which raises the cheeks and tightens the lower eyelid). What might this mean? Under the influence of alcohol, subjects may appraise the stressor as being less threatening and thus not react in anticipation of it. They may be less threatened by their imminent display of affect and thus less likely to try to control it. Or they may be less concerned with trying to put up a brave front and thus less likely to smile falsely for their own benefit or for the benefit of the experimenter.

As previously indicated, in the *shock* window, most all subjects show a variant of the fear expression, which includes contraction of the risorius muscle. Using the strength of the risorius contraction as a simple indicator of the intensity of the fear expression, alcohol reduces the intensity of the fear response (Figure 11). It is important to note that alcohol does not produce facial responses in the shock window that differ *in kind* from those produced by sober subjects; they only differ in intensity. This finding can be interpreted as meaning that alcohol lessens, but does not eliminate, the impact of the shock.

In the *reaction* window, alcohol reduces the occurrence of reactive facial behaviors. Figure 12 shows the reduction in the occurrence of "felt" or genuine smiling (Ekman and Friesen [7] describe this as smiling that includes contraction of both zygomatic major and orbicularis oculi). This finding can be interpreted as indicating that at higher doses, subjects may have built up less tension and dread in anticipation of the stressor, and thus they would have less need to reduce tension by smiling after the stressor was over. Alternatively, at higher doses, subjects could be

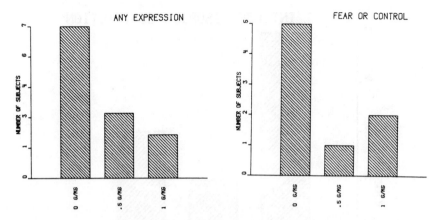

Figure 10. Effects of alcohol dose on facial expressions in anticipatory window preceding shock stressor. Alcohol reduces overall facial expressiveness, and in particular,
signs of fear and attempts at emotional control.

less amused by their own reactions to the shock. This may be because
they had shown less of a fear response, because they were less aware of
their response, or because they were more accepting of their response.

This microanalytic dissection of emotional responding fits nicely with
our other findings that have been presented on the effects of alcohol on
reactivity. Looking at the facial data, alcohol lessens the overall impact of
a stressful event. The shock or the speech comes and goes, and the
intoxicated subject responds with the expected, albeit somewhat diminished, facial expression associated with fear. But that is the extent of the
damage. In contrast, the duration of the stressor is extended for sober
subjects; it begins with a period of anticipatory arousal, continues during the stressor proper, and then spills over into the period after the
stressor has been terminated. Again, the effects of alcohol are positive
and reinforcing. The world is made less disruptive, more manageable,
and less a matter for concern.

CONCLUSIONS AND IMPLICATIONS

We have now reviewed all of the findings we have obtained to date
concerning the effects of alcohol on state and reactivity variables drawn
from response systems that span the brain, self-disclosing behavior,
mood, the ANS, and emotional facial expressions. At each juncture, we

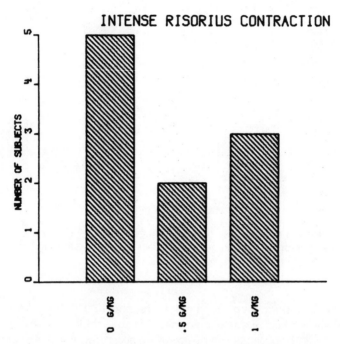

Figure 11. Effects of alcohol dose on facial expressions to shock stressor. Alcohol reduces number of subjects showing high intensity contraction of risorius muscle (pulls lip corners back horizontally).

have presented the case that could be made that these effects are positive and reinforcing. Admittedly, in some instances the argument has been more speculative than we would have liked, but taken together, the bulk of the evidence clearly indicates that nonalcoholic drinkers can derive a number of positive, beneficial, and reinforcing short-term consequences from moderate drinking. This should come as no surprise given the high incidence of drinking in our society.

Because our work is done in the laboratory and not in the field, we are essentially limited to studying these acute, short-term consequences of alcohol consumption. Thus, many of the negative, chronic, and long-term effects escape our inquiry. Nonetheless, there are several negative acute consequences of alcohol consumption that we could have studied but have not (e.g., negative effects on cognitive and psychomotor performance). In addition, the timing of our experiments is such that we are more likely to detect effects associated with the ascending limb and plateau phases of alcohol absorption. Some of the descending limb effects on mood are undoubtedly far less positive. Still, given our concern with better understanding why people drink, the short-term, immediate, positive consequences are probably of greatest importance.

Again, risking stating the obvious, it is no great mystery why people continue to drink, once addictive processes of dependence and tolerance begin to act. The challenge for the behavioral sciences is to understand what it is about alcohol consumption in the short-term that makes it worth running the risk of the negative outcomes that are associated with long-term alcohol consumption. To adopt a single metaphor, such as saying that alcohol consumption is "tension-reducing," greatly oversimplifies and unfairly minimizes the variety of outcomes that can be associated with the early stages of drinking.

There are many questions that remain to be answered. At a very basic level, we need to better understand the relations between alcohol's effects on the ANS and on emotional expressive response. We know from our ANS data that the cardiovascular responses of intoxicated subjects are diminished compared to those of sober subjects, but the grain of measurement for these data has been too coarse (20 or 30 second averages) to allow precise determination of exactly where the cardiovascular

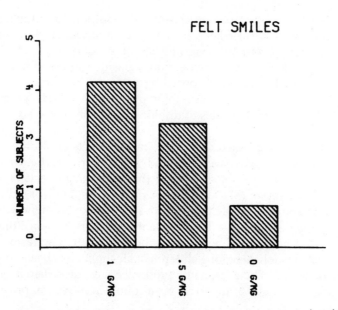

Figure 12. Effects of alcohol dose on facial expression in reaction window following shock stressor. Alcohol reduces the number of felt smiles.

dampening effect begins and ends. The ANS undeniably has inherently longer "time-constants" than the facial expressive system, but we would predict that a precise second-by-second analysis of these data would reveal that the effects of alcohol on cardiovascular reactivity parallel the effects on facial responding in the three windows of reactivity that have been described. Such fine-grained analysis of physiological data would greatly enhance our understanding of the effects of alcohol on physiological responses to stress.

Another issue for which we will soon be able to provide an answer is whether there are consistent gender differences in the effects of alcohol. Our recently completed dose-response study was the first of our studies to include female, in addition to male, subjects.

And finally, we have speculated (22) that the effects of psychological expectancy may be more pronounced at the moderate 0.5 g/kg dose than at the higher 1 g/kg dose, where we have consistently failed to find any effects attributable to expectancy. We will find out whether this speculation is true when the data analyses from the dose-response study are completed.

Individual Differences: Do Some Drinkers Get "More Bang for the Buck"?

As noted at the start of this chapter, in addition to studying what alcohol does, we have also been studying how individuals differ in these effects. Inherent in our thinking has been the notion that if the short-term effects of alcohol are overwhelmingly positive and reinforcing, then any individual who was predisposed by nature or by nurture to experience an extra increment of these reinforcing effects would be much more likely to engage in higher rates of drinking behavior. But, who are these people?

Our studies of individual differences in the effects of alcohol are currently in midstream. We have been studying two groups that we believe may be predisposed to obtain more of the reinforcing effects of alcohol than do other people: (a) the children of alcoholics; and (b) individuals who fit a personality profile that includes traits of outgoingness, impulsiveness, aggressiveness, and antisociality. There is evidence that both groups are at heightened risk for alcoholism. A genetic factor in the incidence of alcoholism among children of alcoholics has been extensively studied (10, 11). The personality profile we have described is one that has been shown to be at high risk for alcoholism in several prospective studies (17, 24, 27).

When this research is completed, we will have studied both of these risk groups in terms of the full range of state and reactivity variables described in this chapter. Thus far, we have completed studies of the personality risk factor that compared subjects who met this profile with those who did not in terms of alcohol's effects on resting ANS levels, and on ANS reactivity to the shock and speech stressors. The results have supported our hypothesis concerning individual differences, in that subjects who matched the high-risk personality profile had the most pronounced cardiovascular stress response dampening at the 1 g/kg dose (29). Thus, these subjects are seen as deriving a larger portion of this potentially positive and reinforcing consequence of alcohol consumption. We believe that this may be an important factor in mediating their heightened risk for alcoholism, especially if it turns out that they are receiving similarly greater amounts of the other reinforcing consequences of alcohol as well. We should know in the next year or so whether this is true, and also whether the children of alcoholics show a similar pattern.

REFERENCES

1. Carpenter JA: Effects of alcoholic beverages on skin conductance: An exploratory study. Quarterly Journal of Studies on Alcohol 18:1–18, 1957
2. Child JS, Kovick RB, Levisman JA, et al: Cardiac effects of acute ethanol ingestion unmasked by autonomic blockade. Circulation 59:120–125, 1979
3. Coopersmith S: Adaptive reactions of alcoholics and nonalcoholics. Quarterly Journal of Studies on Alcohol 25:262–278, 1964
4. Davis PA, Gibbs FA, Davis H, et al: The effects of alcohol upon the electroencephalogram (brain waves). Quarterly Journal of Studies on Alcohol 1:626, 1941
5. Devenyi P, Robinson GM, Roncari DA: Alcohol and high-density lipoproteins. Canadian Medical Association Journal 123:981–984, 1980
6. Doctor RF, Naitoh P, Smith JC: Electroencephalographic changes and vigilance behavior during experimentally induced intoxication with alcoholic subjects. Psychosomatic Medicine 28:605, 1966
7. Ekman P, Friesen WV: Felt, false and miserable smiles. Journal of Nonverbal Behavior 6:238–252, 1982
8. Engel GL, Rosenbaum M: Delirium III: Electroencephalographic changes associated with acute alcoholic intoxication. Archives of Neurology and Psychiatry 53:44, 1945
9. Exner JE: The self-focus sentence completion: A study of egocentricity. Journal of Personality Assessment 37:437–455, 1973
10. Goodwin DW, Guze SB: Heredity and alcoholism, in The Biology of Alcoholism, vol 3: Clinical Pathology. Edited by Kissin B, Begleiter H. New York, Plenum, 1974
11. Goodwin DW: Genetic determinants of alcoholism, in The Diagnosis and Treatment of Alcoholism. Edited by Mendelson JH, Mello NK. New York, McGraw-Hill, 1979
12. Gorlin R: Coronary Artery Disease. Philadelphia, WB Saunders, 1976
13. Greenberg LA, Carpenter JA: The effect of alcoholic beverages on skin conductance and emotional tension: I. Wine, whisky, and alcohol. Quarterly Journal of Studies on Alcohol 18:190–204, 1957
14. Hennekens CH, Rosner B, Cole DS: Daily alcohol consumption and fatal coronary heart disease. American Journal of Epidemiology 107:196–200, 1978
15. Holmberg G, Martens S: Electroencephalographic changes in man correlated with

blood alcohol concentration and some other conditions following standardized ingestion of alcohol. Quarterly Journal of Studies on Alcohol 16:411, 1955
16. Hull JG, Levenson RW, Young RD, et al: The self-awareness reducing effects of alcohol
   consumption. Journal of Personality and Social Psychology 44:461–473, 1983
17. Jones JC: Personality correlates and antecedents of drinking patterns in adult males.
   Journal of Consulting and Clinical Psychology 32:2–12, 1968
18. Kannel WB, Gordon T: Some characteristics of the incidence of cardiovascular disease
   and death: Framingham study. 16-year follow-up. Washington, DC, US Government
   Printing Office, 1970
19. Knott DH, Beard JD: Changes in cardiovascular activity as a function of alcohol intake,
   in The Biology of Alcoholism, vol 2: Physiology and Behavior. Edited by Kissin B,
   Begleiter H. New York, Plenum, 1972
20. Kotani K: EEG studies on endogenous psychoses and alcohol intoxication. Bulletin of
   the Osaka Medical School. Suppl 12:11, 1965
21. Lehrer PM, Taylor HA: Effects of alcohol on cardiac reactivity in alcoholics and nonalcoholics. Quarterly Journal of Studies on Alcohol 35:1044–1052, 1974
22. Levenson RW, Sher KJ, Grossman L, et al: Alcohol and stress response dampening:
   Pharmacological effects, expectancy, and tension reduction. Journal of Abnormal Psychology 89:528–538, 1980
23. Lienert GA, Traxel W: The effects of meprobamate and alcohol on galvanic skin response. Journal of Psychology 48:329–334, 1959
24. McCord W, McCord J: Origins of Alcoholism. Stanford, CA, Stanford, 1960
25. Newman HW: The effects of alcohol on the electroencephalogram. Stanford Medical
   Bulletin 17:55, 1959
26. Obrist PA: Cardiovascular Physiology. New York, Plenum, 1981
27. Robins LN, Bates W, O'Neal P: Adult drinking patterns of former problem children, in
   Society, Culture and Drinking Patterns. Edited by Pittman DJ, Snyder R. New York,
   Wiley, 1962
28. Rohsenow DJ, Marlatt GA: The balanced placebo design: Methodological consideration. Addictive Behaviors 6:107–122, 1981
29. Sher KJ, Levenson RW: Risk for alcoholism and individual differences in the stress
   response dampening effect of alcohol. Journal of Abnormal Psychology 91:350–367,
   1982
30. Thornton J, Symes C, Heaton K: Moderate alcohol intake reduces bile cholesterol
   saturation and raises HDL cholesterol. The Lancet 2:819–822, 1983
31. Varga B, Nagy T: Analysis of alpha rhythm in the electroencephalogram of alcoholics.
   Electroencephalography and Clinical Neurophysiology 92:933, 1960
32. Wallgren H, Barry H: Actions of Alcohol, vol I & II. New York, Elsevier, 1970
33. Wilson GT, Abrams DB, Lipscomb TR: Effects of increasing levels of intoxication and
   drinking pattern on social anxiety. Journal of Studies on Alcohol 41:250–264, 1980

13

Anxiety and Control Issues in Substance-Abusing Veterans

STEVEN PASHKO and KEITH A. DRULEY

Sixty-two substance-abusing veterans who were admitted to our VA Medical Center's Substance Abuse Treatment Unit received a computerized battery of tests. The tests examined tension reduction correlates of substance abuse from the perspectives of overt anxiety, style of stress reactivity, perceived locus of control, and coping styles. Results describe our patients as mildly trait anxious, non-Type-A personalities the majority of whom feel as if they themselves manage their own lives. They are mistrustful, emotionally distant but needy, impulsive, and somewhat depressed. Only 21 of our 62 patients scored in the "alcoholic" range of the MacAndrew scale. A subset of patients (n = 26) scoring high on external locus of control showed significantly elevated levels on tension, anxiety, and MacAndrew scales. These latter results support a Tension Reduction Hypothesis for our patients who perceive themselves as being controlled by external forces. In the future, issues relating to desirability of control will be addressed so as to clarify further control issues as they relate to anxiety in our alcoholic veterans.

INTRODUCTION

The Tension Reduction Hypothesis of alcohol abuse postulates that people drink alcohol for relief from anxiety, tension, or stress (1). By extension, the point has been made that alcoholic consumption of ethanol may be related to high levels of stress (1, 2). The duration and intensity of the stress state should relate directly to alcohol consumption patterns if alcohol is a major means of relieving stress. In as much as individuals may relieve stress through other means, alcohol consumption may be decreased given effective alternative coping mechanisms.

In an attempt to examine the Tension Reduction Hypothesis, we became interested in three issues essential to stress/tension: (1) the duration and intensity of the state; (2) the perception of control over life events; and (3) the personality characteristics that have developed and may be used as a defense against stressful situations. These three factors may identify the background or setting in which drinking takes place, describe a characteristic personality style that develops due to years of chronic stress where effective coping mechanisms other than alcohol consumption have been unsuccessful, and elucidate a way of successfully coping with a stressful environment.

Spielberger (3) has made the distinction between the anxiety of long duration that, in a sense, has embedded itself into the personality of the individual (e.g., trait anxiety), and the anxiety of an acute reaction (e.g., state anxiety). This viewpoint has advanced an aspect of the term "anxiety" from one on an equal footing with "tension" to one connoting the need for long-range coping typically associated with "stress." If the state-trait anxiety distinction is tenable, it may perhaps be used as a tool to investigate the affective setting in which alcohol consumption might take place. Support for a Tension Reduction Hypothesis of alcohol use would be gained if alcoholics showed high levels of trait anxiety compared to the general population.

There exists a body of literature that supports the view that the perception of control over a situation may ameliorate its impact (4). In alcohol rehabilitation units like the one at Coatesville, alcohol relapse prevention strategies are in part based on the patients assuming control over their life style through structured objectives and positive long-range goals. Indeed, Alcoholics Anonymous (AA) uses numerous strategies whereby the alcoholic learns to take charge of his life through structured objectives (e.g., attendance at 90 meetings in 90 days). Taking control over life objectives typifies many therapeutic regimes. Where control can be gained, it may help to lessen anxiety. There are instances, however, where a person may not be able to exert effective control over his surroundings. The Tension Reduction Hypothesis would support the view that where control is insufficient, increased anxiety and drinking would follow. If, in fact, alcoholics have high levels of trait anxiety, it would be interesting to know how they choose to cope with chronic anxiety, in ways other than drinking.

Individuals who experience chronic anxiety may attempt to cope with it in a variety of ways (e.g., recreation). Earlier, we mentioned the tactic of achieving environmental control over a situation through increased attendance at AA meetings. Alternatively, one may become invested in a hard-driving, competitive, and impatient style of life that characterizes a Type-A personality style (5). In so doing, control might be gained through exaggerated alertness to perceived threats because an early response may increase one's chances of overcoming the stressor.

The Type-A personality is certainly not the only way in which individuals attempt to gain control over their life, however it is one of great interest because of its connection with heart disease. If there are other common styles by which alcoholics attempt to cope with life stressors, without the use of alcohol, an understanding of them would be valuable because treatment approaches could be directed at developing more successful types.

A number of factors came together at this medical center that allowed us to examine some of these treatment and theoretical issues. Firstly, we were developing a conference that dealt with stress, coping, and substance use. As with most research, we had an interest in this field before we had data that addressed these issues. Secondly, Coatesville was one of the earlier VA Medical Centers to become centrally computerized. Fortunately, the Substance Abuse Treatment Unit was one of the first services to come on-line. An integral part of the computerization effort was the implementation of a core package of software that permitted patients to self-administer a variety of selected psychological tests at terminals located on our admission/evaluation unit. Finally, we wanted to see if patients were willing to become computer friendly.

When patients come to our unit, they take paper and pencil forms of the MMPI, Beck Depression Inventory, and Shipley-Hartford Scale. This information is primarily used to decide whether the patient would benefit from any of our five inpatient rehabilitation programs and, if so, from which—the fast track drug, fast track alcohol, chronic alcohol, psychiatric illness with substance dependence, or alcohol research treatment program. As related to this project, we also ask them to take computerized tests that address anxiety or tension, style of reactivity to stress, and the perceived locus of control of their health and life events.

In sum, this paper examines the Tension Reduction Hypothesis in alcoholics from three perspectives: (1) the duration and intensity of the anxiety or tension state; (2) the perception of control over life's stressful events; and (3) the characteristic personality style of alcoholics as it may relate to a defense against stressful situations.

METHODS

Sixty-two veterans, who sequentially sought treatment primarily for alcohol abuse/alcoholism in 1983, were used for study; one of the veterans was female. Their average age was 35 years. They had an average level of intellectual functioning, as measured by the Shipley, and all received a positive discharge from military service.

All tests were taken on the Substance Abuse Treatment Unit's admission/evaluation ward. Computerized tests taken were:

1. The State-Trait Anxiety Inventory (STAI) (6)
2. The Symptom Check List-90 (SCL) (7)
3. The Profile of Mood States (POMS) (8)
4. The Jenkins Activity Scale (JAS) (9)
5. The Rotter Internal-External Locus of Control Scale (IEQ) (10)
6. The Multidimensional Health Locus of Control Scale (MHLA) (11)
7. The Minnesota Multiphasic Personality Inventory (MMPI) (12)

During the data analysis, the MacAndrew Alcoholism Scale (MAC) (13) was extracted from the MMPI so as to give us another measure of alcoholism. Once MAC data were extracted, raw scores in the "alcoholic" range (> 23) were separated from raw scores in the "normal" range (≤ 23) (13) across individuals. In this manner, these two groups were compared across their other test scores (e.g., IEQ, JAS). Additionally, STAI-State and IEQ test scores were subdivided into Low (percentile scores 1–49) and High (percentile scores 50–99) categories for comparisons between these subgroups and the average of all 62 veterans. Only Subscale 5 (tension) of the SCL and the anxiety subscale of the POMS were used from these two tests.

RESULTS

MMPI results show our patients to be mistrustful, emotionally distant but having great needs for attention and affection, impulsive, and somewhat depressed (see Table 1). Their scores are consistent with others

TABLE 1
Average of 62 Veterans Entering the
Substance Abuse Treatment Unit

MMPI T-Scores												
48	69	48	68	79	67	80	65	71	73	82	72	56
L	F	K	Hs	D	Hy	Pd	Mf	Pa	Pt	Sc	Ma	Si

who come in for treatment because of a situational crisis. They tend to blame others for causing their problems and resist interpersonal demands placed on them.

Table 2 reveals the overall means of our patients across seven tests. Of note, we found that our patients had mildly elevated STAI-Trait anxiety scores, average STAI-State anxiety and Jenkins activity scores, but low MacAndrew alcoholism, POMS anxiety, and SCL tension scores in comparison to normative groups.

Our patients' personality trait characteristics, according to JAS subscales (A = Type-A personality, I = Impatience, C = Competitive), indicate that they are not the typical Type-A personalities. They are not hard-driving, impatient, or competitive.

In terms of locus of control, our patients consistently lean towards the perception that they have internal control over life (IEQ) and health (MHLA) events. There is a consistent trend across all MHLA subscales (i.e., Internal-External, Powerful Others, and Chance) indicating a perception of internal control.

The MacAndrew subscale of the MMPI, which reportedly discriminates alcoholics from nonalcoholics, shows our veterans to match with MacAndrew's nonalcoholic standardization group.

Results of the inter-test Pearson correlations (Table 3) show high positive correlations between STAI-State, STAI-Trait, SCL tension, and POMS anxiety scores. Additionally, all three MHLA subscales were highly correlated with SCL tension, POMS anxiety, and the IEQ scores. Of note was that neither POMS anxiety, SCL tension, nor STAI subscales correlated well with either JAS subscales or the MAC alcoholism scale.

When we selected a subsample of our veterans ($n = 21$) on the basis of their scoring high (i.e., alcoholic) on the MAC, the scores on the other tests all changed toward a perception of external control (IEQ and MHLA) and more anxiety (SCL, POMS, STAI-State and Trait). These results were not significantly higher than that of the entire group's re-

TABLE 2
Average Scores Across Tests From 62
Sequential Admissions to the
Substance Abuse Treatment Unit

Scale	Score	SD
STAI-state	53.0 percentile	32.2
STAI-trait	60.0 percentile	27.6
SCL	39.0 T-score	23.6
POMS	39.0 T-score	22.2
JAS-Type A	− 0.1 Standard score	8.5
JAS-impatience	2.1 Standard score	9.4
JAS-competitive	1.1 Standard score	8.4
IEQ	41.0 T-score	22.4
MHLA-internal	44.0 T-score	24.7
MHLA-powerful others	41.0 T-score	25.2
MHLA-chance	45.0 T-score	25.8
MacAndrew	19.0 Raw score	9.3

sults. However, the fact that all the anxiety scales went in the direction of increased anxiety is significant at $p<.20$ by the Sign test. Interestingly, all of the locus of control scores increased toward the direction of externality in this group. A Sign test shows this to be significant at $p<.20$.

The selection of a subsample of patients ($n=26$) who perceived they were externally controlled (e.g., IEQ T-Score >50) formed a subgroup of patients who were more anxious, as demonstrated by increased STAI-State ($p<.01$) and Trait ($p<.05$), SCL tension ($p<.01$), and POMS anxiety ($p<.001$) scores, as determined through single sample t-test statistics, than the overall group average (cf. Tables 3 and 4). All JAS scores in this group were increased insignificantly, while MAC scores remained the same as that of the larger group from which these patients were sampled.

DISCUSSION

We began this study with the intention of learning about a number of factors. We needed hands-on experience with a package of computer software that can administer and score psychological tests which could be used to develop psychological profiles for our patients. In working with this system, we decided that a group of tests relating to anxiety, personality style, and perceived locus of control might help us to better

TABLE 3
Correlations Among Test Scales Across 62 Patients

	STAIS	STAIT	SCL	JASA	JASI	JASC	IEQ	MHLAI	MHLAP	MHLAC	POMS	MAC
STAIS	1.00											
STAIT	.87	1.00										
SCL	.50	.47	1.00									
JASA	.17	.24	.21	1.00								
JASI	.44	.55	.25	.63	1.00							
JASC	.07	.17	.16	.56	.39	1.00						
IEQ	.48	.41	.78	.13	.12	.10	1.00					
MHLAI	.40	.31	.81	.10	.10	.01	.77	1.00				
MHLAP	.49	.45	.75	.03	.17	.01	.76	.81	1.00			
MHLAC	.51	.46	.80	.09	.13	.06	.87	.84	.87	1.00		
POMS	.67	.61	.85	.20	.35	.17	.82	.82	.82	.89	1.00	
MAC	.00	-.05	.06	-.15	.06	-.11	.05	.11	.22	.14	.05	1.00

TABLE 4
Average Scores Across Tests From
a Subgroup of Patients ($n = 26$)
Who Scored High on
External Locus of Control

Variable	Mean	SD
STAIS	67.3 percentile	27.6
STAIT	70.9 percentile	23.5
SCL	48.7 T-score	17.4
JASA	1.7 Standard score	9.6
JASI	3.1 Standard score	10.0
JASC	2.1 Standard score	9.5
IEQ	49.0 T-score	6.9
MHLAI	52.7 T-score	11.6
MHLAP	51.4 T-score	18.1
MHLAC	60.7 T-score	12.1
POMS	50.2 T-score	10.1
MAC	18.4 Raw score	10.4

understand the patients who seek substance abuse services from our unit.

As it turns out, we did learn a great deal about our patients, our interactive testing system, and the tests we administered. Our patients genuinely enjoyed working at the computer terminal, taking tests. They would rather sit at a monitor than watch television in our lounge. They tired after an hour and a half, especially if they were on a long version of the MMPI with 566 true and false questions. They would prefer a series of shorter tests if they had their choice. Generally, they looked on the computerized testing as a fun thing to do to break the relative boredom of a detoxification ward.

With reference to anxiety levels, our data suggest that we may be measuring a trait type of anxiety and not a situational type of anxiety reactivity. This result seems surprising because we thought veterans on a detoxification ward would be acutely anxious and tense, if not because of the new and strange environment at least because they were withdrawing from alcohol and/or drugs. It may be that the structured environment—being in the hands of caring professionals, talking with individuals sincerely interested in their well-being, and mixing with patients who share their problems—allows them to feel comfortable and secure. They may also be less anxious because they have removed themselves or been removed from the addictive cycle. High trait anxiety levels, however, were not surprising in that they were predicted by the Tension Reduction Hypothesis. At this time, we cannot say whether high trait anxiety has resulted from environmental factors or whether it was caused by the long-term effects of alcohol (14).

Interestingly, state anxiety scores on the STAI showed our patients to have average degrees of anxiety. In contrast, POMS and SCL anxiety and tension subscales showed our patients to have significantly below average degrees of anxiety or tension. From the evaluation of this data we can conclude that there is no simple one-to-one correspondence between degree of anxiety and the abuse of alcohol. Our patients come into treatment for alcohol abuse/alcoholism but do not show marked degrees of anxiety on our testing. Although these tests are used to report degree of anxiety, an examination of the reason for the differences among the reported scores from our patients needs to be undertaken. This will be an important task, in that the foundation of the Tension Reduction Hypothesis rests on a clear definition of tension. In elucidating a specific type of tension reduction produced by alcohol (e.g., a decrease in muscle potentials vs. a decrease in a number of unwanted thoughts), we may better proceed towards an evaluation of the hypothesis.

While the veterans may have elevated levels of trait anxiety, they do not seem to manifest this trait in any Type-A like behaviors or activities (e.g., impatience, hard-driving nature, or competitive traits). They fall well within the average range on all Jenkins dimensions. They seem to be neither impatient or competitive nor slothful and lazy. Perhaps as the MMPI data suggest, much of the way they deal with trait anxiety may be through the projection of blame onto others. Their elevated Scale 4 and 6 scores support this view.

As to how our patients might manage slightly elevated levels of trait anxiety but not display any Type-A like symptoms, we looked into the literature on locus of control. The results of our locus of control scales suggest that the majority of our patients strongly believe they control their own fate. It may be that our alienated, distant, impulsive, trait anxious, Type-B veterans feel as if they can and must maintain control of their own life events through the use of various psychoactive, usually mood-depressing and tension-reducing, drugs. These drugs usually take effect quickly. Thus, the user would generally be able to associate his use with some resulting anti-anxiety effect. The immediacy and degree to which a substance user might require a change in his mood may strongly relate to his perceived locus of control (15).

A review of the locus of control literature, however, led us to examine other and perhaps most important factors in regard to the control of one's life direction and mood. The other factors are the loss of control and the unpredictability of stressful life events (4, 15). We hope to address these issues in the future.

For the time being, patients who score high on external locus of control uniformly provide data that suggest they are significantly more anxious than their internal locus of control counterparts. In these patients, we may be encountering a specific subgroup of alcoholics who fit the tension reduction model quite well. They abuse alcohol, show markedly high scores on anxiety and tension scales, and feel they have no control over their life or health events.

With this information come questions regarding anxiety and control in this subgroup. Do the anxiety and control issues relate to each other (i.e., loss of control leading to increased anxiety), or are they independent events? Do these patients desire control over their life and health events, or are they comfortable with this type of projection? If our patients do desire control over these events, then it may be that the anxiety and control issues are very much interrelated. We will attempt to tease apart these dimensions with further studies that will include desirability of control measures (4).

Also, our plans regarding the characterization of an individual's substance abuse problem (e.g., loss of control) are to include multiple measures of problems in life areas due to substance abuse. We have been working on the computer interactive version of the Addiction Severity Index (16), since it obtains information from a number of life areas (e.g., medical, social, psychological, financial, and employment problems) and relates them to the quantity, frequency, duration, and type of substances used.

Finally, we are left with an interesting problem. The MacAndrew alcoholism scale, one that is reported to discriminate alcoholics from nonalcoholics, did not pick up all of our subjects as being "alcoholic." Only 21 out of 62 patients were so identified (34%). This seems odd since our patients typically enter our unit to seek inpatient services for substance abuse. MacAndrew (17) and Apfeldorf and Hunley (18) have addressed the issue of false positives. This group is characterized as "secondary alcoholics" (17) and psychiatrically ill patients who drink alcohol (18).

We fully recognize that our veteran population may represent a highly select subsample of substance abusers (e.g., veterans, many with good premorbid histories, multiple treatment episodes, coming from urban centers, at least average IQ). In contrast with MacAndrew (17), results suggest that our veteran patients scoring low (e.g., nonalcoholic) on the MacAndrew scale are by far less disturbed psychiatrically than are those scoring in the alcoholic range. Our low scoring patients seem to fit the character orientation outlined for primary alcoholics as "geared to an impulsive, often ill-considered form of reward seeking" (17). The high scoring group "seem to be more geared to punishment avoidance" (17).

In the future, we plan on breaking down MAC scores into the emotional tension and depression factors MacAndrew outlined in his 1982 paper (19). These factors will be correlated with locus of control and desirability of control measures for a more complete description of our veteran patients.

REFERENCES

1. Cappell H, Herman C: Alcohol and tension reduction: A review. QJSA 33:33–64, 1972
2. Marlatt GA: Alcohol, stress and cognitive control, in Stress and Anxiety, vol. 3. Edited by Sarason IG, Spielberger CD. New York, Wiley, 1976
3. Spielberger CD: Theory and research on anxiety, in Anxiety and Behavior. Spielberger CD. New York, Academic Press, 1966
4. Burger JM, Cooper HM: The desirability of control. Motivation and Emotion 3:381–393, 1979
5. Suls J, Gastorf J, Witenburg S: Life events, psychological distress and the Type A coronary prone behavior pattern. J Psychosom Res 23:315–319, 1979
6. Spielberger CD, Gorsuch RL, Luschene RE: State-Trait Anxiety Inventory. Palo Alto, Consulting Psychologists Press, 1983
7. Derogatis LR: The SCL-90 Manual I: Scoring Administration and Procedures for the SCL-90. Baltimore, Johns Hopkins University School of Medicine, Clinical Psychometrics Unit, 1977
8. McNair D, Lorr M, Droppleman L: Profile of Mood States. New York, Educational and Industrial Testing Service, 1971
9. Jenkins CD, Friedman M, Roseman RH: The Jenkins Activity Survey for Health Prediction. Chapel Hill, NC, Univ of North Carolina, 1965
10. Rotter JB: Generalized expectancies for internal vs external control of reinforcements. Psychological Monographs 80: (whole No 609), 1966
11. Wallston K, Wallston B, Devellis R: Multidimensional health locus of control scales. Health Education Monographs 6(2):160–170, 1978
12. Hathaway RS, McKinley JC: The Minnesota Multiphasic Personality Inventory Manual (Revised). New York, The Psychological Corporation, 1967
13. MacAndrew C: The differentiation of male alcoholic outpatients from nonalcoholic psychiatric outpatients by means of the MMPI. QJSA 26:238–246, 1965
14. Vaillant G: The Natural History of Alcoholism. Cambridge, Harvard Univ Press, 1983
15. Dembroski T, MacDougall J, Musante L: Desirability of control versus locus of control. Health Psych 3:1–11, 1984
16. McLellan AT, Luborsky L, Erdlen F, et al: The addiction severity index: A diagnostic/evaluative profile of substance abuse patients, in Substance Abuse and Psychiatric Illness, Edited by Gottheil E, McLellan AT, Druley K. New York, Pergamon, 1980

17. MacAndrew C: What the MAC scale tells us about men alcoholics. J Studies on Alcohol 42:604–625, 1981
18. Apfeldorf M, Hunley P: The MacAndrew scale: A measure of the diagnosis of alcoholism. J Studies on Alcohol 42:80–87, 1981
19. MacAndrew C: An examination of the relevance of the individual differences (A-Trait) formulation of the tension reduction theory to the etiology of alcohol abuse in young males. Addictive Behavior 7:39–45, 1982

14

Initiation of Social Support Systems—A Grass Roots Perspective

DONALD J. OTTENBERG

The author reviews his involvement as a consultant with four very different groups—the homeless street people, Parents of Murdered Children, the Peace Corps, and Major League Baseball. His experience suggests that members of these dissimilar groups experience a common failure of connectedness and a sense of powerlessness. Specific strategies must be developed to meet the special needs of each group. However, all will benefit from the type of intense, nurturing social support available in mutual self-help groups. The author suggests that all professionals need to reassess the importance of such systems in providing support for their clients/patients during high stress periods. Self-help groups can provide something "different from," but mutually complimentary to, the services provided by professionals.

When I first was invited to speak at this conference, I demurred on the sound basis that I have done no investigative work in this field and would have little to present that would be original research and of general interest. However, I felt that I could at least speak from my own actual experience. Perhaps the freshness of a newly acquired way of reflecting on that experience might compensate in some degree for my lack of predetermined paradigm.

My professional career has taken a sharp turn in the past year or so. Having just retired from a leadership position which I had held for 16 years at Eagleville Hospital, I found myself free to exploit opportunities I previously could not pursue. In the past year, this has included participation in four activities that may be of interest in the context of the conference topic.

The first activity involves working with homeless and street people in Philadelphia, where I have been associated with the SELF Center, Inc., on North Broad Street. The Center provides emergency shelter and basic services to people who live on the street in the city.

The second activity is as a friend of the group and participant with Parents of Murdered Children. A chilling name, and in many ways a chilling activity. This is a self-help or mutual help group that came into being as many mutual help groups do, when people in great need can find no other way to help themselves except to band together and do whatever they can to support one another.

The third activity was some training that I did in Africa for about five weeks at the invitation of the Peace Corps. This was in Malawi, a country most of you have probably never heard of. It is a small country about the size of Pennsylvania in south-central Africa. That was a delightful experience and one of considerable interest with regard to the subject we are addressing here.

The last involvement is as a consultant to Major League Baseball. It is no news to those who follow sports that baseball does have some problems with drugs and alcohol. I was invited to work with a joint committee made up of representatives of the players' union, the Players Association, and Club owners. Their purpose was to put together a policy and program based on common ground of agreement so that baseball could attempt to do something meaningful about this problem.

Now we can scrutinize these four activities for the role and consequences of stress and in this regard I asked four questions:

1. What part, if any, does stress play in the problem or issue? And, if present, what is the character of the stress?
2. What is the response to the stress and was drug or alcohol abuse part of it?
3. What could be done—and ought to be done—to solve or mitigate the problem?
4. What do we learn from this experience?

The homeless and street people of Philadelphia are not a homogenous population, even though much that is reported about them in the popular media seems to imply that they are. There are two major categories, and under each several subcategories. One category, the homeless, are really not on the street as a matter of choice. A significant portion of this group are fallouts from the mental health system. Many are persons who were in psychiatric institutions where they achieved some level of stability on psychotropic medication before being discharged to the community in the wave of deinstitutionalization that occurred in the 1960s and 1970s. A large proportion of this group fell away from the treatment they required, and the community-based mental health system was not properly prepared to provide the needed services. As increasing numbers of persons released from institutions decompensated, it became more and more difficult to get them back into any institutional settings where they could benefit from intensified care. Many of the beds formerly occupied by this population are no longer available, having been closed down as part of the reduction of inpatient capacity in the state system.

The street became home for many of these people, and a variety of meager and largely uncoordinated public and private crisis services became their survival system. In the last couple of years, a more integrated approach to the problems of the homeless has been attempted in the Philadelphia area; but the response has been far from satisfactory, as anyone who follows the communication media can attest to.

Others in the category of homeless are displaced persons and families. Some are caught in the tide of increased unemployment; others are bumped off welfare by changes in the eligibility rules; still others are evicted from housing they can no longer pay for. Some hit the street when fire destroys their living space; some are temporarily without a place to live while they are being deloused and their living quarters fumigated on order of the health department.

A smaller group descend to the street after the loss of a particular person—spouse, sibling, parent, or child—who was the stabilizing anchor of their life.

The street people who make up the other major category do in some sense choose to be there. Now, there are two age groups: middle-aged and older persons who have been on the street for quite a while and have learned somehow to eke out a subsistence, and young people as well. The different age groups have different motives and needs. They, too, are a heterogeneous population.

Some have chosen to live outside the boundaries of conventional society, even to the extent of having no address and no permanent shelter. Some would like to have a warm place to sleep, but cannot—or will not—pay society's price for it. Some are incapable of maneuvering the bureaucratic system on which they have reason and right to be dependent. For example, even though it is difficult to imagine more convincing evidence of destitution than being homeless and penniless on the street, one needs to have a residential mailing address in order to qualify for public assistance.

It has been interesting to contrast the situation of today's homeless and street people with the residents of Skid Row 20–25 years ago, when I first became involved in the field of alcoholism. The population has changed quite a bit. We have made some interesting progress, if you want to call it that. Now the homeless population is racially integrated, whereas the Skid Row population was almost entirely white. The current age spread is much greater, with bimodal, even trimodal, age distribution reflecting three generations that are mingled on the street. The occupants of Skid Row were heavily clustered in the middle-age category. And should we be glad or sorry that homelessness that once was exclusively a male domain now knows no gender bias? In our locality, there are almost as many women as men living on the street.

We have abolished most of the missions, flop houses, and cheap hotels that once characterized Skid Row. Now we have a kind of Skid Row without buildings, one that is not rooted in any single place, a kind of floating Skid Row.

What is the nature of the stress for the people who inhabit our streets? Most obvious is the physical stress resulting from exposure to cold, dampness, rain, snow, inadequate clothing, and lack of shelter. Another type of stress reflects the impact on physiological processes of insufficient food, inadequate toilet facilities, lack of sleep, minimal opportunities for washing, bathing, cleaning, or changing clothes. The psychological and emotional responses are more individualized, with considerable variations in feelings of rejection, humiliation, defeat, worthlessness, hopelessness, etc.

For many of the street people, especially the young, there is also a kind of existential stress. Hans Selye, in an interview (1, p. 69), reminds us that every era has had its prevailing anxieties. He believes that "most old stresses have simply been replaced by similar new ones." He cites as an example the fact that there was no threat of nuclear war a few hundred years ago, but there was the real and terrible danger of bubonic plague, which decimated populations. Then he goes on,

> But there is one type of social stress that I think has particularly increased in our time. This is a loss of motivation, a spiritual malady that has assumed almost epidemic proportions among the young. And with it, naturally, come desperate attempts to escape

the dilemma by any spastic effort. I believe that a large part, if not the major part, of violence, alcoholism, and drug addiction is due to a loss of the stabilizing support of constructive goals. (1, p. 69)

And I think that we can say that street people, almost without exception, share the characteristic of being without constructive goals.

What is the response to the stress? I find it remarkable that people who live on the street are able to tolerate as much stress as they do. They endure cold, wetness, hunger, filth, discomfort, fatigue, and a variety of illnesses. Many are suspicious, even paranoid, about people who approach them and attempt to change them. Many have their pride intact; many are still quite capable of resisting what they do not want to be pulled into. It is not a group that is easily pushed around. Even the police have a difficult time on some of the coldest nights in getting people to enter a van in order to be taken to some warm place so as not to be left at risk of freezing out on the street. Many of the homeless and street people do not like being corralled in that way in a police sweep, even if it is intended to protect them from harsh weather.

And yet, surprisingly, I've encountered little depression in this group. Perhaps a truly depressed person cannot survive on the street. Certainly, many show evidence of other mental illness; quite a few of them are schizophrenic.

Are alcohol and drugs a factor? I believe many in this population drink when they can get it. I think I would, too. But there is not a lot of drug taking, except in the younger group, and even here I do not believe more than 15–20% are really drug dependent persons or that drugs are the primary reason why they are on the street. Perhaps a quarter of the older people on the street now are alcoholics. On Skid Row in the past, that proportion used to be up around 50–75%.

Is there a street community? People out there certainly know one another and at times acknowledge one another. They may sit and talk, share food and drink sometimes, and some even allow one another to share space on an air vent in extremely cold weather. But essentially, they are not a community, being too isolated and psychologically separate from one another to be linked by any common intentional purpose.

Occasionally, we see couples who live together on the street. Some of these relationships are very tight and durable. In working with street people, one must learn how to work with couples who refuse to be separated. This simply makes a difficult job harder.

The metaphor that comes to mind for these people is shipwreck. They are like people shipwrecked, or cast away, each on a little island that marginally sustains life. Barely enough food, water, shelter to stay alive. I can imagine survival on a tiny atoll would be a similar monotonous succession of days—it rains, the sun comes up and sets, the seasons turn. There is nothing but time, and time is occupied by nothing but survival. This is ontologic stress.

Homelessness is no more to be defined as the lack of a home than unhappiness can be defined as the absence of happiness. Homelessness is unaffiliation or disaffiliation, rejection, alienation, the state of being invisible except when being stepped over, the condition of having lost one's substantiality. The stress of the homeless is not so much having no place to live as it is having no place to fit in. In a society that cannot accommodate everybody there are leftover people.

What could be done and should be done? I trust that many of you who live in this area know about Trevor Ferrell. He is the 11-year-old boy who lives in Philadelphia who goes out every night, taken by his parents or his father, to visit various places in center city Philadelphia to give out food, coffee, blankets, and clothing and in some fashion provides help to the homeless on the city streets. This is the private sector response that I think the President was asking for, at least in the heart of one young boy who saw the homeless depicted on television and said to his parents, "How can people let somebody sleep on the street that way? Aren't they cold? Aren't they hungry? Can't we do something?" To the credit of the Ferrell family, they are doing something about it.

But homeless people, including the street people, require a hierarchy of services and facilities tailored to their special needs and capabilities. They need emergency shelter and accessible showers and delousing, if necessary. They need immediate medical and psychiatric care and stabilization in a protected and accepting environment. They need treatment services and day programs and rehabilitation opportunities and transitional supports while moving toward self-sufficient independent living. They also need the concern and encouragement of people who are willing to get to know them and to work with them patiently, in order to find out how to help them move toward a better way of living without violating some part of them that cannot fit into conventional society, the way most of us do.

What we have is far from this simple, incomplete account of what is needed. I shall not go into the ways in which our current programs are impeded by petty squabbling and jealous conflict between different departments of city government, and between people working in the public and the private sectors; I shall not attempt to detail just how fragmented, uncoordinated, and in many ways unfeeling, our efforts are. We seem to be trying to address a societal problem that is complex and deeply rooted with the manners and motives of a kind of charity that is obsolete in our time. We are suspended ineffectually between guilt and indifference. Many of us feel distress, knowing that thousands of people have no place to live except the street and that some die of exposure and neglect; no doubt, many others share an unspoken belief that these people cannot be worth much anyhow or they would not be sleeping on the street.

Despite the unceasing flow of information in the media about the homeless and the widespread clicking of tongues about their plight, homelessness, and the material and spiritual destitution it expresses, is not a high priority item on the current American agenda.

Parents of Murdered Children is a group I got involved with a couple of years ago through a couple who live in Philadelphia whose daughter was murdered. That 20-year-old young woman was an addict who was just about at the point of accepting professional help when she was killed. I learned from a newspaper article that she had been about to enter Eagleville Hospital for treatment. I talked to her parents by phone and then went to visit them. We found a lot that we could talk about, and it seemed to be helpful to them to have someone to talk to.

This couple was instrumental in starting a chapter of Parents of Murdered Children in the Philadelphia area. When this horrible event occurred in their lives, they found themselves unable to get solace from anyone. People around them were obviously touched and sympathetic, but they could not find people they could communicate with in a meaningful way about what was happening to them. They could not find people to whom their situation made sense, or to whom they could make sense, or who could share this experience with them. They heard about Parents of Murdered Children, which had started in Cincinnati five or six years earlier by a couple whose daughter was murdered. After communicating with the couple in Cincinnati, the Philadelphia couple set about organizing a group of this kind in this area. (At the present time, I think there are about 50–60 chapters of POMC scattered around the country.)

I became involved at the urging of the Philadelphia couple and began to attend their monthly meetings. My participation is simply as someone who is a friend of the group, available to help facilitate a bit but without interfering in any way, if I can help it, with the process that depends on their interaction, not mine.

The distress I see there is like nothing I have been involved with previously. It is sudden, unexpected, overwhelming loss and agony that will not go away. It is a unique and terrible assault on defenses that have never been tested in this way, an onslaught of feelings: guilt, anger, rage, emotional torment. The psychological and physiological reactions are numerous: insomnia, terrifying dreams, fear of the dark and of being alone, fear of something happening to one's other children—all irrational and almost constant. Loss of appetite, bowel problems, dizziness, vertigo, weakness, and menstrual dysfunction are all common, as are irrational thoughts and disturbed interpersonal relations. These involve: spouses, children, parents, other family members, and close friends; husbands and wives in painful push-pull interactions, clinging to one another, not being able to help one another, hurting one another; close friends not able to look the grieving family straight in the face, failing to understand that they really are not called upon to say anything if they could just be there. But in the face of this kind of tragedy, not many people can be there.

People do get help from physicians and clergy, but it is narrow, limited help. Physicians offer sedation and treatment of acute conditions of one kind or another. But this is not the kind of help that can carry someone through this terrible experience.

People who suffer this kind of loss tend to focus on the criminal who committed the crime and the processes that have to do with the criminal. This has a useful effect and a counterproductive effect. The usefulness is in supplying a target for much of the intense feeling. If people did not have that, I do not know what they would do to release emotion. There is a constant concern with the status of the criminal justice procedures. Have they caught the guilty person? If they have, what is the stage of the legal process, what kind of evidence is there, what kind of a case can be made? Has there been an arraignment? Has the trial date been set? How will I know when the trial takes place?

One learns that the parents of a murdered person have no formal rights in the court proceeding. The state is the plaintiff and many times the parents are left out of the process. The district attorney may not want to be bothered by the family. The police cannot see every murdered child as they would their own child and have the feelings one would have about the life of someone loved cut off in a senseless and often brutal way. And, of course, that is exactly the response that the parents are looking for, need, and cannot possibly get, except from others who have experienced the same tragedy.

The counterproductive part of this intense focusing on the crime itself and what is happening to the criminal is that the grief process stops and waits until all this is over. People need to get through the sequence of shock, denial, depression, anger, and eventual acceptance as they do with other kinds of grief and loss. This just does not proceed while all the issues of the criminal justice process are unresolved, and a person may remain suspended in the crisis for months, or even years, unable to do very much to change anything and unable to forget it, put it behind, or incorporate it in some way in order to move past the process of mourning toward recovery of equilibrium and going on with life.

Survival and identity are threatened. Some experience suicidal ideation. Some of the effects are very subtle; some people realize that the part of themselves they most admire is threatened by this event. They feel hatred and a wish for retribution. Some people who had been very liberal in their outlook, who had been staunchly against capital punishment, for example, now feel disturbing conflict. They know that they could not trust themselves if they could lay hands on the person who committed this crime—and they do not want to feel such an urge to violence.

The metaphor is a tidal wave—suddenly being torn away from all moorings by a force against which ordinary defenses are impotent.

What could and should be done? I shall not attempt to touch the many issues that have to do with prevention, except to state my belief that for this we all bear responsibility.

For those who are the surviving victims of these crimes—parents, grandparents, children, siblings—Parents of Murdered Children supplies what many need and cannot seem to find in any other way. Here there is the possibility of sharing pain, grief, anger, inadequacy, and all the other powerful feelings that cannot be turned off and for the release of which there are so few opportunities. Interacting with others in POMC provides reassurance that one is not "going crazy" and that one can get through this and even survive intact. The group provides real instrumental help with many practical matters, offering information, advice, referral, and actual assistance, such as accompaniment during court procedures. Members of POMC go to court to support one another. They want the judge, the jury, and the other principals to see that there are those who are interested. Some members express the feeling that they are there to represent the person who cannot be there—the murdered victim.

POMC exerts its influence in another way when members and others they can persuade speak out for improvement of police and judicial procedures and support legislation that addresses the needs and rights of surviving victims of this type of crime.

I have not been aware of much alcohol or drug abuse as a complicating part of the problem. Occasionally, a husband or wife expresses some concern that the partner is drinking a lot more, or relying heavily on sedation. This has been a prominent feature in those I have had a chance to observe—and the Philadelphia POMC group includes some 60–70 members.

I went to Africa for the Peace Corps on their invitation to do training of volunteers. The training was of three types: training of trainers, training in group dynamics and process, and training of persons who were going to conduct COS or close of service programs. In the Peace Corps, over the years it has been observed that the serious culture shock among Peace Corps volunteers does not occur when they leave home and take up work and residence in some small village in the countryside of a foreign country, but rather when the volunteers go home after two or three years when they have finished their service. The COS program was created to prepare people for going home and to buffer the nega-tive—and sometimes deleterious—aspects of that experience.

The culture shock associated with returning home has to do with all sorts of things—size, scale, noise, the pace of life, the impersonal move-ment of people in crowds, the apparent indifference of everyone. There is a clash of values of the small tribal community that the volunteer has been part of with the ego-centered, self-seeking, competitive, and ag-gressive norms of many people in the United States. It has to do with disappointment at home. People returning from the Peace Corps—and most of them are quite young—come home full of all experience that has been quite remarkable. They want to bring the experience home with them and share it with family and friends. Time after time they find that people will listen only for a few minutes, until the awaited evening TV program comes on. In no way is the acceptance commensurate with the offering. Few listen, few are interested, few understand—or even try to understand. There is disappointment and disillusionment when a mar-velous experience is not recognized, and in a way validated, by their own families.

The Peace Corps volunteers are wonderful people. I have traveled a lot around the world and at times when being an American made one an automatic target of criticism. Sometimes I have squirmed when I had to accept the criticism as valid. The Peace Corps experience was very differ-ent. Here was something useful, with real generosity in it, good for those who gave and for those who received. And I was very gratified by an opportunity to be involved in it even to a small extent.

The daily life of the volunteer in the Peace Corps is full of meaning and purpose. One could postulate their life experience as the very antithesis of the vacuity and rudderless drift of young street people, many of whom are the same age as the Peace Corps volunteers and some of whom could have sat at adjacent desks in school just a few years before. The lost and rootless character of the street person's life must engender shock and sadness in the returning Peace Corps volunteer, but I doubt that there is any sense of identification. I can imagine there would be more difficulty understanding and accepting the obscured purpose in the busy lives of many young middle-class Americans who, far from having dropped out, are speeding through life in the fast channels of the main stream. No homelessness here—everyone seems able to afford a good home and an expensive car. What a contrast this must be for the returning volunteer. How could he or she fail to make the comparison between this frenetic contest, which is the everyday life of many young Americans, and the simple life of service in an African village, every day of which was infused with gratifying, clear purpose?

Reconciling the discrepancy between these two life styles—with all the attendant implications of value and meaning—is the painful challenge, and the source of stress, that confronts many returning Peace Corps volunteers.

The metaphor here is "you can't go home again," which I suppose is true for most of us. I find it sad that some of these fine young people end up suspended between two worlds. We should take comfort in the fact that many of them eventually manage a transition and find paths in our own country that satisfy their wish to live useful lives.

I am not aware of substance abuse as a problem in the Peace Corps, certainly not among volunteers overseas. I do not know whether volunteers use more drugs and alcohol after returning to the United States. It is an area of research interest that ought to be explored.

Very little help is going to returning Peace Corps volunteers. The Close of Service Program at least forewarns them and provides practical help in preparing curriculum vitae, finding jobs and opportunities in education, etc.

What is needed is a support group made up of former Peace Corps volunteers who could provide the transitional support that many need. There is a Peace Corps "Alumni" Office in Washington. When I visited there a year or so ago, the staff numbered two, and they seemed to have much more contact with paper than with people. This is not a moment in our history when honest concern and generosity on a person-to-person basis count for much in our international relations. That the Peace Corps continues at all is a bit of a miracle. Perhaps we do well not to call attention to it.

The last involvement I would like to look at is Major League Baseball. There my role as a consultant has been to assist in arriving at policies that would help baseball protect its good name, protect the players from harmful effects of drug and alcohol abuse, and protect the owners from the loss of literally millions of dollars that are at risk when a very expensive ballplayer does in fact lose his effectiveness because of a drug or alcohol problem. It was interesting for me to begin to understand the nature of the stress in baseball.

It begins as soon as one is called up to baseball, which is usually to be chosen for the Minor, not Major, League, and it continues almost inescapably throughout a career. The principal reaction is fear—fear of failure; fear of not measuring up, not making the team; fear of losing what one wants most and having to go home in shame and defeat; fear of disappointing parents, siblings, friends; fear of letting the high school coach and teachers down.

Most of the players just getting into baseball are youngsters in their late teens or early 20s, still making their way out of adolescence. A few may come from New York City, Chicago, or Los Angeles, but most are from small towns and villages. We are talking about Webb City, Missouri, Barboursville, Virginia, and Westlake Village, California; also San Pedro de Macoris, Dominican Republic, and Juana Diaz, Puerto Rico. Not many of us have been to these places recently.

When a high school star gets a tryout in big league baseball, even the Minor League, and leaves his home in Waxahachie, Texas, it's news. His name is in the paper, maybe his picture, too, and a lot of hometown folks from that day on follow his progress through press and radio. Word filters back. His success in baseball qualifies as news. Unfortunately, so does his failure. And with 26 Major League teams, each of which is allowed 25 players on its active roster, there are 650 slots—while there are 5,000 or 6,000 players in the Minor League who want to fill those slots. That leaves room for a lot of disappointment.

There are other fears and uncertainties—anxiety about being alone and away from home; for many this is the first time. Feeling inadequate, not quite knowing how to play the role of professional ballplayer—off the field as well as on. Fear of not being accepted by the older players, of being ridiculed and rejected, of being left out by peers.

These are the stresses in the initial phases of a baseball career. If one manages to stay in and moves to the Majors, the stress does not stop, it simply changes. Now you are in the rat race for real. The prestige rat race, the celebrity rat race, the statistics rat race.

What is your batting average? Against right-handed pitchers? Left-handed? Early and late in the season? How do you hit with men on base? How many games have you won with a hit? What's your slugging average? Runs batted in? How many men have you stranded on base? How's your fielding? Baserunning? How many bases have you stolen? How many times thrown out?

Literally dozens, maybe hundreds, of measures are used to judge and track your proficiency and ability—all weighed against every other player and against what you did last week and last year.

The computer, with its endless outpouring of statistics, can be a nightmare to a ballplayer. I ask myself how I would feel if my professional performance was evaluated and rated by 50 or 60 different measures every working day of my life. And not only for the edification of me and my employer, but to feed the avaricious appetite of a huge public. That is what goes on in baseball.

Money may be the worst rat race, because in this field money is the yardstick of value. If you want to know how you are rated against everyone else on the team, and everyone else in the league, you look at the dollars. And I am confident that most outsiders would not guess within 100,000 dollars that the *average* salary of a Major League ballplayer today is over $300,000. For established stars, the figure is closer to, and sometimes over, $1 million.

Having come from a modest background myself, I feel that I know that very few, if any, 19 and 22 year olds have any concept of what that kind of money means. Such lofty numbers have an unreal quality to them. And yet numbers are the ego satisfiers; they tell you where you are on the competitive scale.

How about other payoffs? Personal satisfaction, respect from teammates, joy of playing the game. When I remember baseball from my youth and learn about its past from books, I know that joy of playing the game was high on the list. From what I have seen recently, I do not think it is now. Joy and satisfaction from the fame itself are overshadowed by other motives and compensations.

What does one do when the ballgame is over? The game ends at 10:00 or 10:30 at night or 4:30 or 5:00 in the afternoon. Then what? Do you cuddle up in your hotel room with a good book? Does the team go together to a nice restaurant and have a few beers and dinner and then go back to the hotel to catch Johnnie Carson on TV? Some do, maybe. Sometimes.

Others are looking for something else. Some come out of backgrounds where the mark of achievement is to spend money, not just have it. To spend it on all the things that indicate "the good life": parties, women, cocaine. And bees do not target on pollen faster or more accurately than purveyors of "the good life" hone in on celebrity professional athletes who show the slightest evidence of being susceptible. There are plenty of helpers around.

This is star system stress, a paradoxical byproduct of "success." A suitable metaphor might be "lost at sea." Not shipwrecked and alone, but on a beautiful yacht in the company of beautiful people doing beautiful dope and booze—and all going around in circles, lost without a compass.

What could be done and ought to be done in this sad situation? I have given a lot of thought to this question. After all I am being paid to do so, I can report few conclusions firmly arrived at, except the primary fact that there are no easy answers.

For drug and alcohol problems, one could hardly design a worse prognostic matrix than the naturally occurring situation of big league ballplayers. They are young and strong and think they are going to live forever; they are celebrities at an early age, which frequently tends to get heads turned into funny positions; and they are rich, which never did help to prevent or cure addiction. They also are caught in a whirlwind of attention generated by a culture that seems always hungry for excitement and stimulation.

Need one add that some of the more susceptible players may be lonely and may be frightened and not too comfortable with something about themselves under all the glitter of a hip-macho veneer?

In stating that few conclusions have been reached about what would be useful in baseball, I am not implying that there are not a lot of suggestions being offered. At times, it seems that almost everybody knows what to do about baseball's drug problem, except those who have the responsibility of doing something about it. Sportscasters and commentators, fans who write letters to the newspapers, law enforcement personnel, coaches and trainers—all have ideas about how to solve the problem.

Some team owners want to "get tough"; they favor harsh punitive measures, believing that strict policing and severe punishments will be an effective deterrent. Others prefer a more moderate concept, not only to support the approach to drug and alcohol dependence as a medical/health problem, rather than a police matter, but also in the hope of averting polarization of baseball, with owners and managers on one side and players with their supporting union on the other side in an intensifying conflict.

Major League baseball is trying to find a position in the middle ground. Owners and management, players, and the Commissioner with his staff, are all searching for policies and procedures they can jointly create and support. The program is in an incipient stage, so it is not appropriate to say much about it. I can report that the policy adopted views drug and alcohol abuse as treatment issues, unless an individual is found guilty of some criminal charge or is proved to distribute drugs or to use them on the premises of a ball club. The program includes a neutral panel of three professionals qualified in the drug/alcohol field who provide consultative support to the program and assist in mediating disputes that arise when a player denies the use of drugs and management feels that it has "reason to believe" the player is involved.

In concluding this scrutiny of a disparate collection of people that includes homeless and street people, the parents of a murdered child, the returning Peace Corps volunteer, and the Major League ballplayer in danger of losing everything he worked so hard to attain, I want to ask what, if anything, do these troubled people have in common?

It does not stretch a point artificially, I believe, to say that all of them have experienced a failure of *connectedness*. They have lost, or never had, or something serious has happened to, an essential connecting relation with a sustaining person, family, or community. Another characteristic in common is a feeling of vulnerability and *powerlessness* against the very force that separates them from the support they need, be that circumstance abject poverty, complicated by alienation or psychotic aberration, fear of failure in the midst of success, or being a stranger among family and friends by virtue of an experience that cannot be kept or shared.

I believe that all these troubled people also have in common a likelihood of benefiting from the kind of social support, intense and nurturing, that is available in what we have learned to call "mutual help groups." These are simply people with a common problem coming together to share their experience in order to support and help one another. Participating in such a group reconnects a person with other persons and offers the solace of knowing that others suffer like you, understand what is happening to you, and care about you. The group can provide a candid reflection of you, as in a faultless mirror, without denying you unqualified acceptance as a person. The process reawakens hope and restores confidence that one can move beyond the present moment of agonizing incapacity.

Witnessing the struggle of others reflects accountability back to oneself, gently and without judgment reinforcing the idea that others can help but ultimately you are responsible for yourself. Your concern for the well-being of others evolves as a complement to the support others give you. The cumulative shared experience of the group is a reservoir of helpful information and protective buffering. In the process of lending strength to someone else, almost without realizing it, you strengthen yourself. The very act of being an anchor another person can grasp to keep from being swept away, reminds us that one's own life has value, even in the midst of adversity, and needs to be sustained.

I believe that the self-help movement, which is tolerated or acknowledged in an almost contemptuous way by some professionals, may be one of the more important movements of recent history. Literally thousands of different self-help groups exist throughout the country. In Philadelphia, the Self-Help Clearing House lists over 3,000 groups representing several hundred different problems. Just about every disease or human health problem that provides a challenge people have difficulty meeting is likely to result in the formation of a self-help group. We know, of course, that Alcoholics Anonymous is the ancestor of all of them.

I believe that professionals—and as a physician I speak most directly to them—are not properly equipped to practice if they do not understand and make use of the mutual-help resource. Mutual help supplies something different and complementary to what professionals offer. People frequently need both kinds of help. This is clearly evident and well documented in the addictions, but I know it is true for many other human problems. This is a resource that deserves more than passive acknowledgement. We should have no hesitancy in our efforts to help people learn how to help themselves and one another.

REFERENCE

1. Cherry L: On the real benefits of Eustress: Hans Selye, interviewed by Laurence Cherry. Psychology Today 11(10):60–70, 1978

15

The Large-Group Social Support Network in the Treatment of Substance Abuse: Naturalistic and Experimental Models

MARC GALANTER

A naturalistic investigation of two sects and an experimental study of a self-help treatment group are presented. Results indicate that such large-group interactions exert a potent social influence. This mechanism can be used to enhance the effectiveness of other treatment modalities by generating the social support network required to assist the substance abuser during the process of recovery.

Cohesive and ideologically oriented large-groups have been influential in altering patterns of substance abuse in a variety of settings. Until this century, religious conversion, typically in a group context, was one of the few vehicles open to the substance abuser for relinquishing a pattern of addiction. Alcoholics Anonymous, also based on mutuality and commitment, has emerged in this century as the most widespread modality in the relief of addictive illness. Relatively little in the way of research findings, however, is available with regard to the mechanisms underlying these vehicles for social influence. In addition, we have as of yet done little to adapt these techniques for persuasion to institutional treatment.

This research was supported in part by a grant from the Commonwealth Fund.

225

With these issues in mind, this chapter will address two examples of the relationship between the psychology of large-groups and patterns of substance abuse. The first is an empirical study on two naturalistic settings, each a contemporary religious sect which has borne a profound influence on substance use and abuse among its members. The second is an experimental treatment program which I have developed in order to draw on the same sources of social influence within the large-group context; it is based in an institutional treatment setting for alcoholism.

NATURALISTIC STUDIES ON SECTS

A number of new religious sects emerged in recent years which appeal primarily to late adolescents and young adults. Many of these groups offered a life style which was closely organized around group norms and relatively austere. Most discouraged the use of drugs among their members. In order to gain some understanding of the role that large, cohesive groups such as these can play in altering drug use patterns, levels of drug use among sect members were examined on the basis of systematic self-reports.

This work was conducted over the course of several years. Extensive interviews within two sects, the Divine Light Mission (DLM) and the Unification Church (UC), were used as a basis for developing self-report research instruments, which were then applied to large cohorts of members and potential members. Our reports (1–3) dealt with the effects of membership on an individual's psychological and social adjustment. In addition, however, these studies were also directed at patterns of social intoxicant use, that is, alcohol and marijuana (3–5). The following experimental subject groups were studied: long-standing members of the Divine Light Mission and the Unification Church and persons undergoing recruitment into the Unification Church.

Subjects were studied by means of interviews conducted by the author and his colleagues, followed by questionnaire administration. The studies were undertaken with agreement of the respective national organizations which conduct administrative matters for each of the sects. Because of this, assistance was available during administration from members, who were trained and supervised by the author. Respondents were specifically instructed by the assistants to answer frankly and factually. Because of the willingness of members to cooperate with officially sanctioned activities, questionnaires were carefully filled out and items which were unclear were individually reviewed.

Members of the DLM were surveyed at a national religious festival. A sample of 119 initiated members were selected in a random fashion at the time of registration. Two hundred twenty-seven American-born UC members were studied in large church residences in the New York area. Because of the residential policies of the UC, these members originally came from all parts of the United States. The third population studied consisted of 104 nonmembers who in 1978 began three-week residential workshop sequences which can lead to joining the UC.

Questionnaire items addressed a number of demographic, psychological, and social issues. Subjects were also asked to assess their level of drug use during different 2-month periods, along a 5-point quantity-frequency scale ("not at all" to "more than once on most days"). The long-standing members were asked to respond to a series of eight items which reflected their feelings of social affiliation toward different groups of people inside and outside the religious sect. These were derived from items originally developed by Schutz (6) for studying feelings of group cohesiveness.

As indicated, long-standing members in both groups were asked to report on the 2-month period prior to contact with the sect during which they consumed the most alcohol and the most marijuana, the 2-month period prior to joining the sect, the 2-month period right after joining, and the last 2-month period. The incidence of any use at all of alcohol and marijuana among members of the DLM was calculated for each of the four 2-month periods to ascertain the effects of membership on social intoxicant use, and a decline in incidence was found, as indicated in Table 1.

TABLE 1
Social Intoxicant Use Relative to
Joining the Divine Light Mission

		Respondents using drugs (%)				
		Most before joining	Right before joining	Right after joining	Last 2 months	Q Value*
Marijuana	ever used	92	82	44	42	129.7
	daily use	65	45	0	7	154.2
Alcohol	ever used	86	71	29	33	140.9
	daily use	17	13	1	0	47.7

*Cochran Q Test, all comparisons significant $p < .001$.

Affiliative feelings toward the sect were considered in relation to the decline in use of alcohol and marijuana. First, reported levels were examined in the DLM for the two 2-month periods immediately before introduction to the sect and immediately after joining. Using the quantity-frequency rating scale, the mean decline in scores on this scale was 43% for marijuana and 32% for alcohol. Second, responses on the social affiliation scale were then examined to demonstrate relative affiliative ties of members both inside and outside the sect. Members' mean responses to affiliation scale items reflected closer ties toward both the members they saw most often (mean=4.31) and the membership overall (mean=4.07) than toward the nonmembers they saw most often (mean=3.31). These comparisons of group means were highly significant ($p<.001$). Finally, the declines in scores on the alcohol and marijuana scales were used as dependent variables in two stepwise multiple regression analyses. The cohesiveness items served as independent (predictor) variables. The resulting multiple correlations showed that cohesiveness items were significant predictors of decline in alcohol and marijuana use (accounting for 15% and 14% of the variance, respectively).

With regard to contemporaneous use, UC members were also polled for marijuana and alcohol consumption at the time of the study. A small number used some marijuana or alcohol during the most recent 2-month period, and each of the two drugs was used on a daily basis by only one (0.4%) of the UC members during the most recent 2-month period.

Let us now consider some implications of these findings. The mechanisms by which society exercises control over social intoxicants may be divided into two types: formal social controls, which reflect explicit social regulation and legal codes, and informal social controls, which operate by consensus and by the pressure inherent in social relations. In our own society, examples of formal controls include laws against unlicensed liquor production, legal restraints on the sale of marijuana, and codes involving physicians' prescribing of certain drugs subject to abuse. Informal controls include parental pressure on teenage children, disapproval by strangers of public drunkenness, and pressure from coreligionists to conform to codes for proper behavior. Significantly, the informal controls are generally conceded to carry out the principal weight of the regulation of drug use (7). In a setting in which religion is influential, religious norms may then assume a primary role in the network of informal social controls.

Based on these controlled studies and related observations, I concluded that "large-groups" such as these are characterized by the following traits: They have a *large membership*, larger than the traditional therapy group. Individuals have *strong cohesive ties* toward the overall membership; unlike persons participating in traditional therapy groups, members' affiliativeness and shared responsibilities extend outside their experience in the group's formal meetings. Members have strongly held *consensual beliefs*, beliefs which may be compared in their unifying role to the strongly avowed abstinence orientation of AA. By means of multiple regression statistics, we also found that a member's *affective status* is positively correlated with both the intensity of his cohesiveness toward the group, and his ascription to the group's beliefs. These relationships between affective status and both cohesiveness and acceptance of group beliefs form a basis for the operant reinforcement of members' compliance with group behavioral norms. Compliance is implicity perceived as assuring the maintenance of emotional stability. It is these models for social influence in large-groups which served as a basis for developing the experimental treatment. The specific nature of the experimental model which we studied will be described below.

The large-group phenomena described here apparently exerted considerable influence in altering members' behavioral norms. A related model may provide assistance in gaining a better understanding of the considerable potency and cost-effectiveness of Alcoholics Anonymous (AA). Given the observations reported here, the following traits of large-group therapy for the alcoholic may apply both to self-help groups and religious sects: large-group size vs. small therapy-group size (such as large chapter meetings); high level of social cohesiveness and a shared support system; intense, nonrational or antirational belief systems; members' psychological well-being correlated with cohesiveness and a consensual belief system; major behavioral norms, such as those for drinking, determined by the group; and an explicit system of rituals (such as the Twelve Steps of AA).

SELF-HELP TREATMENT FOR ALCOHOLISM

While these studies were under way, I decided to draw on the principles of large-group psychology observed in freestanding self-help (SH) treatments for addictive illness, such as Alcoholics Anonymous and the drug-free therapeutic communities, as well as these very religious sects. Both AA and the sects effect changes in addictive behavior by means which are qualitatively different from the usual hospital-based therapy. By adapting a model of social influence from these large-groups, I hoped to tap a therapeutic paradigm different from the typical small therapy group, drawing instead on a broader base of mutual support and leadership among patients of a large, cohesive population of the clinic overall.

In the experimental self-help treatment approach, certain therapist functions are placed in the hands of the patient population, so that stabilized patients play an active role in providing care for more recent admissions, and a feeling of community, shared commitment, and mutual responsibility is encouraged. The program also introduces the option of patients' strong identification with, and cohesiveness toward, a treatment network of many more than 8–10 patients in the usual therapy group; it encourages affiliative feelings among the full complement of self-help patients, providing an experience of a large, cohesive group with shared goals and ideals. This is promoted by therapeutic contact with a number of stabilized patients who are involved in the therapy groups; by program-wide patient-run activities, such as the orientation groups open to patients in crisis; and in monthly large-group meetings, also open to all patients. This broader identification forms the bulwark of the self-help orientation.

An outcome study on this treatment model will be outlined here as a vehicle for delineating the experimental approach. The study was conducted to ascertain whether this experimental self-help model could achieve patient retention and visits comparable to the typical outpatient treatment format, while using *half* the counseling staff.

The treatment approach was developed in a multimodality alcoholism unit, part of a general medical care teaching hospital. The alcohol unit itself consists of 20 beds and 500-patient outpatient unit. The patients treated at this hospital are predominantly unmarried (81%) and unemployed (83%) men (76%). The majority are high school dropouts (59%) and members of ethnic minorities (47% black, 26% Hispanic). Because these patients are largely unemployed, with limited social stability and resources, they carry a relatively poor prognosis.

The control treatment and the experimental self-help program operate simultaneously and independently in the outpatient department. Principal differences between the two programs are outlined below.

The first area considered is peer therapy. Patients in the control group are encouraged in group therapy to be supportive of each other, but there is no expectation that they assume responsibility for the needs of their peers, particularly outside the group. Self-help patients are made aware that the primary source of support in the clinic is derived from the peer group. New patients are encouraged to seek out peers and senior patients who will be available to assist them through the program. Senior patients are supervised in assisting with crises, where judged clinically appropriate by the primary therapist. Most of these exchanges take place in the large, unpartitioned self-help therapy area, around the time of therapy meetings.

A Senior Patient Program was also established in the group. Potential members are screened for sobriety and social stability, and assist in management of the program for a time-limited period. Those who serve as group leaders meet weekly as a group with the primary therapists, focusing on their therapeutic functions in the unit. Under supervision of the therapists, they direct orientation, therapy, and activity groups. Their interventions in more difficult patient problems are reviewed with the primary therapists, and they refer self-help patients to their respective primary therapist for more troublesome problems. Other Senior Patients have administrative functions in the program.

Meetings of the full patient group are also held for the self-help group, but not for the controls. A monthly meeting open to all self-help patients serves as a focus for group esprit and as a context for organizing recreational activities. The meetings are run collaboratively by staff and senior patients, with program-wide activities and patients' progress as the focus. Socialization around the time of these meetings may focus on the status of patients' recovery. The experimental self-help program is characterized by an early exposure to the self-help format while on the ward. This takes place in the orientation groups which meet three times a week and are conducted primarily by the self-help Senior Patients, rather than by staff. Inpatients are thereby apprised of the more active patient role in the ambulatory program and meet the Senior Patients and other self-help outpatients in the orientation groups. Senior Patients express interest in the post-discharge plans of these inpatients, for example, indicating that they would be working with them after discharge.

The following study was designed to examine the outcome for patients treated in the SH program, with half the counselor-to-patient ratio as the control program. More specifics on the study are published elsewhere (8).

There were two *inpatient* control groups in the study. The first ($N=32$) operated contemporaneously with the self-help program. A second control group ($N=31$) served as a contrast for both self-help ($N=32$) and the first control. Data on the second group of controls were drawn from a continuous series of inpatient admissions during a comparable period one year prior to the institution of the experimental format. For this second control group there was no association with outpatients in orientation groups during the hospital stay, although they did meet with their outpatient therapist before discharge. This group therefore highlights the differential role of early acquaintance with outpatients in a transitional orientation group (used for the self-help and first control), so as to enhance patient retention. In the *outpatient* program 70 self-help and 70 control patients were followed for a period of one year after admission.

For the *inpatients,* who constitute 40% of the sample, engagement into outpatient treatment after discharge from the ward was considered. Those in the self-help cohort were found to be engaged in treatment better than the control groups. A higher rate of retention was maintained by the self-help cohort, so that the percentage of inpatients who made outpatient visits in the year after ward discharge was greater for the self-help than the first and second control cohorts (84%, 63%, and 52%, respectively, $\chi^2 = 9.16$, $p < .02$). There was, however, no significant difference between the three cohorts for the mean number of either group therapy or individual therapy visits over the course of the first year among those subjects who made at least one visit. The mean number of outpatient visits for discharged patients was 8.0, 21% of them for individual counseling.

For those patients who entered the program as *outpatients,* equivalent retention rates were observed in the self-help and control groups. There was no significant difference in the number of SH and control outpatients who returned to the clinic each month over the course of the year studied. After the 1st month, for example, 55% and 49% returned, respectively, 25% and 21% after the 6th month, and 23% and 13% on the 12th month. There was also no significant difference between the self-help control cohorts in the mean number of visits for the first year of treatment (11.3) or the fraction of visits which were for individual counseling (16%).

EPILOGUE: APPLICATIONS

The development of more cost-effective models in the alcoholism field is of considerable importance. In a recent federal survey, the total economic cost of alcoholism on a national scale was reported to be greater than that of both addiction and general mental illness combined; despite this, less funds are actually allotted to the treatment of alcoholism than either of the other two illnesses (9). This problem is further accentuated by the fact that only a modest portion of alcoholics in the community are actually treated.

Given a need for increased treatment services, it is important to note that social workers and counselors constitute 66% of the staffing in all federally assisted alcoholism treatment facilities, which constitute the bulk of publicly supported programs. We must consider whether such counseling staff is used in the most effective way. One problematic aspect of this is observed in the finding of Paredes and Gregory (10), i.e., in alcoholism treatment programs, the amount of economic resources invested in alcoholism treatment is not positively correlated with outcome. They concluded that the type and quantity of therapeutic resources invested are related to the characteristics of the agencies themselves rather than a treatment strategy conceived for optimal cost-effectiveness.

We have therefore considered two areas of study—the naturalistic investigation of two sects and the experimental study of a self-help treatment. What emerges from this is a conception of the potent social influence available through the large-group model. By using this mechanism, it may be possible to enhance our effectiveness in treating alcohol and drug abuse by generating the means of social support necessary to assist the substance abuser through the process of recovery.

REFERENCES

1. Galanter M, Buckley P: Evangelical religion and meditation: Psychotherapeutic effects. J Nerv Ment Dis 166:685–691, 1978
2. Galanter M, Rabkin R, Rabkin J, Deutsch A: The "Moonies": A psychological study. Am J Psychiatry 136:165–170, 1979
3. Galanter M: Psychological induction into the large group: Findings from a contemporary religious sect. Am J Psychiatry 137(12):1574–1579, 1980.
4. Galanter M: Sociobiology and informal social controls on alcohol consumption: Findings from two charismatic sects. J. Stud Alcohol 42:64–79, 1981
5. Galanter M, Buckley P, Deutsch A, Rabkin J, Rabkin R: Large-group influence for decreased drug use. Am J Alcohol and Drug Abuse 7(3):291–304, 1980
6. Schutz WC: The Interpersonal Underworld. Palo Alto, CA, Science & Behavior Books, 1966
7. Amar AM: Social Control as a Factor in Non-Medical Drug Use. Symposium of the World Health Organization, Toronto, 1977, pp 113–139
8. Galanter M: Self-help large-group therapy for alcoholism: A controlled study. Alcoholism: Clin and Exper Res 8:16–23, 1984
9. Vischi TR, Jones KR, Shank FL, Lima LH: The Alcohol Drug Abuse and Mental Health National Data Book. Washington, DC, US Department of Health and Human Services, 1980
10. Paredes A, Gregory R: Therapeutic impact and fiscal investments in alcoholism services, in Currents in Alcoholism, vol IV. Edited by Galanter M. New York, Grune & Stratton, 1979.

SECTION IV

Newer Conceptions and Theoretical Developments

16

Alcohol and Tension Reduction: What's New?

HOWARD CAPPELL

The recent literature concerning the hypothesis that alcohol reduces tension (the TRH) is mixed in its support for the TRH. This is notwithstanding the considerable advances in methodological and theoretical sophistication that have been achieved during the last decade. The best interpretation for the continuing disarray in this literature is that alcohol has tension-increasing effects at doses that are not much higher than those that reduce tension. This argument is supported in a comparison of the "margin of safety" between anxiolytic and stressful doses of alcohol and the class of drugs (benzodiazepines) that has been developed precisely for its effectiveness in reducing tension.

In 1972, Cappell and Herman (1) published a review of what was at the time the most prominent psychological theory of voluntary alcohol consumption. A few years later, Cappell (2) fleshed out this theory and accorded it upper case recognition as the Tension Reduction Theory, or TRT. "Tension" was defined as the "generic construct best summarizing such constructs as fear, anxiety, frustration, etc., all of which share in common that they denote hypothesized aversive states which can control behavior" (1, p. 33). The TRT is founded on two tenets: (1) alcohol reduces tension, and (2) alcohol is consumed for its tension-reducing properties.

In these reviews, the TRT was recognized for its plausibility but criticized because the breadth of its reach went considerably beyond the scope of its empirical support. Today, the TRT as originally stated seems unsophisticated in the extreme, but nonetheless it has been the engine of a great deal of research. In the last decade or so, our research methods have become better and our approach to the research questions in this area more elaborate (the latter development constituting a mixed blessing for writers of reviews). My purpose here is to review what has become of the TRT; in order to constrain its size, the review will be restricted primarily to data concerning the TRH (i.e., the hypothesis that alcohol reduces tension). Although this means that the important literature on alcohol self-administration will not be considered, inclusion of that literature would not alter the essence of what follows.

The question of this paper is "What's new?" The answer could come in both short and long versions. The short version will be offered here. Research using both human and animal subjects will be considered. To conclude, I will compare alcohol to the prototypical class of tension-reducing drugs (benzodiazepines) in an attempt to give a pharmacological account of why support for the TRH can inevitably be expected to be inconsistent. I will not confront the issue of defining stress or tension precisely.

RESEARCH WITH HUMANS

In principle, it should be simple to determine whether or not alcohol can reduce tension in man. One need only administer alcohol and measure the consequences for various indicators of tension level. In practice, however, there has been anything but simplicity in the human literature. Consider the study by Steffen, Nathan, and Taylor (3), in which correlations among blood alcohol level (BAL) and two indices of tension were computed. The subjects in this study were alcoholics who drank over 12 consecutive days in a laboratory setting. When tension level was assessed electromyographically, the correlational analysis supported the TRH. However, the correlations between BAL and "subjective units of disturbance" supported a contrary view. This led Steffen and his colleagues to conclude that "relations among level of intoxication, tension level, and level of subjective disturbance are . . . more complex than previously believed" (p. 546).

Steffen et al. argued that the use of a chronic drinking regime was a virtue of their study, providing for more valid results. In contrast, Sher and Levenson (4) took the opposite position that results contrary to the TRH based on chronic drinking should be viewed with caution. Their concern was that studies of chronic drinking typically do not involve the explicit application of a stressor, but instead determine the effect of alcohol on the resting state. They incorporated both self-report and psychophysiological measures in their studies, in which subjects were administered a dose of 1 g/kg. Evidence consistent with the TRH was obtained with the psychophysiological measures, but somewhat less so with self-report of anxiety. Beverage expectation (cf. later on in this paper) had no effect on the outcomes, but an interesting individual difference variable, "risk for developing alcohol problems," did. Alcohol was effective in dampening the effects of a stressor for "high risk" subjects, but not for those assessed as "low risk." Individual differences continually emerge as important qualifiers of the TRH in the recent literature.

One of the most influential developments in psychology in recent years has been the rediscovery that belief, expectation, and cognition can influence behavior. This has been increasingly incorporated into experimental designs involving the TRH. Complex factorial designs have become the order of the day, with interesting but often frustratingly complex results. For example, Polivy, Scheuneman, and Carlson (5) manipulated anxiety prior to administering what subjects were led to believe in some cases to be alcohol and in others to be vitamin C. Although there was evidence that the actual ingestion of alcohol reduced subjective reports of anxiety, the *belief* that alcohol had been consumed had quite the opposite effect. Polivy et al. had to develop an elaborate explanation for these results, and concluded that the anxiogenic effect of alcohol might have had something to do with previous negative experience with alcohol in their population, which consisted mainly of light drinkers. In support of this argument, they cited Williams' (6) observation that even in heavy social drinkers, the initial reduction of anxiety that occurred during a drinking episode was reversed at higher doses.

Further elucidation of the importance of dose and subject considerations is contained in a study by Lipscomb, Nathan, Wilson, et al. (7). This study included the independent variables of tolerance, dose (0.5 or 1.0 g/kg), a stress manipulation of what might be called social anxiety, and a variety of dependent measures of tension. Only psychophysiological measurements supported the TRH, and this support was qualified in various ways. Although it did appear that alcohol mitigated the effect of a social stressor using one indicator of stress, subjects who were classified as tolerant enjoyed this benefit only at the higher dose.

Some investigators have included measures of approach to a feared stimulus in tests of the TRH. Rimm, Briddell, Zimmerman, et al. (8) found that a dose of 0.5 g/kg did not affect subjects' willingness to approach and handle a 4-foot boa constrictor, although it did reduce self-reported fear of the snake. In this instance whether subjects were led to believe that their drink was alcohol or a placebo had no effect on approach or self-report. Lindman (9), however, had better luck with approach behavior, finding that subjects were less reluctant to expose themselves to electric shock after consuming 0.9 g/kg. However, a measure of skin conductance failed to show any effect of alcohol in the same study. Lindman (9) also found that subjects were more willing to handle a mouse in a bottle after drinking alcohol; of some clinical interest was the finding that training in behavioral coping was equally effective in producing approach behavior in the absence of alcohol.

Subsequent experiments failed to confirm findings reported by others. Compared to the actual ingestion of alcohol, expectancies were not critical in facilitating approach behavior. Additionally, when skin conductance was used to measure the effect of anticipating a confrontation with the feared rodent, alcohol appeared to reduce baseline tension before the threat became imminent, but had the opposite effect as the time to approach the mouse grew near. In a final set of experiments, Lindman studied the effect of low (0.45 g/kg) and high (0.90 g/kg) doses of alcohol on eye contact during a social interaction. The only strong result was that after the high dose, females avoided eye contact with other females who were sober. This was interpreted to be inconsistent with the TRH.

Superficially, the findings of Rimm et al. (8) and Lindman (9) appear at odds as far as actual approach behavior is concerned. However, to the extent that the TRH fared better with mice than with snakes, perhaps it was because Lindman used double the dose of alcohol than the subjects of Rimm et al. enjoyed. As for the ability of alcohol to increase tension in Lindman's work, he could only appeal to (unspecified) "factors in the experimental setting" (cf. also to 5).

Although the introduction of cognitions and expectancies has been an important theoretical and methodological development in the alcohol literature generally, recent support for the TRH would probably be less ambiguous if this development had not occurred. For example, Wilson, Abrams, and Lipscomb (10) produced relatively straightforward support for the TRH when heart rate was used as an index of tension during a social interaction task; although a dose of 0.5 g/kg was relatively ineffective, 1.0 g/kg substantially attenuated the increase in heart rate that was seen during the task in placebo and low dose conditions. However, the effect of expectancy could not even be assessed because dose and expectancy could not be manipulated orthogonally. This study also called into question the utility and validity of self-report measures of tension states, since they were not sensitive to the dose manipulation.

Other studies from the same laboratory (11, 12) give a different picture of expectancy effects. In the earlier one (11), the mere belief that subjects had consumed alcohol attenuated the increase in heart rate that otherwise occurred in a stressful social situation, but there was no direct effect of alcohol on the same response. This general pattern of results was corroborated by self-ratings of anxiety and by observer ratings. In the later study (12), subjects' belief about the beverage they had consumed was the only effective manipulation, but the results contradicted those reported earlier. Although the subjects reported in advance that they *expected* alcohol to reduce anxiety, the psychophysiological index suggested the opposite and the self-report index was simply negative. The most obvious difference between the two studies was that males were subjects in the earlier one and females in the other, and the most obvious explanation for the discrepancy between the studies was that females were more wary than males in a social situation in which they thought they had been drinking. There is some consistency between this result and the one reported for females by Lindman (9) in a comparable test situation.

The difficulty in finding consistent evidence concerning the TRH continues in the work of Keane and Lisman (13). In contrast to Wilson and Abrams (11), they found that the TRH was contradicted in experiments involving a social interaction test even in male subjects. One study employed subjects rated low in social anxiety and the other subjects rated high on this dimension. The contradiction occurred with both performance and psychophysiological indicators of tension. A manipulation of expectation had little effect on any outcome, and the results of self-report were generally negative. For added measure, Bradlyn, Strickler, and Maxwell (14) failed to find any effect of alcohol or expectancy on self-report or physiological measures of tension in a public speaking task. Like Wilson et al., they had some trouble in manipulating expectancy cleanly. On the other hand, Steele, Southwick, and Critchlow (15) reported that alcohol (2 ounces of vodka) attenuated cognitive dissonance, which is generally accepted as an aversive motivational state; this was taken as support for the TRH. However, the pendulum swings back again in considering the finding of McCollam, Burish, Maisto, et al. (16) that alcohol (0.5 g/kg) had no effect on self-report of anxiety or on a physiological index.

A final word on expectancies and the TRH is in order. The manipulation of expectancy has not had consistent effects where laboratory experiments are concerned. However, there is remarkable consistency in self-reports of alcohol-related expectancies across a wide variety of populations. Generally speaking (17–22), people believe that alcohol relieves tension, notwithstanding that this belief does not always translate into predictable behavior in the laboratory. In 1975, Cappell (2) may have anticipated this discrepancy in the comment that the failure of the tension-reduction model "is perplexing since the rationale underlying the TRH seems so plausible and so consistent with commonplace experience" (p. 202). Perhaps what is important is that commonplace experience is usually elicited by simple questions and reported in a general way; it does not come packaged in a $2 \times 2 \times 3$ factorial version.

RESEARCH WITH ANIMALS

Generally, the more recent findings of animal research are crystal-clear compared to data from humans. In this section, I will review recent data on alcohol and compare these with results from research on benzodiazepines. This is an important comparison because benzodiazepines are tension-reducers *par excellence*. This comparison will be used to pave the way for a pharmacological hypothesis about why the TRH has continued to be a source of contradiction.

In an early study, Ellis (23) found that alcohol raised plasma corticosterone levels in rats in a dose-related manner. This would at first blush seem to be contrary to the TRH. More recently, however, results more supportive of the TRH have begun to emerge. Brick and Pohorecky (24) showed that alcohol (0.5 g/kg in rats) attenuated the elevation of corticosterone and plasma free fatty acids (FFA) produced by footshock. This pattern was confirmed when other stressors (e.g., restraint) were applied. In a particularly important experiment, Brick and Pohorecky (24) found that the serotonin depleter para-chlorophenylalanine (PCPA) and a relatively high dose (1.5 g/kg) of alcohol each were capable of elevating plasma FFA. Nonetheless, alcohol still attenuated the elevation produced by PCPA alone. This suggests that the background of stress into which alcohol administration is introduced figures importantly in its net effect. This result was not replicated with plasma corticosterone.

Other investigators (25) have also obtained results consistent with the TRH using biochemical indicators of stress drawn from the brain. Vogel and Deturck (26) reported that a low dose (0.5 g/kg) exerted a protective effect against a stressor without altering biochemical responses by itself.

They were also able to breed strains of rats that were either "low" or "high" responders to immobilization stress. Alcohol had little effect on the biochemical responses of low responders, but did attenuate the stress response in high responders. This dovetails nicely with the suggestion from work with humans (4) that individual difference factors need to be taken into account in predicting what effect alcohol will have on the response to stress.

The parallels between alcohol and benzodiazepines are very much worth considering in this context. As Vogel and Deturck did with alcohol, File and Peet (27) found that chlordiazepoxide (5 mg/kg) attenuated the elevation of plasma corticosterone caused by stress, but had no effect in unstressed rats. Lahti and Barsuhn (28) found another interesting parallel in that low doses of benzodiazepines attenuated the corticosteroid response to stress in rats, whereas high doses produced an elevation in unstressed rats. Interestingly, the drug-induced elevation waned with chronic administration, but the ability of the benzodiazepine to protect against a stress-induced elevation did not. This differential feature of the acute and chronic effects needs to be investigated with alcohol.

A potential mechanism for interpreting the relationship between drugs and stress was suggested in the work of Lahti and Barsuhn (28). They showed that low doses of phenobarbital protected against corticosteroid elevation by a stressor, moderate doses did not, and higher anesthetic doses did. They hypothesized that the depressant effects and ataxia produced by CNS depressants are stressful. Low doses do not have such effects and can therefore be protective, intermediate doses have such effects and are consequently stressful, and high doses that produce anesthesia are protective because stressful stimulation does not "register," nor does behavioral disturbance (such as ataxia) occur. Thus, a feedback mechanism based on the dose-related consequences of drug administration can be suggested to account for otherwise paradoxical findings.

What of the comparison of alcohol and benzodiazepines at the level of behavioral action? Benzodiazepines are without pharmacological peer with respect to anxiolytic action (cf. 29). With remarkable consistency, they restore behavior in rats that has been suppressed by punishment in the "anti-conflict test." Interestingly, tests involving approach-avoidance conflict have provided the best support for the TRH in animal studies (2). A direct comparison of alcohol and chlordiazepoxide (CDP) using the same methodology for assessing conflict is fortunately available (30, 31). This comparison showed that both alcohol and CDP were effective in restoring responding that had been suppressed by punishment with shock. However, CDP was effective at a wide range of doses that had minimal effects on motor coordination, whereas the higher doses of alcohol that restored punished behavior also produced significant motor impairment. In fact, the most potent dose of CDP in relieving conflict was one that had no effect on motor impairment, and that dose was a more potent anti-conflict agent than any dose of alcohol tested. There was no dose-response curve for alcohol and the anti-conflict effect, but there was one for CDP; Breese et al. (31) suggested that the overlay of motor impairment by alcohol might be responsible for the flat dose-response relationship with alcohol. Since alcohol was found to be a less effective anxiolytic than CDP, they suggested that other differences in drug action, particularly in relation to general impairment, might underlie the superiority of CDP (cf. 28). It is worth noting here that the doses of alcohol (0.5 g/kg) that have been found effective in blocking the biochemical consequences of stressors are ones that have very little effect on motor behavior in rats.

TOWARDS A PHARMACOLOGICAL ACCOUNT OF THE INCONSTANCY OF SUPPORT FOR THE TRH

The comparison between alcohol (a so-so anxiolytic) and benzodiazepines (fairly good anxiolytics) forms a good basis for a hypothesis that can address the continued failure to obtain solid support for the TRH. Advancing the hypothesis requires a comparison in animals of dose-response curves for degrees of impairment and toxicity produced by alcohol and benzodiazepines. The idea for such a comparison was provided by Boisse and Okamoto (32). The actual data are taken from Irwin (33) and are based on orally effective doses in rats. Note that the dose-response curve for CDP and diazepam in Figure 1 are relatively flat over a wide dose range. The significance of this is that proportionally large increases in dose are required to move from the range of anxiolytic effectiveness to the range of behavioral toxicity and ultimate lethality. In contrast, the "margin of safety" between anxiolytic activity and impairment for alcohol is very slim, and much more of a balancing act is required to achieve the former without the expense of the latter.

If it is accepted (28) that drug-induced impairment is stressful in itself, this may explain why the window of alcohol's tension-reducing potential is very narrow. The small margin of safety would go a long way toward explaining the enormous variability in human response by pointing to the possibility for "errors" of self-regulation of dosing. The relatively

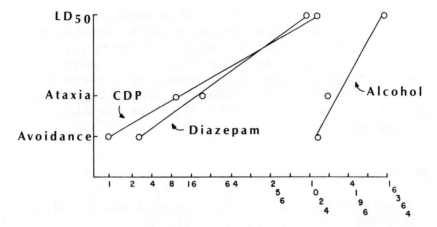

Figure 1. Dose-response curves for chlordiazepoxide (CDP), diazepam, and ethanol. The ordinate gives effective doses for reduction of avoidance responding, production of ataxia, and lethality. The abscissa gives doses in mg/kg p.o. in the rat. Adapted from Irwin (33).

narrow dosage gap from which tension reduction slips into the opposite can, for example, explain how an individual might begin drinking with the expectation of reducing tension but end by experiencing an increase as the dose approaches and exceeds the threshold for impairment (cf. 34 for some interesting data on this point in alcoholics).

With a little imagination, testable hypotheses can be derived from this speculative approach. Considering individual differences, it generates the prediction that the tension-reducing effects of alcohol will be greatest for those individuals who display relatively flat dose-response curves for motor impairment, but relatively steep ones for anxiolytic action. Such a relationship among dose-response curves would characterize heavy drinkers if tolerance to motor impairment is greater than tolerance to tension-reduction. Without such a configuration of dose-response curves, increases in tension would begin to occur even at the lower doses which are most effective for tension-reduction, and thus obscure a genuine capacity of alcohol to reduce tension.

In conclusion, despite much improvement in the quality of effort that has been brought to bear on the TRH, it remains clear that it is not tenable as a generally true hypothesis. It does seem fair to say that alcohol possesses the capacity to reduce tension, and even fairer to say that most people believe in this property of alcohol to some degree.

However, there are many conditional variables affecting when the TRH applies in man. Although the pharmacological hypothesis advanced here is only one among many, the suggestion that the margin of safety between tension reduction and toxicity is very narrow for alcohol offers a very parsimonious account for the continued disarray in the human literature on the TRH. Moreover, this pharmacological hypothesis suggests that it is unlikely that the TRH will ever enjoy consistent experimental support.

REFERENCES

1. Cappell H, Herman CP: Alcohol and tension reduction: A review. Q J Stud Alcohol 33:33–64, 1972
2. Cappell H: An evaluation of tension models of alcohol consumption, in Research Advances in Alcohol and Drug Problems, vol 2. Edited by Gibbins RJ, Israel Y, Kalant H, et al. New York, John Wiley & Sons, 1975
3. Steffen JJ, Nathan PE, Taylor HA: Tension-reducing effects of alcohol: Further evidence and some methodological considerations. J Abnorm Psychol 83:542–547, 1974
4. Sher KJ, Levenson RW: Alcohol and tension reduction: The importance of individual differences, in Stress and Alcohol Use. Edited by Pohorecky LA, Brick J. New York, Elsevier Biomedical, 1983
5. Polivy J, Scheuneman AL, Carlson K: Alcohol and tension reduction: Cognitive and physiological effects. J Abnorm Psychol 85:595–600, 1976
6. Williams AF: Social drinking, anxiety, and depression. J Pers Soc Psychol 3:689–693, 1966
7. Lipscomb TR, Nathan PE, Wilson GT, et al: Effects of tolerance on the anxiety-reducing function of alcohol. Arch Gen Psychiatry 37:577–582, 1980
8. Rimm D, Briddell D, Zimmerman M, et al: The effects of alcohol and the expectancy of alcohol on snake fear. Addict Behav 6:47–51, 1981
9. Lindman R: Alcohol and the reduction of fear, in Stress and Alcohol Use. Edited by Pohorecky LA, Brick J. New York, Elsevier Biomedical, 1983
10. Wilson GT, Abrams DB, Lipscomb TR: Effects of intoxication levels and drinking pattern on social anxiety in men. J Stud Alcohol 41:250–264, 1980
11. Wilson GT, Abrams DB: Effects of alcohol on social anxiety and physiological arousal: Cognitive versus pharmacological processes. Cog Ther R 1:195–210, 1977
12. Abrams DB, Wilson GT: Effects of alcohol on social anxiety in women: Cognitive versus physiological processes. J Abnorm Psychol 88:161–173, 1979
13. Keane TM, Lisman SA: Alcohol and social anxiety in males: Behavioral, cognitive and physiological effects. J Abnorm Psychol 89:213–223, 1980
14. Bradlyn AS, Strickler DP, Maxwell WA: Alcohol, expectancy and stress: Methodological concerns with the expectancy design. Addict Behav 6:1–8, 1981
15. Steele CM, Southwick LL, Critchlow B: Dissonance and alcohol: Drinking your troubles away. J Pers Soc Psychol 41:831–846, 1981
16. McCollam JB, Burish TG, Maisto SA, et al: Alcohol's effects on physiological arousal and self-reported affect and sensations. J Abnorm Psychol 89:224–233, 1980
17. Brown SA, Goldman MS, Inn A, et al: Expectations of reinforcement from alcohol: Their domain and relation to drinking patterns. J Consult Clin Psychol 48:419–426, 1980
18. Christiansen BA, Goldman MS: Alcohol-related expectancies versus demographic/

background variables in the prediction of adolescent drinking. J Consult Clin Psychol 51:249–257, 1983
19. Christiansen BA, Goldman MS, Inn A: Development of alcohol-related expectancies in adolescents: Separating pharmacological from social-learning influences. J Consult Clin Psychol 50:336–344, 1982
20. Farber PD, Khavari K, Douglas FM IV: A factor analytic study of reasons for drinking: Empirical validation of positive and negative reinforcement dimensions. J Consult Clin Psychol 48:780–781, 1980
21. Rohsenow DJ: Drinking habits and expectancies about alcohol's effects for self versus others. J Consult Clin Psychol 51:752–756, 1983
22. Southwick L, Steele C, Marlatt A, et al: Alcohol-related expectancies: Defined by phase of intoxication and drinking experience. J Consult Clin Psychol 49:713–721, 1981
23. Ellis FW: Effect of ethanol on plasma corticosterone levels. J Pharmacol Exp Ther 153:121–127, 1966
24. Brick J, Pohorecky LA: The neuroendocrine response to stress and the effects of ethanol, in Stress and Alcohol Use. Edited by Pohorecky LA, Brick J. New York, Elsevier Biomedical, 1983
25. Kuriyama K, Kanmori K, Yoneda Y: Preventive effect of alcohol on stress-induced alterations in metabolism and function of biogenic amines and gamma-aminobutyric acid (GABA) in neuroendocrine system, in Stress and Alcohol Use. Edited by Pohorecky LA, Brick J. New York, Elsevier Biomedical, 1983
26. Vogel WH, Deturck KH: Effects of ethanol on plasma and brain catecholamine levels in stressed and unstressed rats, in Stress and Alcohol Use. Edited by Pohorecky LA, Brick J. New York, Elsevier Biomedical, 1983
27. File SE, Peet LA: The sensitivity of the rat corticosterone response to environmental manipulations and to chronic chlordiazepoxide treatment. Physiol Behav 25:753–758, 1980
28. Lahti RA, Barsuhn C: The effect of various doses of minor tranquilizers on plasma corticosteroids in stressed rats. Res Commun Chem Pathol Pharmacol 11:595–603, 1975
29. Cook L, Sepinwall J: Behavioral analysis of the effects and mechanisms of actions of benzodiazepines, in Mechanism of Action of Benzodiazepines. Edited by Costa E, Greengard P. New York, Raven Press, 1975
30. Vogel RA, Frye DG, Wilson JH, et al: Attenuation of the effects of punishment by ethanol: Comparisons with chlordiazepoxide. Psychopharmacology 71:123–129, 1980
31. Breese GR, Frye GD, Vogel RA, et al: Comparisons of behavioral and biochemical effects of ethanol and chlordiazepoxide, in Stress and Alcohol Use. Edited by Pohorecky LA, Brick J. New York, Elsevier Biomedical, 1983
32. Boisse NR, Okamoto, M. Ethanol as a sedative-hypnotic; comparison with barbiturate and nonbarbiturate sedative-hypnotics, in Alcohol Tolerance and Dependence. Edited by Rigter H, Crabbe JC Jr. Amsterdam, Elsevier Biomedical, 1980
33. Irwin S: Anti-neurotics: Practical pharmacology of the sedative-hypnotic and minor tranquilizers, in Psychopharmacology: A Review of Progress, 1957–1967. Edited by Efron DH. Washington, DC, US Government Printing Office, 1968
34. Stockwell T, Hodgson R, Rankin H: Tension reduction and the effects of prolonged alcohol consumption. Brit J Addict 77:65–73, 1982

17

Stress as a Factor in Alcohol Use and Abuse

ROBERT J. POWERS

A Stress Reduction Hypothesis (SRH) is presented as an alternative to the Tension Reduction Hypothesis (TRH). The SRH explains some of the contradictory evidence generated by the TRH. The SRH invokes a Stress Manifold and a Stress Response Manifold in a model designed to explain stress relief drinking. The stress manifold is composed of an array of external, internal, physical, mental, conscious, and unconscious stressors impacting on the individual simultaneously or in very close sequence. Stress includes major negative stimuli (distresses), major positive stimuli (eustressors), and mesostressors (i.e., daily hassles, annoyances, performance demands, minor uplifts, and maintenance of defenses). The Stress Response Manifold includes varied physiological, cognitive, affective, and behavioral responses to stressor stimuli experienced simultaneously or in very close sequence. Using this model, drinking for stress relief is viewed by the author as a highly complex behavior. A semistructured clinical interview based on the SRH was administered to normal subjects and abstinent alcoholics. Results suggest that subjects can distinguish between the three forms of stressful stimuli and can indicate when alcohol consumption is directed towards reducing the specific type of stressor. In general, results suggest that equal numbers of alcoholics and normals drink to relieve mesostressors and eustressors. However, alcoholics may be more prone to consume alcohol when confronted with major negative stressors. The author outlines factors that may play a role in causing habituation and dependency including intermittent reinforcement and modeling. Finally, it is suggested that this model provides an outline for helping the alcoholic patient clarify the ways he uses alcohol in his life.

Stress has long been considered important in the use and abuse of alcohol. Nonproblem "social" drinkers, and especially alcohol dependent individuals, have frequently identified stress relief as a primary motive for drinking (1, 2, 3). Initial experimental research also supported the role of stress relief in alcohol use and abuse. In animal studies, Masserman and Yum (4) and Conger (5) found evidence for what has been termed the "Tension Reduction Hypothesis" (TRH). The TRH achieved considerable prominence and, in many respects, was viewed as defining the relation between stress and alcohol. According to the TRH, alcohol use serves to reduce tension, and the reduction of tension from drinking reinforces and increases the drinking response (6).

Relatively recently, however, a number of investigators have observed that the TRH has not been well supported by the research data (6, 7, 8). In particular, alcohol has been found in many instances to result in an increase, rather than a decrease, in anxiety or tension (9, 10). In other instances, increased anxiety or tension has not been found to result in higher rates of drinking (11, 12). The tenuous evidence for the TRH has challenged the traditional assumption of a strong relation between stress and drinking.

The TRH, however, appears limited conceptually in representing the relation between stress and alcohol. Powers and Kutash (13) point out that the TRH in practice has frequently limited investigation of stress to one form of stress response, tension or anxiety. Regrettably, such terms as stress, tension, anxiety, and other dysphoric states, have often been used interchangeably (6). Powers and Kutash (13) suggest exploration of a Stress Reduction Hypothesis (SRH), in place of the Tension Reduction Hypothesis. The SRH posits that drinking may occur for the relief of varied stress states individually and/or in combination, e.g. anxiety, depression, and resentment, and that stress-relief drinking may contribute to increased usage and to eventual habituation and dependence.

Examination of the SRH involves more variables and is a more complex undertaking than exploration of the TRH. In the present study, an attempt is made to advance the investigation of the SRH through a reconceptualization of the constructs: stress, stressors, and stressor responses. Additionally, efforts are made, through clinical studies, to identify important parameters in stress-relief drinking and in the relation of stress-relief drinking to habituation and dependence.

STRESS DEFINED: DISTRESS, MESOSTRESS, EUSTRESS

In the past 50 years, there has been great progress in identifying the forms of stress and their varied effects. In the 1930s, Selye (14) adapted the term stress from physics to refer to the "wear and tear" on the body, and later used the term to refer to the "non-specific response of the body to any demand." Selye (14) observed that the term stress is often used to denote distress or negative stress. He pointed out that stress can also be experienced as positive or beneficial. He termed positive stress "Eustress" or "good" stress (Eu = Greek for good), as distinguished from distress or "bad" stress (Dis = Latin for bad).

Phenomenologically, however, stress is very frequently experienced as not particularly good or bad, positive or negative. Most of the events of everyday life are subjectively experienced as neither especially distressful or eustressful, yet in combination they may create considerable "wear and tear" on the individual. Unfortunately, this common, intermediate form of stress is often overlooked or ignored, especially in studies of substance abuse.

Mesostress is a term offered here to refer to the intermediate form of stress, which is a "middleground" between eustress and distress. Meso (from Greek, Mesos, middle) is a combining word meaning intermediate or in the middle (15). Schematically, the general construct stress may be viewed as composed of three subconstructs: eustress, mesostress, and distress.

The term mesostress refers to events that are experienced as not particularly good or bad, as well as events that are considered mildly positive or mildly negative. The term eustress denotes stress events ranging from mildly positive to extremely positive, and distress refers to events ranging from mildly negative to extremely negative or catastrophic (Figure 1). Ratings of degrees or levels of eustress, mesostress, and distress may be made with ordinal rating scales and statistically analyzed with ordinal level statistics (16).

Mesostress may involve a wide variety of intermediate demands upon the individual, including, most prominently: (1) performance of a multi-

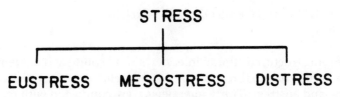

Figure 1. Three forms of stress.

tude of common daily tasks, where there is little positive or negative affect; (2) confronting minor frustrations or "hassles"; (3) appreciating minor accomplishments or "uplifts"; and (4) maintaining psychological defenses against internal or external conflicts or threats, both conscious and unconscious.

Mesostress, in the form of the "wear and tear" of common daily tasks, has been frequently overlooked or ignored in stress research, particularly in research on alcohol and drug use. Attention is most often focused on major life events (17) or on relatively intense and emotionally arousing stressors, such as electric shocks (18) and social evaluation (19). Many individuals, however, have reported a relation between the cumulative stressful effects of "everyday" demands and stress-relief drinking. A businessman, for example, may routinely have a few drinks at lunch to "ease the pressures of the day," without feeling especially bad (distress) or good (eustress). Homemakers, similarly, may have one or more drinks at dinner to "unwind" after a busy day of child care. Shopworkers, on a Friday evening, may have several drinks to "put the week behind them."

Other forms of mesostress, daily hassles and uplifts, have begun to receive attention from Kanner, Coyne, Schaefer, et al. (20). Although those investigators have developed a scale to measure the stressful impact of hassles and uplifts, no efforts as yet appear to have been made to use the scale in relation to stress-relief drinking.

Further sources of mesostress—psychological defenses—have, of course, received considerable attention, particularly in the psychoanalytic literature (21). The frequent wearing or "draining" effects of maintaining psychological defenses has been well recognized (22). When defenses, such as repression, are working well, an individual may experience little subjective discomfort or emotional arousal. Yet the psychological demands of maintaining such defenses against internal and external threats may well be considerable. To date, little attempt appears to have been made to relate stress-relief drinking to stress resulting from maintaining defenses.

CLINICAL DATA ON FORMS OF STRESS-RELIEF
DRINKING

Sixty semistructured clinical interviews were conducted to identify the relative occurrence of three forms of stress-relief drinking: distress, mesostress, and eustress. Thirty interviews were conducted with male alcohol dependent patients in an Alcohol Treatment Program, in a Veterans Administration Medical Center; and 30 interviews were conducted with male, nonproblem or "social" drinkers, who were patients on medical wards of the Center. The average ages of the two groups of patients were 47.6 years and 53.4 years respectively.

Each patient was read the following definition of stress and its three forms, and also was shown Figure 1.

> Stress consists of life demands and the reactions or responses to those demands. Stress may be experienced as negative, as positive, or as not particularly positive or negative, depending on how the life demands are evaluated and responded to. There are three primary forms of stress. *Distress* involves negatively evaluated life experiences, ranging from extremely negative, such as death of a child, to moderately negative, such as loss of a job. *Eustress* entails positively evaluated demand experiences, ranging from moderately positive, such as a promotion, to extremely positive, such as a marriage engagement. *Mesostress* consists of many demands that range from mildly negative "hassles," such as a flat tire, through daily tasks, such as grocery shopping, to mildly positive "uplifts," such as friends unexpectedly stopping over for dinner. Different persons may experience similar life demands very differently, depending upon how they evaluate them and respond to them. One individual could experience a job promotion as eustressful (positive), as providing greatly desired new responsibilities, money, and prestige; and another individual could view a promotion as distressful (negative), because of increased work loads; while a third person could consider a promotion as mesostressful (not especially positive or negative), because it had been expected and already adjusted to.

Discussion or amplification of the stress definitions was provided, as appropriate. Each patient was then asked whether he had ever drunk alcohol to try to relieve any of the three forms of stress and, if so, was asked to describe the circumstances or provide an example.

The semistructured interviews are an initial step in a program of research to explore the three forms of stress-relief drinking. The data provide preliminary information on whether individuals can meaningfully distinguish three different general forms of stress and stress-relief drinking. Also, the data provide initial information on the rank order of the occurrence of the three forms of stress-relief drinking. Results of the interviews, discussed below, should be viewed in terms of their heuristic value. Efforts are currently in progress to develop a questionnaire that will determine more fully the frequency and amount of forms of stress-relief drinking.

In the present interviews, the patients appeared to have little difficulty comprehending the distinctions among the three forms of stress and making judgments regarding stress-relief drinking. The patients' responses, of course, represented their conscious memories of the motives for their drinking. The conscious memories are highly important in that they represent how the patients view themselves and how they tend to perceive drinking situations. In this respect, the patients' responses can be considered self-statements of one major motive for drinking—stress relief. Patients may have engaged in stress-relief drinking for unconscious or preconscious motives and failed to report the drinking as related to stress relief. The self-reports of patients in the present study thus are conservative regarding stress relief. Considerable additional stress-relief drinking may have occurred of which the patients were consciously unaware. In other studies, attempts should be made to determine the occurrence of unconscious motives for stress-relief drinking, possibly through psychodynamically oriented interviews/psychotherapy sessions and/or use of projective assessment instruments.

Results of the interviews showed mesostress to be the most common form of stress-relief drinking for both nonproblem drinkers and alcohol-dependent individuals. For the 30 nonproblem drinkers, 18 (60%) individuals reported mesostress relief drinking as compared to 12 (40%) for eustress, and only 4 (13%) for distress. For the 30 alcohol-dependent individuals, 16 (53%) patients acknowledged mesostress relief drinking, *before* alcohol began to cause problems, compared to 12 (40%) for eustress, and 12 (40%) for distress. For the same 30 individuals, 25 (83%) indicated mesostress-relief drinking, *after* alcohol had begun to cause them problems, as contrasted with 24 (80%) for distress and 14 (47%) for eustress. It should be remembered that the above self-reports are based on conscious awareness and recall. It is quite possible that additional stress-relief drinking occurred that was not available to consciousness or not recalled.

Statistical analyses with the chi-square test (16) showed that a significantly greater number of alcohol-dependent patients indicated distress-relief drinking than did nonproblem drinkers, for both the periods before ($p < .05$) and after ($p < .01$) alcohol had begun to cause problems. Also, a significantly ($p < .05$) greater number of alcohol-dependent patients reported distress-relief drinking after alcohol had begun to cause problems, as compared to before the problems.

The above findings confirm that mesostress-relief drinking is a very common form of stress-relief drinking for both nonproblem drinkers and alcohol-dependent individuals. As noted above, alcoholism researchers have generally overlooked or ignored intermediate forms of stress, in focusing on more salient forms of distress and, in some cases, eustress. Further attention clearly needs to be given to intermediate stress forms. Investigation of daily "hassles" and "uplifts" in respect to drinking would be a good starting point, possibly utilizing Kanner et al.'s measures (20) for those forms of stress.

The finding that alcohol-dependent individuals reported more distress-relief drinking than nonproblem drinkers has implications for treatment interventions. Distress-relief drinking may serve as a marker for identifying individuals with a heightened potential for problem drinking. Individuals acknowledging distress-relief drinking could be offered particular assistance in clarifying the role of alcohol in their lives, especially in respect to possible progression in the amount and/or frequency of drinking and in the development of a variety of alcohol-related problems. To more firmly establish distress-relief drinking as an identifying sign for problem drinkers, the present study needs to be replicated with a wide range of populations.

A greater number of alcohol-dependent patients reported distress-relief drinking from the period before compared to the period after alcohol had begun to cause problems. It may be that stress-relief drinking contributed to the development of alcohol problems and to eventual alcohol habituation and dependence. It may also be, however, that drinking for reasons other than stress relief also contributed to the development of alcohol problems and that these problems, in turn, resulted in more stress-relief drinking.

Eustress- and mesostress-relief drinking may be important contributors in the development of distress-relief drinking and in the progression of alcohol dependence, but the data are correlational, and no judgments may be made yet on possible causal effects. Eustress- and mesostress-relief drinking may provide an opportunity to "practice" or directly experience stress-relief effects of alcohol, just as marijuana use may provide "practice" or experience in altered psychoactive states that is strongly associated with the development of other drug use, such as heroin abuse (23). In both stress-relief drinking and marijuana use, it is important to document strong associations to other alcohol and drug use. But it is equally important to recognize that eustress- and mesostress-relief drinking do not constitute necessary and sufficient conditions for distress-relief drinking or the development of alcohol dependence, just as marijuana use does not constitute such conditions for other drug use. As a guide to further investigation of the association between stress and alcohol, the Stress Reduction Hypothesis will now be examined, particularly in respect to stress-relief drinking and progression in drinking behaviors.

STRESS REDUCTION HYPOTHESIS

The Stress Reduction Hypothesis (SRH) described above must be refined in respect to clinical findings. Individuals clearly may drink for the relief of some forms of stress (e.g., mesostress), but not others (e.g., distress and eustress). The SRH, as revised, may be stated: Individuals may drink for the relief of some forms of stress and perhaps not others, and the relief of those forms of stress through drinking tends to perpetuate the drinking behaviors. The SRH recognizes, implicitly, that varying stressors may impact the individual over time, and that the total or combined effects of the stressors and stressor responses may have differing effects on stress-relief drinking. In different settings, especially drinking situations, over a period of time, there may be important changes in the total sets of stressors and stressor responses experienced by the individual.

In order to better understand the varying sets of stressors and stressor responses influencing the individual, it is helpful to consider two terms—stressor manifold, and stressor response manifold. In a previous clinical study, Powers and Kutash (24) proposed the term "Stressor Manifold" to represent the array of stressors impacting an individual simultaneously or in very close sequence. The term stressor here refers to all stimuli—external and internal, physical and mental, conscious and unconscious—that elicit stressor responses. As an illustration, a stressor manifold for a "composite" alcohol-dependent patient is presented in Figure 2. The stressors chosen for illustration are a composite from different alcohol-dependent patients treated by the author in individual psychotherapy. The manifold identifies salient stressors that could impact upon a patient at any one moment. Undoubtedly, for an individual patient, other stressors that were unperceived or unreported by the patient and/or the therapist would be having additional impacts.

The term "Stressor Response Manifold" was proposed (24) to refer to

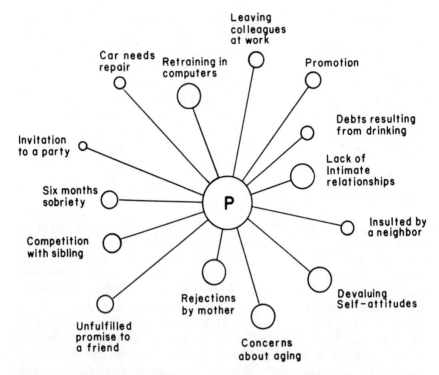

Figure 2. *Stressor Manifold* illustrating possible stressors having an impact on an individual simultaneously or in close sequence. *P* represents a person, and each circle represents a stressor. The larger the circle, the more intense the stressor.

the varied responses to stressors that an individual may experience either simultaneously or in very close sequence. The term "stressor response" refers here to the wide variety of physiological, cognitive/affective, and behavioral responses that may be experienced by an individual. As an example, Figure 3 represents the partial stressor response manifold corresponding to the stressor manifold of the composite patient referred to above, in Figure 2.

An individual's appraisal of stressors is crucial to the stressor responses and forms of stress experienced (25). As illustrated in the composite case above, an individual may perceive the opportunity for retraining in computers and the accompanying promotion as a very great stressor, but as basically very positive (eustress). Other individuals could well perceive such a stressor as just another work demand (mesostress), while still others could view it as very disruptive and basically negative (distress).

Stress is an ongoing process, not simply a single, discrete event. An individual may begin to drink for relief of one form of stress, such as mesostress in attending an office party. Then, as new stressors are experienced, such as receiving word at the party that his/her promotion had been denied (distress), he/she may continue to drink for relief of eustress and may or may not begin to drink to relieve the other forms of stress. For individuals with alcohol problems, there is the added possibility that drinking for one form of stress, such as mesostress, can quickly result in other forms of stress, such as distress from the disapproval and rejection by a spouse or other persons.

The effects of stress-relief drinking are thus likely to be quite variable, due to changes in the stressor and stressor response manifolds. At times, he/she might experience stress relief; at other times, with increased stressors during the drinking, he/she may very well experience increased stress.

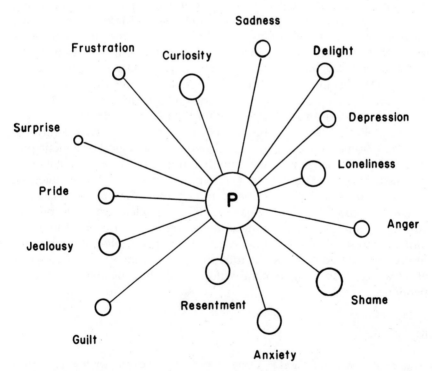

Figure 3. *Stressor Response Manifold* illustrating possible stressor responses experienced simultaneously or in close sequence. *P* represents a person, and each circle represents a stressor response. The larger the circle, the more intense the stressor response.

In stress-relief drinking, many factors may help reinforce drinking and contribute to habituation and dependence. Intermittent reinforcement may be especially important. As has been noted, drinking may at times result in a decrease in stress, but at other times may result in no change or an increase. Intermittent reinforcement, as Skinner (26) among others has well documented, is generally more powerful as a conditioner than continuous reinforcement. Paradoxically, then, the SRH, when viewed from a perspective of intermittent reinforcement, would predict a more powerful conditioning effect than would be predicted for continuous reinforcement. Thus, the fact that at times individuals do not experience expected stress relief when drinking could result in a greater reinforcement of drinking behaviors than if they experienced stress relief each time.

Modeling effects may also play a role in perpetuating stress-relief drinking. An individual may observe others drinking for stress relief and may consciously or unconsciously try to imitate them (27). Advertising may be especially influential in modeling effects. Many television ads, for example, portray drinking for relief of mesostress or eustress. A series of Budweiser ads, for instance, shows different workmen, at the end of a hard day, gathered in a tavern for a few relaxing beers (mesostress relief). Several Michelob ads show persons competing hard at various sports for a few social drinks (eustress relief). However, no ads that I know of portray or promote drinking for the relief of distress.

Stress relief, of course, is but one of many factors that may contribute to habituation and dependence on alcohol. Physiological or genetic predispositions (28, 29) may be particularly influential. Environmental influences, such as peer pressure, may also play a role (30, 31). Psychological issues, such as deficits in self-esteem, additionally may be related to increased alcohol use and abuse (32, 33). It is clear from the present study that stress-relief drinking is quite common, in each of its three forms: distress relief, mesostress relief, and eustress relief. It remains for future studies to determine the full extent of the roles of the three forms of stress-relief drinking as contributors to alcohol habituation and dependence.

REFERENCES

1. Farber P, Khavari K, Douglas F: A factor analytic study of reasons for drinking: Empirical validation of positive and negative reinforcement dimensions. J Consult Clin Psychol 48:780–781, 1980
2. Deardorff CM, Melges FT, Hout CN, et al: Situations related to drinking alcohol: A

factor analysis of questionnaire responses. J Stud Alcohol 36:1184–1195, 1975
3. Wanberg K: Prevalence of symptoms among excessive drinkers. Int J Addict 4:169–185, 1969
4. Masserman JH, Yum KS: An analysis of the influence of alcohol on experimental neuroses in cats. Psychosom Med 8:36–52, 1946
5. Conger JJ: The effects of alcohol on conflict behavior in the albino rat. Q J Stud Alcohol 12:1–29, 1951
6. Marlatt GA: Alcohol, stress, and cognitive control, in Stress and Anxiety, vol 3. Edited by Sarason IG, Spielberger CD. New York, John Wiley & Sons, 1976
7. Cappell H: An evaluation of tension models of alcohol consumption, in Research Advances in Alcohol and Drug Problems II. Edited by Gibbins RJ. New York, John Wiley & Sons, 1975
8. Williams AF: The alcoholic personality, in The Biology of Alcoholism, vol 4: Social Aspects of Alcoholism. Edited by Kissin B, Begleiter H. New York, Plenum, 1976
9. Mendelson JH, LaDou J, Soloman P: Experimentally induced chronic intoxication and withdrawal in alcoholics, part 3, psychiatric findings. Q J Stud Alcohol Supplement 2:40–52, 1964
10. Vanicelli M: Mood and self-perception of alcoholics when sober and intoxicated. Q J Stud Alcohol 33:341–357, 1972
11. Holroyd KA: Effects of social anxiety and social evaluation on beer consumption and social interaction. J Stud Alcohol 39:737–744, 1978
12. Miller PM, Hersen M, Eisler RM, et al: Effects of social stress on operant drinking of alcoholics and social drinkers. Behav Res Ther 12:67–72, 1974
13. Powers RJ, Kutash IL: Stress and alcohol. Int J Addict 20:461–482, 1985
14. Selye H: The stress of life. New York, McGraw Hill, 1956
15. Websters Third New International Dictionary. Springfield, MA, G & C Merriam Company, 1976
16. Siegel S: Nonparametric statistics for the behavioral sciences. New York, McGraw Hill, 1956
17. Morrissey ER, Schuckit MA: Stressful life events and alcohol problems among women seen at a detoxication center. J Stud Alcohol 39:1559–1578, 1978
18. Vogel-Sprott M: Alcohol effects on human behavior under reward and punishment. Psychopharmacologia 11:337–344, 1967
19. Wilson GT, Abrams DB, Lipscomb TR: Effects of intoxication levels and drinking pattern on social anxiety in men. J Stud Alcohol 41:250–264, 1980
20. Kanner AD, Coyne JC, Schaefer C, et al: Comparison of two modes of stress measurement: Daily hassles and uplifts versus major life events. J Behav Med 4:1–39, 1980
21. Freud A: The ego and the mechanisms of defense. New York, International Universities Press, 1966
22. Fenichel O: The psychoanalytic theory of neurosis. New York, W W Norton & Co, 1945
23. Platt JJ, Labate C: Heroin addiction: Theory, research, and treatment. New York, John Wiley & Sons, 1976
24. Powers RJ, Kutash IL: Alcohol abuse and anxiety, in Handbook on Stress and Anxiety. Edited by Kutash IL, Schlesinger LB. San Francisco, Jossey-Bass, 1981
25. Lazarus RS: Psychological stress and the coping process. New York, McGraw Hill, 1966
26. Skinner BF: The behavior of organisms. New York, Appleton Century, 1938
27. Bandura A: Social learning theory. Englewood Cliffs, NJ, Prentice Hall, 1977
28. Rodgers DA: Factors underlying differences in alcohol preferences of inbred strains of mice, in the Biology of Alcoholism, vol 2, Physiology and Behavior. Edited by Kissin B, Begleiter H. New York, Plenum, 1972
29. Winokur G: Alcoholism III: Diagnoses and familial psychiatric illness in 259 alcoholic probands. Arch Gen Psychiatry 23:104–111, 1970
30. Madsen W: The American alcoholic: The nature nurture controversy in alcoholic research and therapy. Springfield IL, Charles C Thomas, 1974

31. Cahalan D, Cisin IH: Drinking behaviors and drinking problems in the United States, in The Biology of Alcoholism, vol 3, Social Aspects of Alcoholism. Edited by Kissin B, Begleiter H. New York, Plenum, 1976
32. Clare AW: The causes of alcoholism, in Alcoholism in Perspective. Edited by Grant M, Gwinner P. Baltimore, University Park Press, 1979
33. Heinemann ME, Smith-DiJulio K: Assessment and care of the chronically ill alcoholic person, in Alcoholism: Development, Consequences, and Interventions. Edited by Estes NJ, Heinemann EM. St Louis, CV Mosby Company, 1977

18

Stressful Events and Human Drinking Behavior: The Role of Contextual Variables

JALIE A. TUCKER

Research concerned with stress-reduction accounts of human alcohol consumption suggests that an adequate description of how stressful events influence consumption requires consideration of the context within which the event and the consumption occurs. A conceptual framework based on behavioral theories of choice is presented within which the notion of drinking contexts may be formulated. This approach points to changing constraints on access to valued activities as an important property of stressful events with respect to the relationship between such events and drinking behavior. Research derived from this approach is presented, and implications for accounts of human alcohol consumption are discussed.

The notion that enthanol reduces aversive internal states, such as tension or anxiety, has been a directive framework within which much research has been conducted on the effects and determinants of human alcohol consumption. Several reviews (1, 2, 3) of this substantial empirical literature, however, have clearly indicated that a straightforward Ten-

Manuscript preparation was supported in part by Grant Nos. 1-P50-AA05793 and 1-R01-AA06122 from the National Institute on Alcohol Abuse and Alcoholism.

sion Reduction Hypothesis of human drinking behavior is unlikely to be adequate. Consistent empirical support has not been obtained for the related hypotheses (a) that alcohol consumption decreases various self-report, physiological, and behavioral measures of stress, anxiety, or other negative emotional states, and (b) that human or animal subjects self-administer ethanol in response to event occurrences that presumably induce such states.

Despite the equivocal support obtained for tension-reduction formulations, it seems clear that stressful events and negative emotional states bear some relationship to human alcohol consumption, at least on some occasions for some individuals. Several studies of the determinants of alcoholic relapse after treatment (4, 5, 6, 7) implicated negative emotional states or the occurrence of stressful events in 40%–50% of reported relapse occurrences. Laboratory analogue studies on the determinants of human alcohol consumption (8, 9) have also observed increased enthanol intake in response to stressful interpersonal events. However, similar laboratory studies that employed other types of stressful events (e.g., threat of electric shock or intellectual performance evaluation) did not consistently demonstrate increased consumption (10, 11, 12). Conversely, studies of the effects of alcohol administration on various self-report and physiological indices of anxiety or stress found evidence supporting either stress-reducing (13), stress-inducing (14), or no effect on subjects' levels of stress or anxiety (15). The variable results of these latter studies generally suggested that different drinking or experimental situations elicited different emotional responses to alcohol administration.

This body of research further suggests that relationships between stress and alcohol consumption are difficult to explicate unless the surrounding environmental conditions, or context, is also considered. This notion is certainly not new in the alcohol or drug literature (15, 16, 17). To date, however, concern with context variables has often been post hoc when experimental findings have been inconsistent with predictions based on tension-reduction or related hypotheses. Or, attention has been focused on the effects of environmental variables on some internal mediational state of the drinker, as in cognitive labeling explanations of the effects of alcohol (15, 18).

The remainder of this paper describes an alternative approach based on behavioral theories of choice (19) that is directly concerned with the role of contextual variables in human drinking behavior. Data are presented from a program of research (20, 21, 22), conducted collaboratively with Rudy E. Vuchinich, that is aimed at applying these concepts to an analysis of the determinants of alcohol consumption.

The impetus for pursuing this approach arose from the previously noted inconsistencies in studies concerned with the role of stressful events or negative emotional states as determinants of human alcohol consumption. Although many individuals appear to consume alcohol in response to stressful events or negative emotional states, these same persons clearly do not do so in response to all stressful event occurrences, despite the ready availability of alcohol in most environments. Thus, it seemed reasonable to ask: What dimensional properties of event occurrences other than their emotional consequences might also be related to individuals' choice of consuming alcoholic beverages over other available behavioral alternatives? Although the emotional consequences of events certainly appear to correlate with drinking behavior under some circumstances, this relationship is an imperfect predictor at best. Other dimensional qualities of events might both better predict alcohol consumption and reflect the controlling variables of individuals' drinking behavior.

At a general level, our approach to this issue has focused on developing a way to characterize the circumstances, or context, surrounding event occurrences that do and do not lead to alcohol consumption. As summarized in Vuchinich and Tucker (20), we assumed that like all reinforcing events capable of maintaining behavior—including basic ones such as food and water—alcohol consumption will be reinforcing only under certain circumstances, or contexts, that are defined by the conditions that surround consumption. The task at hand, then, is to distinguish those contexts in which alcohol will and will not be a reinforcer.

In the previous literature concerned with the reinforcing value of alcohol consumption, the dimensions typically used to define the contexts in which alcohol consumption will be a reinforcing event have been heavily influenced by neobehavioral learning theories (23) and their extension to areas of clinical importance (24). Specifically, those contexts usually have been defined along dimensions that involve various internal states of the drinker that are modified by alcohol at the time of consumption. The Tension Reduction Hypothesis of alcohol consumption is perhaps the best known example of this approach, but there have been many other internal states postulated to provide the context within which alcohol consumption will be a reinforcing event. Examples of these include states of increased self-awareness (3), decreased personal power (25), and decreased personal control (2).

The important point here, however, is that the available research does not favor one particular state hypothesis over the others. In many respects, this is unfortunate because our task would be considerably simplified if we could reliably measure characteristics of individual drinkers, such as their levels of anxiety or stress, to account for their drinking behavior, instead of having to concern ourselves with a characterization of the seemingly myriad events and environments that surround consumption. Equally important, the neobehavioral views of reinforcement that underlie these state hypotheses of drinking behavior have been seriously questioned in recent years in the basic experimental literature (19, 26), and these changes are exemplified by work on behavioral theories of choice (19, 27). The research summarized here (20, 21, 22) applied this strategy to an analysis of the determinants of human alcohol consumption.

Behavioral theories of choice are generally concerned with providing a molar account of how an organism's behavior is allocated among a set of available activities as a function of parameters of the contingencies of reinforcement associated with those activities. The subject's allocation of behavior to the alternative activities is related to parameters of the consequences, such as the type and amount of reinforcer, and to the constraints imposed to gain access to the consequences, such as the response requirement and the delay of receipt of the consequences. The relative amount of behavior allocated to gain access to a particular behavioral alternative is considered a measure of its reinforcing value.

As applied to human alcohol consumption, the task at hand becomes one of distinguishing those contexts in which alcohol emerges from among the totality of available activities as the preferred activity. This approach further suggests that an analysis of those contexts might begin by defining them along two dimensions. The first pertains to the direct constraints imposed on access to alcohol. Several studies have shown, for example, that consumption decreases when the response requirement or "cost" to obtain it increases (28). The second concerns activities other than alcohol consumption that are available and the constraints imposed on access to them. This second class of variables has received less research attention, but, as articulated by Vuchinich and Tucker (20), an argument can be made that they may be the more important set of determinants. In most natural environments, there seem to be few, relatively minor direct constraints on access to alcohol, such as the time and money required to obtain and consume it. Thus, the situation may be characterized as involving relatively minor and invariant constraints on access to alcohol, but substantial variability in alcohol consumption both within and across individuals. This generally suggests that reinforcers other than alcohol and constraints on their access may be critical variables to investigate.

Two variables that have been found to influence choice behavior are (a) amount of reward available per unit of behavioral allocation, and (b) the delay in receipt of reward from the time of choice. The probability of choice of a given behavioral alternative increases with amount and decreases with delay (27). Choices between a small, immediately available reward and larger rewards available after a delay have provided a useful scheme for investigating self-control, and alcohol consumption is readily cast within this framework: Alcohol is viewed as the smaller reward that is immediately available, whereas rewards gained from other activities, such as income from employment, are viewed as the larger, delayed rewards. Thus, individuals' preference for alcohol should increase as the latter rewards become smaller, less accessible, or more delayed.

We investigated these hypotheses in two laboratory experiments with normal drinkers (20, 21) and have completed a field study from this perspective on the determinants of relapse in alcoholics after their discharge from inpatient treatment (22). In both laboratory studies, 50–60 male normal drinkers participated individually in a single experimental session that involved a choice situation with two behavioral alternatives; one produced access to alcohol consumption, and one produced access to money. By responding on an operant, button-press task with a change-over key that registered points on two separate response counters, subjects could respond to earn points that were delivered on two concurrent variable-interval 20-second schedules of reinforcement. One counter registered points earned for alcohol consumption, and the other counter registered points earned for money. In both experiments, any alcohol chosen was available during the session following the 20-minute choice procedure, and constraints on access to it were held constant.

Both experiments manipulated two independent variables in a 2×3 factorial design that involved constraints on access to money. In the first study, the independent variables were (a) amount of money available per unit of behavioral allocation (either 2 cents or 10 cents) and (b) delay in receipt of the money from the time of choice (either no delay, 2-week delay, or 8-week delay). Points earned on both the alcohol and money counters were directly related to the amounts received of each commodity. In the second study, an identical design and method were used except for one change in the independent variable manipulation of money amount. Instead of responding on the button-press task to receive direct access to money, subjects responded to earn points towards subsequent opportunities to win money on a second, probabilistic dice-throwing task, to which they had been exposed before the choice procedures. The number of points earned on the money counter determined the number of dice rolls the subjects received after the choice procedure. Outcomes on the task were manipulated at two probabilistic levels (20% or 80%

probability of a "win"), as dictated by certain combinations of dice roll outcomes. The three levels of the delay of receipt of any money received were the same as in the first study. In both studies, the primary dependent measure was the proportion of subjects' responses that were allocated to gain access to alcohol consumption. It was predicted that preference for alcohol consumption would vary negatively with the amount of money available and positively with the delay of receipt of the money.

The results of Experiment 1 supported both hypotheses, as evidenced by significant main effects for both the amount and delay variables on the measure of subjects' preference for alcohol. Consistent with the hypotheses, subjects' preferences for alcohol were negatively related to the amount of alternative reward available and positively related to the delay of receiving the reward from the time of choice. In Experiment 2, the results for the delay variable were replicated, but the predicted effects for the probabilistic amount of money variable were only marginally significant ($p = .10$), though the means were in the predicted direction.

These findings support the present analysis of the determinants of drinking as involving choices between an immediately available, "small" reward (alcohol consumption) and "larger," more delayed rewards that can be gained by engaging in alternative behavioral activities. The somewhat discrepant findings in the two studies for the different amount manipulations suggest that certain, rather than probabilistic, outcomes are of greater reinforcement value, as measured by subjects' relative preferences at the two levels of the different amount manipulations.

In addition to the main choice findings, in both studies we collected self-report measures of subjects' emotional state using the Mood Adjective Check List (29), which yields 12 mood factors including an anxiety factor. Analyses of subjects' mood ratings, which were obtained before and after the experimental procedures, failed to yield results that would suggest that a tension-reduction or frustration-reduction process may have mediated their choice behavior. Correlational analyses between subjects' mood scores and their alcohol preference scores also failed to substantiate a tension-reduction formulation.

We also have completed a clinical study of the determinants of alcoholic relapse from this perspective, which yielded correlational data relevant to this type of analysis. The study involved 6-month follow-up procedures with 26 alcoholics after their discharge from an abstinence-oriented inpatient treatment program at the Gainesville Veterans Administration Medical Center. Prior to their discharge from treatment, subjects were interviewed using the Drinking Problem Scales developed by Cahalan (30) to assess the degree to which subjects' past drinking behavior had disrupted their functioning in the life-health areas of (a) intimate relations, (b) family relations, (c) social relations, (d) vocational functioning, (e) finances, and (f) physical health. After discharge, subjects kept daily records for 6 months of any alcohol consumed, the number of situations they encountered in which alcohol was available, and the occurrence of life-events. From the perspective of behavioral theories of choice, the main hypotheses were: (a) relapses would be associated with entry into situations in which alcohol was immediately available; (b) relapses would likely be associated with event occurrences that signalled a decreased probability of rewards in life-health areas that had previously been disrupted by alcohol consumption; and (c) relapses associated with events that signalled decreased availability of future rewards would be relatively more severe than those associated with mere alcohol availability.

During the 6-month study period, the 26 subjects reported 271 events and 133 relapse episodes. Independent raters classified each relapse episode as either event- or nonevent-related (i.e., one or more life-events did or did not occur within three days of the relapse, respectively); each event occurrence was classified as pertaining to one of the six life-health areas assessed by the Cahalan scales and as being either a positive or negative event. The results of primary interest concern correlations between the portion of event occurrences in each life-health area that were associated with relapses and subjects' pretreatment scores on the six Drinking Problem Scales, which assessed the degree to which alcohol consumption had previously disrupted their functioning in each area. These correlational analyses were significant in the predicted direction in the life-health areas of intimate relations, family-related events, and vocational events; the more disruption in these life-health areas that subjects had previously experienced due to drinking, the greater the probability that, after treatment, events in that area would be associated with a relapse. This relationship was not found for the other life-health classes.

A second result of interest concerned the predicted difference in the severity of relapses associated with events that signalled a decreased probability of receipt of future rewards in a given area of life-health compared to relapses that merely involved an increased availability of alcoholic beverages. For the 15 subjects who reported both types of relapses, comparisons showed that, as hypothesized, relapses were more severe in terms of the quantity and duration of subjects' alcohol consumption for those associated with events that signalled a decreased probability of receipt of future rewards compared with relapses associated only with increased alcohol availability.

Overall, the results from the relapse study provide additional correlational evidence for an analysis of the determinants of human alcohol consumption based on behavioral theories of choice. From the data available, we are encouraged to pursue this approach to characterizing the contexts in which alcohol consumption may emerge from the totality of available activities as the preferred activity. Life events clearly bear an important relationship to drinking behavior; but instead of focusing primarily on their emotional or stress-inducing consequences, we have thus far found it useful to also inquire about the meaning of such events for individuals in terms of what they signal about the availability of future rewards in important areas of life-health functioning. It is not yet clear whether an approach based on behavioral theories of choice will eventually yield a more adequate account of human alcohol consumption than one based on earlier tension-reduction formulations. Nevertheless, this approach appears to provide a useful preliminary framework within which to begin conceptualizing and investigating the role of contextual variables in human drinking behavior.

REFERENCES

1. Cappell H: An evaluation of tension reduction models of alcohol consumption, in Research Advances in Alcohol and Drug Problems (vol 2). Edited by Gibbons RJ, et al. New York, Wiley, 1975
2. Marlatt GA: Alcohol, stress, and cognitive control, in Stress and Anxiety (vol 3). Edited by Sarason IG, Spielberger CD. Washington, DC, Hemisphere, 1976
3. Hull JG: A self-awareness model of the causes and effects of alcohol consumption. J Abnorm Psychol 90:586–600, 1981
4. Chaney EF, O'Leary MR, Marlatt GA: Skill training with alcoholics. J Consult Clin Psychol 46:1092–1104, 1978
5. Hore BD: Life events and alcoholic relapse. Brit J Addict 66:83–88, 1971(a)
6. Hore BD: Factors in alcoholic relapse. Brit J Addict 66:89–96, 1971(b)
7. Marlatt GA: Craving for alcohol, loss of control, and relapse: A cognitive-behavioral model, in Alcoholism: New Directions in Behavioral Research and Treatment. Edited by Nathan PE, Marlatt GA, Loberg T. New York, Plenum, 1978
8. Higgins RL, Marlatt GA: Fear of interpersonal evaluation as a determinant of alcohol consumption in male social drinkers. J Abnorm Psychol 84:644–651, 1975
9. Miller PM, Hersen M, Eisler RM, et al: Effects of social stress on operant drinking of alcoholics and social drinkers. Behav Res Ther 12:67–72, 1974
10. Higgins RL, Marlatt GA: The effects of anxiety arousal on the consumption of alcohol by alcoholics and social drinkers. J Consult Clin Psychol 41:426–433, 1973
11. Holroyd KA: Effects of social anxiety and social evaluation on beer consumption and social interaction. J Stud Alcohol 39:737–744, 1978
12. Tucker JA, Vuchinich RE, Sobell MB, et al: Normal drinkers' alcohol consumption as a function of conflicting motives induced by intellectual performance stress. Addict Behav 5:171–178, 1980
13. Polivy J, Schueneman AL, Carlson K: Alcohol and tension reduction: Cognitive and

physiological effects. J Abnorm Psychol 85:595–600, 1976
14. Dengerink HA, Fagan NJ: Effect of alcohol on emotional responses to stress. J Stud Alcohol 39:525–539, 1978
15. Vuchinich RE, Tucker JA, Sobell MB: Alcohol, expectancy, cognitive labeling, and mirth. J Abnorm Psychol 88:641–651, 1979
16. Pliner P, Cappell, H: Modification of the affective consequences of alcohol: A comparison of social and solitary drinking. J Abnorm Psychol 83:418–425, 1974
17. Tucker JA, Maisto SA, Vuchinich RE, et al: Alcohol and anxiety: The role of drinking context, expectancy, and sex of subject. Behav Psychother 7:75–84, 1979
18. Vuchinich RE, Tucker JA: A critique of cognitive labeling explanations of the emotional and behavioral effects of alcohol. Addict Behav 5:171–178, 1980
19. Rachlin H, Battalio R, Kagel J, et al: Maximization theory in behavioral psychology. Brain Behav Sci 4:371–417, 1981
20. Vuchinich RE, Tucker JA: Behavioral theories of choice as a framework for studying drinking behavior. J Abnorm Psychol 92:408–416, 1983
21. Vuchinich RE, Tucker JA, Rudd EJ: Preference for alcohol consumption as a function of amount and delay of alternative reward. J Abnorm Psychol (in press)
22. Vuchinich RE, Tucker JA, McNeil D, Hoon E: Determinants of alcoholic relapse. Paper presented at the meeting of the Association for the Advancement of Behavior Therapy, Washington, DC, November, 1983
23. Hull CL: Principles of Behavior. New York, Appleton-Century, 1943
24. Bandura A: Social Learning Theory. Englewood Cliffs, NJ, Prentice-Hall, 1977
25. McClelland DC, Davis WN, Kalin R, et al (eds): The Drinking Man. New York, Free Press, 1972
26. Herrnstein RJ: On the law of effect. J Exp Anal Behav 13:243–266, 1970
27. Ainslie G: Specious reward: A behavioral theory of impulsiveness and impulse control. Psychol Bull 82:463–469, 1975
28. Bigelow G, Griffiths R, Liebson I: Experimental models for the modification of human drug self-administration. Federation Proc 34:1785–1792, 1975
29. Nowlis V: Research on the Mood Adjective Check List, in Affect, Cognition, and Personality: Empirical Studies. Edited by Tomkins SS, Izard CE. New York, Springer, 1965
30. Cahalan D: Problem Drinkers: A National Survey. San Francisco, Jossey-Bass, 1970

19

Stress and Stages of Addiction

DAN J. LETTIERI

This paper suggests that both stress and the addiction cycle have their own characteristic form of expression but no particular, specific cause. Any stimulus can serve as a stressor; any stressor can act as a causal factor in propelling the individual through progressive stages of the addiction cycle. Phenomenological models may afford us the most fruition in future research. In treating alcoholism, it is necessary to understand the feedback loops which entrap the user into potentially intractable behavioral repertoires. These loops may entrap the clinician and can diminish therapeutic satisfaction and effectiveness.

In his famed autobiographical novel of 1862, entitled *The House of the Dead*, Dostoevski wrote "acute consciousness is no cure for neurosis." One could easily substitute the words alcoholism or stress for neurosis.

In some respects this paper can be regarded as a prolegomenon to the conceptual links between stages of stress and cycles in addictive behaviors. In turn, it attempts to explore and occasionally dissect three focal

The views expressed herein do not necessarily reflect those of the Department of Health and Human Services, nor the National Institute on Alcohol Abuse and Alcoholism.

conceptions: stress, dedifferentiation, and addiction cycles. In sum, its form is topographic, its demeanor is lucubratory, and its intent, like a haiku, is to carry one's thoughts.

STRESS

For the substance abuse research field, accepting that stress may be the cause of the behavior may not allow us to fully understand, predict, or treat that behavior. Stress is a term with both excess and excessive meanings. It has been used as noun, verb, referent, and object, as well as cause and effect. It is, in fact, an omnibus concept, a catchall term. In many respects, it is a stressful concept.

It can signify antecedent, concomitant, or consequent factors. It is no pun to say it is omnipresent and tautological. The term stress has been used tautologically to refer both to the external stimulus which produces a reaction and to the reaction itself. Consequently, a basic difficulty in working operationally with the term has been how to define it independently of the effects it produces. For Selye (1), among the first to technically define the term, stress referred to a syndrome, i.e., a set of physiological patterns or reactions which prepared the organism for either fight or flight. Specifically, Selye wrote that stress is "the state manifested by a specific syndrome which consists of all the nonspecifically induced changes within a biologic system" (1, p. 54). He remarked that we would have no way of knowing an individual were under stress unless the syndrome and its attendant changes were evidenced. Selye carefully defined the characteristics of the syndrome, such as increased adrenal hormone production, gastrointestinal ulcers, etc. He labeled the syndrome General Adaptation Syndrome or G.A.S. It is critical to understand that the stress syndrome is a specific one in that it is characteristic of stress and only stress, but is nonspecifically induced or caused since any and all forms of stressful stimulation will produce the same syndrome.

In this paper, stress refers to the stress syndrome and resides in the organism; stressors are sources of stressful stimulation. These usually reside outside the organism; however some stressors (e.g., internal hemorrhaging) can be inside the organism. Hence stressors may be either internal or external to the organism and may interact linearly or configurally (Figure 1).

Differentiating internal and external stressors is difficult. Thus, while drinking may diminish an external stressor (i.e., the drinker's perception

Organism   Environment

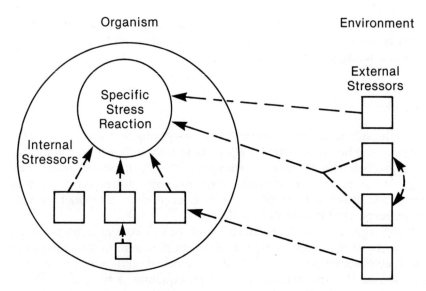

Figure 1. Internal and external stressors.

or recognition of it), drinking may in fact augment and increase internal physiological stressors (2). It is only by differentiating these two types of stressors that one can understand how drinking behavior both reduces and increases stress or tension.

In contrast to this usage of these terms, others (3) have used stress to refer to environmental stimuli and strain to refer to the internal stress syndrome. On the other hand, Lazarus (4) has argued that stress (whether positive or negative) resides neither in the environment nor in the person, although it may be interdependent with both; moreover stress arises from the adaptational relationships as it is appraised by the person. In this regard stress is best seen as a *transaction*. Note the word transaction to imply a mutually reciprocal relation between person and environment, rather than a linear, unidirectional relationship. Viewed as a transaction, both the person and the environment can, at once, be causes and effects of stress.

Finally, what if an individual does not respond to stressors? Does this mean he is resistant to stress or that the particular stressor was not idiosyncratically stressful? The work of Maher (5) shows that when subjects are allowed to define stress in their own way, there are none who do not react to stressors with a stress reaction. Noteworthy is the conclusion that no persons are immune to stress—the differences are presumably phenomenological, idiotropic, and socioenvironmentally determined.

In the language of industry, corporate liabilities resulting from stress are known as the five "As": alcoholism, absenteeism, accidents, apathy, and antagonism.

STAGES OF STRESS

Many experimental studies of stress may be flawed because the stressors are of very short duration. It is not implausible to suggest that (1) the stressors of everyday life go on over longer time periods than those induced in the laboratory, and (2) long-term vs. short-term stress reactions are probably qualitatively different. Selye outlines three stages in his general adaptation syndrome or stress reaction: (1) the Alarm Stage, (2) the Resistance Stage, and (3) Exhaustion. The alarm reaction is of relatively short duration wherein the individual's resources are alerted to deal with the stressors. The resistance stage can be of short or long duration and herein the body mobilizes to alleviate the stressors. If the individual does not reduce the stress and bodily resources are depleted, then Stage 3 ensues, the exhaustion stage, and death may be the inevitable outcome. Recently, Powers and Kutash (6) have adapted the terms to apply to alcohol-dependent persons. They cite three primary stages: (1) the demand stage, where the individual attempts to apply existing coping strategies; (2) the threat stage, where the individual is unable to apply existing coping strategies to meet the demands and attempts to marshal new ones; and (3) the exhaustion stage, in which the individual is unable to cope and experiences feelings of hopelessness and helplessness. At each stage of stress, progressive drinking may occur.

A host of reactions to stress can be observed, but four are of particular relevance here: (1) anger-out, (2) anger-in, (3) anxiety or fright, and (4) no reaction. A common reaction to stress is for the stressed individual to vent his anger out at the perceived cause of his stress; conversely, the anger may be directed inward whereby the stressed person blames himself for his plight. Anxiety and fright, or flight, is another reaction; however, some persons do not appear to react to apparently stressful stimuli. This latter observation demands we systematically describe the event and the individual's phenomenological perception of it before we can fully understand stress reactions and stressors. In fact, future research should examine the linkages between stress, anxiety, sensation-seeking, and self-awareness feedback loops. Some research indicates that persons with high sensation-seeking needs consume more alcohol than those with low sensation-seeking needs, and that there is no relationship between anxiety and alcohol consumption (7). Hull's (8) self-awareness model proposes that alcohol is an inhibitor of self-awareness processing, and as such offers the individual a feeling of psychological relief. More specifically, the model proposes that alcohol interferes with the individual's recognition of cues regarding appropriate behavior and the self-evaluative nature of *feedback* about past behaviors. One can only speculate that if feedback processing is impaired, then sensation-seeking needs may be affected.

The notions of anger-out and anger-in have been used to psychoanalytically explain homicide (viz., aggression turned outward) and suicide (aggression turned inward). But these terms also carry a passing resemblance to the description of alcoholics as passive aggressive.

DEDIFFERENTIATION

In exploring the relationship between stress and alcoholism behavior, it is heuristic to invoke the concept of differentiation. The concept of dedifferentiation has had other names such as psychological myopia or tunnel vision.

The concept of dedifferentiation can serve as an algorithm to resolve metric problems inherent in operationalizing the idiotropic aspects of perceived stress. Quite simply, it may be as utile to count the number of perceived stressors rather than try to scale each one in terms of degree or severity. Or more statistically elegant, to submit an individual's many perceived stressors to factor analytic rotation and reduction and count the number of significant factors as a metric to characterize the individual's generalized degree of differentiation or dedifferentiation.

In suicide research, Lettieri (9) and Neuringer and Lettieri (10) successfully employed such a metric. It was found that as the risk of suicide increased, the number of differentiated cognitive, affective, and attitudinal factors decreased; alternatively stated, suicide risk and dedifferentiation were positively correlated. Recently, in chemical dependency work, Bry, McKeon, and Pandina (11) reported that higher substance use was associated with increased numbers of perceived stressors. If chemical abuse is a coping strategy, it may well be that coping can be assessed by contrasting the number of perceived stressors before, during, and after a substance abuse episode. In a related vein, Gaines (12) noted that women at high risk to problem drinking have an impaired ability to differentiate between different kinds of anxiety-evoking situations.

It is my contention that for chemical dependency research the quintessential conundrums in our models and nosologic schemes have been their dedifferentiation. It is ironic that both the addicted individuals and the explanatory models for their behavior are confronted with essentially the same yoke—namely dedifferentiation.

Substance abuse or chemical dependency is not a unidimensional disorder. In the illicit drug field, this has been easier to accept because the drugs are many, and their psychological and physiological reactions vary widely. Correctly, that field early dismissed the search for a singular addictive model or syndrome. What became commonly accepted was the notion that the user of one class of drugs (e.g., stimulants) had needs, life themes, characteristics, coping styles, and motives different from the user of another class of drugs (e.g., depressants).

Most importantly, the substance user was seen to act as his own psychopharmacologist. One assumed he selected particular drugs at certain times to achieve specific effects, malleations, or realignments in perceived needs and mood states. Implicit in this conceptualization is the acceptance of a phenomenological perspective and its attendant underpinnings.

Particularly noteworthy in this regard is the seminal work of Spotts and Shontz (13, 14, 15, 16) wherein a series of drug-specific and personologic-specific descriptive schema were developed, and distinctions between them were contrasted.

For the alcohol field, the fact that only one chemical substance is in question may have served to retard clarification of a more phenomenological and/or qualitatively differential approach. Certainly Jellinek's work stands as a conceptual hallmark in this regard; however, much other early work sought to class and calibrate alcohol dependency on a quantitative continuum based on quantity measures of alcohol ingestion. Of late, there appears to be a resurgence of qualitative conceptualization as evidenced by the burgeoning popularity of the term "alcoholisms" rather than "alcoholism."

It would seem that to malleate and differentiate our conceptualizations of the alcoholisms, one must dissect the life course or cycle of addictive chemical dependency, as well as examine its interaction with other relevant cycles such as that of stress.

ADDICTION CYCLE

In a compendium of 43 theories of substance abuse, Lettieri, Sayers, and Pearson (17) delineated five theoretical stages in the addiction cycle.

The five stages (initiation, continuation, transition or escalation, cessation, and relapse) can be posed as germinal clinical questions one must answer to achieve a useful explanation or understanding of chemical dependency. These are, in order, (1) Why or how does one begin using,

(2) Why does one continue to use, (3) When and why does use escalate to abuse, (4) Why does one cease use, and (5) Why, how, and when does relapse occur? (Figure 2.)

Upon reviewing the vast array of variables employed to explain addictive behavior (18), one can sort these into seven major domains: (1) euphoria/pleasure, (2) drug knowledge, (3) cognitive factors, (4) tension-anxiety reduction, (5) interpersonal variables, (6) personological factors, and (7) social/environmental factors.

In Table 1, I have tried to summarily lump those variables which seem to capture similar notions.

On examining the listing of terms specifically used by theoreticians (17, 18), one is struck with the veracity of Mc Dougall's famed old saw, in 1910, that many psychological concepts are like old wine in new bottles. In purveying the listing, one can conclude that each of the variables might act as a stressor and hence enormously complicate the study of addictive behavior. Clearly we no longer need to coin new phrases for variables, although we might wish to reissue some of these (Table 2).

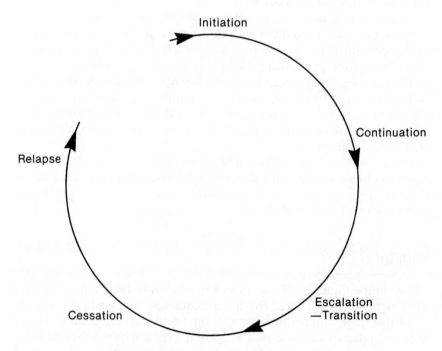

Figure 2. Five stages in the addiction cycle.

TABLE 1
Variables Relevant to Addiction Cycle

1. EUPHORIA/PLEASURE
A. Biological Systems
- biological drive, pleasure as a biological preference system
- metabolic disease, genetic susceptibility, biologic rhythms
- sensory overload, quality of sensory experiences
- narcotic hunger, physical dependence, narcotic blockade
- opioid receptors, endorphins, enkephalins
B. Intrapsychic System
- pleasure/pain balance, abstinence syndrome, withdrawal avoidance, pain relief, euphoria, dysphoria, hypophoria, pain modulation, sense of well being
- pursuit of altered consciousness
- immediate gratification needs
- sensation seeking, stimulation seeking, relief from boredom

2. DRUG KNOWLEDGE
- knowledge about drugs, perceived drug effects, prior drug use, values, cognitive awareness of dependence, attitudes towards drugs, controlled drug use, beliefs

3. COGNITIVE FACTORS
A. Cognitive Variables
- social sanctions, non-normative group expectations
- impaired feedback
- search for meaning
- cognitive style, habit, cognitive set
- self-medication
B. Learning and Reinforcement
- learning, social learning, conditioning, reinforcement, intermittent reinforcement, dependence as a memory function

4. TENSION/ANXIETY REDUCTION
A. Anxiety/Pain/Tension
- anxiety reduction, stress and tension reduction, hypophoria reduction, pain relief, discomfort relief, stimulation avoidance
B. Coping
- cognitive conflict, conflict/aggression reduction
- adaptive/defense function, coping strategies, coping abilities and mechanisms, behavioral styles, affective defense
- lifestyle enhancement

5. INTERPERSONAL VARIABLES
A. Interpersonal Influence
- social pressure, drug-using culture, social control, social acceptance, addict/peer/family/social influence
- normative systems, social rituals, social deviance, conduct norms, cultural modes of decorum
- conformity/nonconformity, conventionality/unconventionality, social orientation
- population density/control
- social isolation

(continued)

TABLE 1
(Continued)

B. Family Factors
• family homeostatic model, family systems, middle-class parent culture, disrupted family-life, family isolation, parental relations, parent-child over-involvement
C. Interpersonal Loss and Trauma
• death/separation/loss, traumatic loss
• role strain/deprivation, social constriction/entrapment
D. Interpersonal Factors
• achievement orientation, achievement/performance competition

6. PERSONOLOGICAL FEATURES
A. Personality Characteristics/Deficiencies
• curiosity, risk-taking
• claustrophobia
• guilt
• low self-esteem, self-concept, self-deprecation, narcissism
• autonomy/independence, locus of control, externalization
• rebelliousness, obedience
• retreatism, escapism
B. Affective States
• emptiness, alienation, fear of separation
• hopelessness, powerlessness, helplessness, depression
• hypersensitivity to stimuli
• rage, emotional/affective deprivation, apathy, affective regression
• feelings of inferiority/superiority
C. Personality Syndromes and Characterological Features
• personality deficiency, inadequate personality syndrome, self-pathology, ego-state alterations, self vs. ideal self, arrested crisis resolution, ego deficiency, pseudo-individuation, super-ego deficits and splits, developmental disturbance
• self-destructiveness, self-care, self-preservation, self-rejecting styles
• delinquency, antisocial personality, tolerance of deviance, sociopathy
• addiction proneness
• present vs. future orientation
• phobic core
• self-perceived behavioral pressures

7. SOCIAL/ENVIRONMENTAL FACTORS
• drug availability, drug distribution
• socioeconomic status, social class, social location

It is my contention that the viciousness of the addiction cycle emanates from the way an individual gets caught up in minifeedback loops. The most resistant to change are those loops which fall between addiction stages—what I shall call interstitial feedback loops (viz., problem drinking loop, compulsive drinking loop). They are difficult to change because they encompass more of the individual's core behaviors and because they have the quality of a closed feedback system. For the therapist to break the loop may well require encouraging the client to (1) regress to a prior stage and (2) probably experience increased stress. Presumably the client moved from one stage to the next as a means of reducing stress from the prior stage (Figure 3).

Thus, for each forward moving therapeutic step, the client may experience it as stressful and backward stepping. Doubtless, this diminishes client satisfaction with the therapeutic process.

What can we conclude? Perhaps both stress and the addiction cycle have their own characteristic form of expression, but no particular, specific cause. Any stimulus can serve as a stressor; any stressor can act as a causal factor in propelling the individual through progressive stages of the addiction cycle. Ultimately, phenomenological models may afford us

TABLE 2

Addiction Stages by Variables

INITIATION
- stress from peer pressure
- drug/alcohol availability
- social status needs
- role modeling
- boredom relief
- early learned coping styles

CONTINUATION
- stress from physiological needs
- partial reinforcement schedule
- intolerance for ambiguity

TRANSITION OR ESCALATION OF USE TO ABUSE
- learn games such as "persecutor," "savior"
- change in social groups and attendant social pressures
- intolerance for ambiguity
- physiological needs
- dedifferentiation coping style
- divergent and/or dichotomous thinking style

CESSATION
- pleasure/pain imbalance
- peer/work group pressure
- physical ails, impairments

RELAPSE
- many of above cited variables

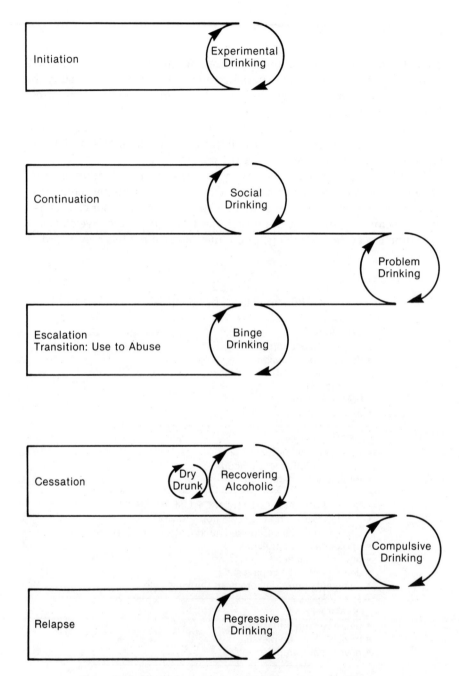

Figure 3. Feedback loops and cycles in the stages of addiction.

the most fruition in future research. Finally, in treating alcoholism, it is necessary to understand the feedback loops which entrap the user into potentially intractable behavioral repertoires. In some ways, these loops entrap the clinician and can diminish therapeutic satisfaction and effectiveness.

Both stress and addiction have specifiable stages, and while they can interact, the overall pattern of stages seems quite robust and constant. In clinical practice, one should aim to short-circuit the client's progression through the stages. Movement through the stages, per se, can have phenomenologically positive value for the client in setting a path, direction and meaning for life, relief of boredom, and a host of other features. At each progressive stage of addiction and intoxication, the client's problem-solving abilities are further impaired, and while each stage is embraced with renewed hope for a solution, those hopes can be quickly dashed and feelings of powerlessness and hopelessness return with increased verve.

REFERENCES

1. Selye H: The Stress of Life. New York, McGraw-Hill, 1956
2. Pohorecky LA: Interaction of alcohol and stress: A review. Neuroscience and Biobehavioral Review 5:209–229, 1981
3. Langer TS, Michael ST: Life Stress and Mental Health. London, Free Press of Glencoe, Collier-Macmillan, 1963
4. Lazarus RS: The Stress and Coping Paradigm, in Models for Psychopathology. Edited by Eisdorfer C, Cohen D, Kleinman A, et al: New York, Spectrum Books, 1981
5. Maher BA: Principles of Psychopathology. New York, McGraw-Hill, 1966
6. Powers RJ, Kutash IL: Alcohol abuse and anxiety, in Handbook on Stress and Anxiety. Edited by Kutash I. San Francisco, CA, Jossey-Bass, 1980.
7. Schwarz RM, Burkhart BR, Green SB: Sensation-seeking and anxiety as factors in social drinking. Journal of Studies on Alcohol 43(11):1108–1114, 1982
8. Hull JG: Self-awareness model of the causes and effects of alcohol consumption. Journal of Abnormal Psychology 90(6):586–600, 1981
9. Lettieri DJ: Affect, attitude and cognition in suicidal persons. Dissertation Abstracts 70-25369, 1970
10. Neuringer C, Lettieri DJ: Cognition, attitudes and affects in suicidal individuals. Journal of Life-Threatening Behavior 1(2):106–124, 1971
11. Bry B, McKeon P, Pandina RJ: Extent of drug use as a function of number of risk factors. Journal of Abnormal Psychology 91(4):273–279, 1982
12. Gaines LS: Anxiety in women at risk for middle-age problem drinking. Bulletin of the Society of Psychologists in Substance Abuse 1(4):163–164, 1982
13. Spotts JV, Shontz FC: Cocaine Users: A Representative Case Approach. New York, Free Press, 1980
14. Spotts JV, Shontz FC: Ego development, dragon fights and chronic drug use. International Journal of the Addictions 17(6):945–976, 1982

15. Spotts JV, Shontz FC: Psychopathology and chronic drug use: A methodological paradigm. International Journal of the Addictions 18(5):633–680, 1983
16. Spotts JV, Shontz FC: Correlates of sensation-seeking in heavy, chronic drug users. Perceptual and Motor Skills 58:427–435, 1984
17. Lettieri DJ, Sayers M, Pearson HW (eds): Theories on Drug Abuse: Selected Contemporary Perspectives. Washington, DC, US Govt Print Off, 1981
18. Lettieri DJ: Drug abuse: A Review of explanations and models of explanation. Advances in Alcohol and Substance Abuse 4(3/4):9–40, 1985

20

Is Sensation Seeking a Predisposing Trait for Alcoholism?

MARVIN ZUCKERMAN

Studies relating substance use/abuse, sensation seeking, and cultural change are reviewed as are the personality characteristics of drinkers, motivation for drinking, and developmental studies.

In the major thrust of the paper, the author postulates that low MAO levels constitute a marker for sensation seeking and alcoholism. The marker seems to indicate a disposition towards impulsive, extroverted, sensation-seeking temperament, which in turn constitutes a risk factor for alcoholism and other kinds of drug abuse. A willingness to take risks for the sake of immediate pleasure or gratification seems to be the behavioral characteristic associated with addiction proneness. A new ''optimal catecholamine system activity theory'' is proposed as the mediating mechanism.

The previous papers I presented at conferences on drugs (1, 2) were primarily concerned with the relationship between the personality trait of sensation seeking and the use of illicit drugs. The sensation-seeking motive in alcohol abuse was minimally treated except for some speculations about the reason that illicit drug use was more highly related to the sensation-seeking trait than was alcohol abuse (2). Despite the rise and fall of fads in illicit drugs, the latest being the rising popularity of cocaine, alcohol remains the king of drugs and the most prevalent health-

and social-problem-producing substance. I will, therefore, concentrate on the personality dispositions that place persons at risk for the development of alcoholic disorders with special emphasis on sensation seeking.

The legality of alcohol and its easy availability make it the first drug used and the more widely used drug (3). Attitudes among students indicate almost universal approval of the legal status of alcohol, less than a majority supporting the legalization of marijuana, and very few approving of legal availability of other drugs (4). The student data reflect the wide acceptance of alcohol in the general community except in certain religious groups. Students are more likely to find parental models for alcohol use in their homes compared to models for use of other drugs (5).

The greater acceptance of alcohol by society probably makes it somewhat less attractive to high sensation seekers than other drugs. The trait of sensation seeking has been defined as " . . . the need for varied, novel, and complex sensations and experiences and the willingness to take physical and social risks for the sake of such experience" (6, p.10). Although almost all persons using illegal drugs start with alcohol, I would expect that the merely moderate sensation seekers stop there while the higher sensation seekers go on to search for the variety of effects provided by other drugs.

Apart from the direct effects provided by the drugs, there is a special risky style of life that is connected with illegal drugs. The added risk of obtaining and using these drugs paradoxically enhances their attractiveness for the high sensation seeker. The results based on our first studies of college students done in the early 1970s suggested that drug use was more related to a generalized sensation-seeking trait that includes sexual activity than was alcohol (7). However, styles and expressions of sensation seeking change. In the previous study (7), there was no correlation between drug and alcohol use among the males, although there was in the females. Subsequent studies indicate that the two college male cultures of the 1970s, the hard-drinking "jocks" and the drug-using "hippies," have blended into one drinking-drug-using (particularly marijuana) group, contrasted with the rarer abstainers and the larger modal group of occasional, light social drinkers. These changes may make sensation seeking a more salient trait in the prealcoholic personality than it has been in the earlier decades.

SENSATION-SEEKING SCALE (SSS)

The first SSS (Form II) (8) was developed in the early 1960s in an attempt to evolve an instrument based on the idea of individual differences in optimal levels of stimulation and arousal (9). It was initially hoped that the measure would predict individual differences in responses to the situation of sensory deprivation. In the 1970s, my program moved away from sensory deprivation research into the broader area of sensation seeking, using the new scale as the nucleus for explorations of putative sensation-seeking phenomena and biological characteristics associated with the trait (10).

The first version of the SSS (8) included only a *General* scale containing items describing diverse activities, that were intercorrelated in a single broad factor. Later forms of the test were based on factor analyses of results from American (11) and English (12) subjects and revealed four factors:

1. *Thrill and adventure seeking.* Items expressing the desire to try risky sports or activities involving elements of speed, movement, and defiance of gravity.
2. *Experience seeking.* Items expressing a desire to expand experience through the mind and the senses, through music, art, travel, and an unconventional style of life with like-minded nonconformists.
3. *Disinhibition.* Items expressing a hedonistic philosophy and an extroverted style, an enjoyment of parties, social drinking, and a somewhat cynical, variety-seeking attitude toward sex.
4. *Boredom susceptibility.* Items expressing a strong aversion to monotony, a preference for unpredictability in activities and friends, and a general restlessness when things are not changing.

Because the scales were moderately intercorrelated, the last published form (V) of the test (12) uses a Total score based on the sum of the four subscales in place of the General scale used in prior versions (II and IV). The Total score shows higher internal reliability (about .85) than most of the shorter component subscales (6). Apart from relationships to drug use (1, 2), the scales have been related to engaging in risky sports (13), habitual driving speeds (14), responses to sensory deprivation and confinement, volunteering for unusual experiments and group activities, gambling, cognitive, perceptual, and esthetic preferences, and many other types of phenomena that involve novelty, complexity, and, in some cases, risk taking (6).

In the area of psychopathology, the SSS has shown relationships to primary sociopathy (15, 16, 17), manic-depressive disorder (17), and manic-depressive tendencies in normal populations (6, 18). These relationships with sociopathy and mania are most prominent with the Disinhibition subscale although they are also apparent with the General and

Total scores. Schizophrenics, particularly behaviorally retarded ones, tend to score low on the SSS (19). Sensation seeking is unrelated to neurosis (14) or neuroticism as a personality trait (6, 20).

PERSONALITY OF YOUNG DRINKERS

Comparisons of diagnosed chronic alcoholics with controls reveal many kinds of personality patterns in the alcoholic groups (21, 22). Many factors may make such data irrelevant for an understanding of the prealcoholic personality. The stress of a long alcoholic history may have produced various neurotic patterns which were not originally part of the personality makeup. Most of these groups have been newly admitted to a treatment program in which there is an implicit demand to present themselves as psychologically "sick."

Zuckerman, Sola, Masterson, et al. (23) found a variety of types of psychopathology in the MMPI's of young male and female drug clients newly admitted to a therapeutic community. However, after 3 to 6 months in the program most of the neurotic and psychotic scores dropped to near normal levels, leaving only the elevations on Scales 4 (Psychopathic Deviate) and 9 (Hypomania) still elevated. On entry to the program, only 21% of the clients showed the classical psychopath profile (4-9) while 40% had neurotic profiles. By the time they reached the reentry phase, 63% (57% of the males and 93% of the females!) had psychopathic profiles and only 4% had neurotic profiles. Although this study was done on drug abusers, there is every reason to suspect that similar results would be found for alcoholics entering similar programs. It should be emphasized that the treatment in this drug program was primarily addressed to the psychopathic problems and only incidentally directed to neurotic problems. It was our belief that the residual psychopathic personality, seen after the stresses of program entry have subsided, really represents the typical preaddictive personality.

For these reasons it would seem better to study the young heavy drinker who is at risk for alcoholism. At this stage, the heavy drinker is seldom ashamed of his drinking and, apart from some academic and job problems, he has not encountered the full stress of an alcoholic existence.

College Students

Table 1 shows the percentage of high and low scorers on the SSS who reported drinking to any extent in two studies (24, 25) done in the early 1970s. The data for marijuana, the strongest drug competition for alcohol

TABLE 1
College Students' Use of Alcohol and Marijuana

	Zuckerman et al. 1970			Zuckerman et al. 1972			
	High SS %	Low SS %	χ^2	High SS %	Med SS %	Low SS %	χ^2
Alcohol (1 to 6 drinks per week or more)	53	13	9.16**	42	44	38	.29
Marijuana (any use)	58	11	18.88**	64	33	31	8.81*

*p<.05
**p<.01

in these years, are also presented. Although the percentage difference between high and low sensation seekers in drinking alcohol was significant in 1970, it was not so in 1972. The reason appears to have been a decrease in the highs using alcohol and a large increase in the lows who were drinking. The data for marijuana show a slightly different change, with the highs increasing somewhat and the lows increasing markedly in marijuana use. However, the differences remained significant for marijuana in 1972. This could illustrate the effect of a drug fad on the personality-drug use relationship. The increase in both alcohol and marijuana use in the low sensation seekers may have been due to social pressures and a perceived diminution of risk in the wider and more open use of alcohol and drugs in the early 1970s. Some of the highs may have switched from alcohol to marijuana and other drugs, while others may have continued to drink while also using drugs.

Segal, Huba and Singer (26) did a large-scale study of personality patterns in relation to alcohol and drug use among college students and navy personnel in the years 1973 and 1974. Among the scales used were measures of psychological "needs," daydreaming and mental "styles," optimal levels of stimulation (the SSS), and perceived sources of reinforcement. All items referring to drugs or alcohol were removed from the SSS before it was administered in order to avoid confounding the scale content with reports of actual substance use.

Subjects were classified into four groups: (1) nonusers of alcohol or drugs, (2) users of alcohol only, (3) users of marijuana only, and (4) polydrug users. Of all the personality variables studied, the sensation seeking scales, particularly the Experience Seeking (ES) and Disinhibition (Dis) subscales, accounted for most of the significant discrimination between the groups. The main difference in results in the college and navy populations was that the Experience Seeking scale was the most discriminating one for college students and the Disinhibition scale was most discriminating for navy men and women.

In the college samples, alcohol-only users scored higher on the General SS and two subscale (ES and Dis) than nonusers of alcohol or drugs, but marijuana and polydrug users scored even higher than alcohol-only users. In the Navy samples, alcohol users were also higher than nonusers on sensation-seeking scales, but for these populations there was little difference between alcohol-only and marijuana-only users. The next significant increment in sensation seeking in the naval groups occurred between marijuana-only and polydrug users. In the course of developing a new form of the SSS using college students, I have noticed that the items referring to a desire to use drugs have moved from the experience-seeking to the disinhibition factor, along with those indicating the use of alcohol.

Increasingly, alcohol and drug use appear to be interchangeable expressions of a common disinhibition trait. The specialized use of drugs instead of alcohol may have been a transient expression limited to the college students in the 1960s and 1970s. Walking the streets around Berkeley in the late 1970s, I noticed a number of aging "hippie" types on the streets drinking alcohol out of bottles concealed in paper bags. In the drug rehabilitation center where I formerly consulted, it was observed that many of the more successful program "graduates" (successful in the sense of no longer using illegal drugs or stealing) were slipping into the kind of heavy drinking that precedes alcoholism. This was particularly true of former hard-drug users. To paraphrase Dorothy Parker, heroin is super but liquor is cheaper (and safer in the legal sense). These results support the concept of an "addictive personality" in which many different kinds of drugs are interchangeable for persons with this particular kind of personality. In reviewing previous studies, we have noted (2, 6) that sensation seeking is more highly related to the variety of drugs used than to the specific drugs used. However, for the polydrug user alcohol may be the last as well as the first drug that is used.

What Motivates Drinking?

A popular theory of alcoholism is that people drink to reduce anxiety and therefore the prealcoholic is likely to be a highly anxious person. It is true that alcohol is the oldest anxiolytic drug and had been shown to reduce fear in mice and men. It is also true that diagnosed alcoholics frequently show elevations on scales measuring anxiety and low self-esteem. However, it is possible that the anxiety that alcohol reduces was originally generated by the stress of alcoholism itself, rather than being part of their prealcoholic personality makeup.

Schwartz, Burkhart, and Green (27) compared an index of alcohol use in college students with measures of sensation seeking (SSS) and anxiety. Using a multiple regression analysis, they found that sensation seeking accounted for 33% of the variance in the index of drinking, while anxiety scales added only an additional 1% to the prediction. All of the SS scales correlated significantly with the drinking index, while only one of the anxiety scales (Physical Danger anxiety) correlated with drinking at a low but significant level; but this correlation was negative ($r = -.15$) rather than positive!

The authors suggest an interpretation of their results with which I am in total agreement:

> For young adults, drinking may serve primarily as an outlet for sensation-seeking needs, whereas, later in life, especially for vulnerable individuals, drinking may come to serve as a coping mechanism for feelings of anxiety and stress. (27, p. 1145)

Segal et al. (26) asked their subjects their motives for drinking. The most frequently given reason in all groups was "just to be sociable." Asked more specifically, most subjects said that drinking "is something people do on special occasions" and that it "makes get-togethers more fun," "helps you relax," "makes you less shy," "makes you feel happier," and "sometimes helps you feel better." These reasons suggest that the primary motives for drinking are the social disinhibition and euphoria-producing effects of moderate social drinking. Other reasons suggesting anxiety-reduction motivation, like "helps you forget your problems," were found in small proportions of the sample.

Another analysis by the authors used canonical correlation to compare the reported motivational factors with the personality variables. These results are interesting, since they indicate more specific connections between motives for drinking and type of personality.

One dimension of reasons for drinking had to do with hot weather and hard work. This might be called "drinking after work to relax and cool off" or the "happy-hour" pattern. Males score higher than females on it. High scorers are high on Disinhibition and Experience Seeking and a similar scale called "Need for External Stimulation." "Happy hour" habitués also tend to report sexual daydreams, have elevated needs for dominance and play, and low needs to avoid harm or be nurtured. The authors interpret the high loading of Disinhibition sensation seeking on this form of drinking as "a means of 'letting go' of reality and constraints" (26, p. 157).

The second factor is the use of alcohol when "feeling under pressure," "having nothing else to do," or "feeling sad." This factor seems to represent a compensation for boredom, frustration, or loneliness, seeking to counteract these states with the euphoria-producing qualities of alcohol. Positively correlated with this factor were external locus of control, experience sensation seeking, absorption in daydreaming, hostility, need for achievement, sexual fantasies, and impulsivity.

The third factor has to do with drinking when having personal problems, feeling lonely, and frustrated by "not getting ahead." Sensation seeking also plays a role here in the form of Disinhibition and Boredom Susceptibility. Also loading on the dimension are needs for affiliation, impulsivity, nurturance, play, and social recognition, as well as many negative daydreaming scales.

The fourth factor is primarily defined by the popular "just to be sociable" reason. The main personality correlates are a high need for social recognition and a low autonomy need. The factor seems to represent people who drink just because others are doing so, and it is the one factor with little or no relation to sensation seeking. Although not determinable from the data, one would guess this represents a group with relatively light consumption of alcohol.

PERSONALITY OF ALCOHOLICS

Using the Personality Research Form, Nerviano (21) reports eight personality types found in a male alcoholic population. Using the MMPI, Skinner, Jackson, and Hoffman (22) defined five personality types. According to these researchers, there is no single type that predominates among alcoholics. I have already pointed out why the finding of diversity among hospitalized alcoholics or those in treatment programs may be misleading in terms of the prealcoholic personality.

Kilpatrick, Sutker, and Smith (28) compared a regular drug user, a problem drinker, an occasional drug and alcohol user (the modal group), and a nonuser group on a battery of personality tests including tests of anxiety and sensation seeking. All subjects were patients in a general Veterans Administration hospital. Considering the criteria used, the problem drinkers were probably all alcoholics, although they were not necessarily hospitalized for that reason.

The problem drinkers were higher than the occasional drug and alcohol users on neuroticism, trait and state anxiety, social-interpersonal anxiety, and fear of failure or loss of self-esteem. Occasional users of drugs or alcohol did not differ from nonusers on any of these scales. Problem drinkers did not differ from occasional users on ego strength, dogmatism, locus of control, or extroversion; nor did occasional users differ from nonusers on any of these scales.

On the SSS, the problem drinkers differed from occasional users on only one subscale—they were higher on Boredom Susceptibility. Occasional users were significantly higher than nonusers on all of the SS scales.

It is interesting that the neuroticism and anxiety scales differentiated alcoholics from occasional users, while the other trait scales such as extroversion and sensation-seeking did so with less success. Of course, the alcoholics were higher than the nonuser group on all of the SSS scales, but only the Boredom Susceptibility scale showed a significant increment beyond the occasional user group.

As noted previously, boredom seems to be a major motive for drinking, so it is not surprising that this particular scale differentiated alcohol use groups so well. Disinhibition may be related to the initial motives for alcohol use but less related to the subsequent motivations that turn a social drinker into an alcoholic.

Maletesta, Sutker, and Treiber (29) compared two groups of chronic alcoholics who were all involuntary admissions to a detoxification facility. One group had a history of chronic public drunkenness with 20 or more involuntary admissions to the facility over three years; the other group had only five or fewer admissions. Both groups were equivalent in age, education, and years of drinking. The chronic public drunkards scored significantly higher than the other alcoholics on all of the SS scales. The authors suggest that sensation seeking plays a role in the life style pattern of drinking, with the high sensation-seeker alcoholics more likely to reject social conventions and violate social norms about display of drunkenness. They are more likely to get into trouble with the law and be arrested.

DEVELOPMENTAL STUDIES

We cannot assume that the characteristics of drinkers, even heavy drinkers, are the characteristics that were part of the prealcoholic personality of the alcoholic. It is estimated that only 5%–7% of drinkers become addicted to alcohol (30). Studies in which data are available from future alcoholics that were obtained years before they became alcoholic are needed to definitively answer the questions concerning the prealcoholic personality. Only a few such studies have been reported.

From the late 1940s until 1962, all entering freshman in many colleges of the University of Minnesota were routinely given the MMPI. Loper, Kammeier, and Hoffman (31) found 32 men admitted to alcoholic treatment centers in Minnesota who had MMPI records from their entry to the university 13 years earlier. These records were compared with a control group of records of 148 of their classmates selected at random. The prealcoholics had higher scores on the F (general response deviancy), Psychopathic Deviate (Scale 4), and Hypomania (Scale 9) scales of the MMPI. They also scored higher on content scales of authority conflict and poor health. The prealcoholics actually scored lower on a Social Maladjustment (Neuroticism) scale than their peers, although the difference did not reach significance. Thus, the prealcoholic personality of these males appears rebellious, impulsive, gregarious, and less conforming than that of their peers. There is certainly no evidence of the neuroticism found in the records of many alcoholics tested after they have become alcoholic.

Jones has reported the personality antecedents of male (32) and female (33) adult "problem drinkers." The data are from a 30-year follow-up of children first studied at the age of 10 in the Oakland growth study. At the time of junior high school, the future male problem drinkers were rated by observers as more rebellious, undercontrolled, hostile, "pushing the limits," manipulative, self-indulgent, sensuous, negativistic, expressive, assertive, talkative, humorous, and "other-directed" than their peers who became moderate drinkers or abstainers. During high school and in early adult life the future problem drinkers were rated as higher on almost all of the same variables. In addition, the future problem drinkers were rated low on dependability, objectivity, calmness, productivity, and acceptance of dependency at all periods in their lives. The total picture is consistent with the impressions of an impulsive or even psychopathic personality disorder in MMPIs of prealcoholics in the Loper et al. (31) study.

The problem drinking women from the same study showed many of the same prealcoholic characteristics as the men, namely unstable, unpredictable impulsivity. However, they also showed some depressive, self-negating, distrustful tendencies not seen in men. Curiously, they resembled the total abstainers on these neurotic traits. Problem drinkers were judged to be sumissive when young but rebellious as adults.

The picture of the male alcoholic from preadolescent years to the beginning of alcoholism is fairly consistent, but the story is not quite as simple for the female prealcoholic. While sharing some of the impulsive personality of the male prealcoholic, the female seems also to have a neurotic component in her personality. In contrast to the woman problem drinkers, the female heavy drinkers seem to be sensation seekers, using alcohol to enhance social hedonism.

Personality and Psychological Motives for Alcoholism

The motives for drinking in the prealcoholic phases are not necessarily the same as those in the alcoholic stage. The opponent-process model of Solomon and Corbitt (34) offers an explanation of the change of motive at the psychological level. According to the theory, the addict first uses the substance because it produces a state that is intrinsically reinforcing (pleasure). This state rewards all behaviors associated with getting and using the substance. However, the initial euphoric process strengthens an opponent process, which produces a state of displeasure or discomfort when an adequate supply of the substance is not ingested. Only the substance can reduce the opponent process and its associated state. Habituation of the first state reaction increases the amount of the substance required to reduce the second process. In a nutshell, the alcoholic begins drinking for pleasure and ends by drinking to reduce discomfort. However, it is not only the discomfort of withdrawal that maintains alcoholism, but it is also the discomfort produced by the stressful consequences of drinking.

For the male, at least, the prealcoholic personality does not seem to be characterized by a neurotic vulnerability to stress. Rather, the prealcoholic seems to be characterized by extroverted, impulsive, and sensation-seeking traits. However, before withdrawal symptoms become a serious problem, the prealcoholic learns, almost incidentally, that alcohol also has marked anxiolytic effects. Narcotization therefore becomes the major way of coping with stress and frustration. Given the personality of the prealcoholic, stress and frustration are almost inevitable, since an impulsive personality often encounters problems in work and relationships even before alcohol becomes the main source of these problems.

If we go back to the reported reasons for drinking in young persons, as assessed in the Segal et al. (26) studies, we find that the need to relax after hard work is given as one of the reasons by high sensation seekers.

Alcohol has been used by working men to relax for centuries. It probably achieves this effect through antagonism of sympathetic system arousal, particularly as expressed in muscle tension.

Another frequent reason given by sensation seekers is boredom or, paradoxically, feeling under pressure. Boredom susceptibility is one of the four primary factors in the general trait of sensation seeking. In the Kilpatrick et al. (28) study of V.A. patients, it was the only subscale differentiating problem drinkers from occasional drinkers. Sensation seekers are interested in and attracted to jobs that provide variety and excitement (6). However, all too often they are limited, because of education or social background, to monotonous, repetitive work. A study of young male industrial workers showed significant negative correlations between job satisfaction and the General, Disinhibition, and Experience Seeking SS scales (35). The SSS predicted job satisfaction better than extroversion, neuroticism, manifest anxiety, or their actual job pay. The General and Experience Seeking scales also predicted the lack of satisfaction with a simulated monotonous job task. Alcohol makes time pass quickly but it is not very good for job performance. Problems on the job end in either dismissal or lack of promotion leading to additional frustration which, of course, leads to increased drinking.

Feeling lonely and sad also is associated with drinking in the sensation seeker. Alcohol has always been used for social disinhibition. Social disinhibition is the reason that alcohol is served at most celebrations or parties. It is strange that the prealcoholic, who generally has fewer social inhibitions than the nondrinker, needs alcohol in order to maximize his or her social enjoyment. "Letting go" certainly is easier for impulsive, sensation-seeking extroverts than for their opposites. Perhaps they simply desire to enhance their natural proclivities. If a little disinhibition is fun, more is better. The low sensation seekers are too threatened by disinhibition to endanger their already effective self-control. The social disinhibition motivation for drinking probably becomes weaker as alcoholism becomes progressive. Almost all alcoholics start as social drinkers but many end as solitary drinkers.

There is another aspect to the use of alcohol to enhance the enjoyment of parties which may also explain why the prealcoholic drinks to cope with stress. There is a biological vulnerability to overstimulation in the high sensation seeker which will be discussed in the next section. Alcohol seems to provide a protection against overstimulation which is provided by endogenous mechanisms in the low sensation seeker. The prealcoholic may drink to "stay cool" in situations of either pleasurable or stressful overstimulation.

BIOLOGICAL BASES OF THE ADDICTIVE PERSONALITY

Genetics

At the fourth Coatesville Conference on Addiction Research, Goodwin (36) summarized the research on the genetics of alcoholism. He presented clear evidence, from both twin and adoption studies, of the strong genetic determination of alcoholism. However, he also noted the failure to find specific genetic markers for alcoholism. This would suggest that alcoholism is inherited as part of a broad disposition probably influenced by polygenetic determination. I will now discuss some specific inherited biological traits that are common to alcoholism and the sensation-seeking trait.

Augmenting-Reducing of the Cortical Evoked Potential (EP)

Individual variation in the cortical response to a range of stimulus intensities has been called "augmenting-reducing." The method developed by Buchsbaum and Silverman (37) has been to present four intensities of light flashes or tones in randomized blocks and to measure the EP amplitude from peak to trough (P1-N1). The slope of the best fit linear regression line between stimulus intensity and EP for an individual defines the person's relative degree of augmenting or reducing. Augmenting is defined by positive slopes and reducing by negative slopes. The differences between extreme augmenters and reducers are generally found at the highest stimulus intensities where the augmenters show increased amplitude EPs and the reducers have marked decreases in EP amplitude. Peripheral factors, such as pupillary diameter changes, have been ruled out as explanations of the phenomena by studies in humans and animals. The method has provided a reliable individual difference measure in humans and cats, and has been shown to be related to a wide range of psychological traits, psychopathology, and behavioral characteristics (10, 38). Sensation seeking has been related to augmenting of the visual EP (39, 40, 41, 42) and the auditory EP (41, 42). The Disinhibition subscale, the one most prominent in antisocial and impulsive personality, and most related to use of alcohol, is also the one that shows the strongest relationship to augmenting.

Augmenting is also typical in alcoholics (43, 44). Among alcoholics, EP augmenting was related to high alcohol acquisition behavior (45). Alcoholics (46) and normals (47) are likely to show reducing of the EP when given alcohol. Reducing is conceptualized as a cortical mechanism that protects the organism against pain or other forms of overstimulation. In this sense, alcoholics and high sensation seekers lack this protection. Alcohol may substitute for whatever endogenous biochemicals mediate the inhibition of cortical reactivity at high intensities, possibly endorphins (48).

Monoamine Oxidase (MAO)

Platelet MAO is another common marker for sensation seeking and alcoholism. Several studies (49, 50, 51, 52, 53) have found low platelet MAO levels in alcoholics. One study (54) also found a tendency toward low MAO levels in relatives of alcoholics. Platelet MAO is a very stable characteristic (55) in humans and is not immediately affected by alcohol ingestion (54). Although long-term ingestion might conceivably alter levels of MAO, there are inconsistent results on this.

Significant negative correlations were found between the General SS scale and platelet MAO in two studies (56, 57) in America and two studies in Sweden (58, 59), although the first of these (59) used its own SS scale, called "Monotony Avoidance." Von Knorring, Oreland, and Winbald (60) also studied MAO and sensation seeking in a sample of 1,120 18-year-old recruits in the Swedish Army. Although the Disinhibition subscale was not used, low MAO subjects were significantly higher than high MAO subjects on the SSS modified Total score, the Boredom Susceptibility scale, and the Swedish Monotony Avoidance scale, as well as a scale of impulsivity. Although the Eysenck scales were used in this study, they were not related to MAO.

The recruits were asked in a questionnaire about alcohol and drug consumption habits, and questions relating to early signs of alcohol addiction (i.e., tolerance, blackouts, morning drinking, loss of control over drinking) were included. More low MAO subjects than highs reported alcohol-induced blackouts and at least one sign of alcohol dependence. More lows also reported using marijuana and none were tobacco smokers. Intelligence proved to be a moderator variable in that the low MAO subjects who were also low in intelligence were more likely to use alcohol or drugs than the more intelligent low MAO types. The latter were more likely to be high on Thrill and Adventure and Experience Seeking scales. In spite of the positive association between intelligence and sensation seeking, there were *more* users of alcohol among the high sensation seekers and more of them were regular users. There was also more evidence of alcohol tolerance developed in the highs and more of them used marijuana. The use of other types of drugs was rare in this population, but the few cases admitting their use were in the medium or high SS groups.

To summarize this interesting study, low MAO levels are associated with high sensation seeking and early signs of alcoholism, and sensation seeking is associated with some of these same signs of alcoholism.

It has been suggested that the prealcoholic is impulsive, extroverted, and sensation seeking. In both monkeys (61) and humans (62), low platelet MAO levels have been associated with high levels of social activity in both sexes. Conversely, high MAO types in both species tend to be inactive and solitary.

Twin studies (63, 64) indicate a high degree of heritability for platelet MAO and augmenting of the EP (65), as well as sensation seeking itself (66). Consistent with the sex differences in sensation seeking and rates of alcoholism, males are lower in MAO at all ages (55).

In sum, low MAO levels constitute a biological marker for sensation seeking and alcoholism. However, low MAO has also been found in bipolar affective disorders, delinquency, and chronic schizophrenia (perhaps due to chronic phenothiazine treatment), so it cannot be regarded as a specific marker for alcoholism. It seems rather to indicate a disposition toward the impulsive, extroverted, sensation-seeking temperament which in turn constitutes a risk factor for alcoholism or other kinds of drug abuse. This personality type is also common in tobacco smokers. The willingness to take risks for the sake of immediate pleasure or gratification seems to be the behavioral characteristic associated with all addiction proneness.

The Monoamines and Addiction

The finding of an association between sensation seeking and MAO led me to speculate about the role of the monoamine systems regulated by MAO in the brain (6, 67). Recently, I have reviewed the comparative literature bearing on the functions of these systems (68, 69). The first idea was that sensation seeking is related to the sensitivity of the catecholaminergic (norepinephrine and dopamine) reward centers in limbic brain. Low MAO levels might mean that there is less metabolic degradation of these neurotransmitters which have been implicated as mediating primary reward on the basis of self-stimulation studies. However, levels of platelet MAO provide no basis on which to predict levels of neurotransmitters in the brain. In actual fact, we have found evidence of a negative relationship between norepinephrine in the cerebrospinal fluid

(CSF) of normal humans and their sensation-seeking scores (70). This finding has suggested the possibility that sensation seekers seek intense and novel external stimulation and use catecholamine-releasing drugs like amphetamine and cocaine in order to activate these systems. In an unstimulated state (producing boredom), high sensation seekers may be below an optimal level of activity in catecholaminergic systems. Low MAO levels may allow these monoamine systems to fluctuate within wide limits. Thus, a period of intense excitement could be followed by a depletion of catecholamines leading to further attempts to stimulate the system.

How does this apply to alcohol use? Does alcohol directly stimulate primary reward receptors, or are the effects of alcohol largely conditioned relaxation responses? Animals will self-administer cocaine, amphetamines, morphines, and short-acting barbiturates, but the results with ethyl alcohol have been spotty and largely unsuccessful in rats (71). However, like cocaine and amphetamines, alcohol consumption increases catecholaminergic activity, particularly norepinephrine turnover (72). But the catecholaminergic turnover is further increased in the withdrawal period where it is accompanied by acute discomfort. According to my new optimal catecholamine system activity (CSA) (69) theory, moderate levels of CSA are optimal and associated with rewarding or pleasurable effects, while very low or high levels are associated with dysphoria. Actually, such a theory is compatible with the effects of increasing doses of alcohol which show mild euphoria and disinhibition at lower doses and increased anxiety and depression at higher doses or after more prolonged drinking. The alcoholic seems to follow the maxim "if a little is good a lot is better." Unfortunately, the central nervous system follows the maxim "moderation and homeostasis in all systems."

REFERENCES

1. Zuckerman M: Drug usage as one manifestation of a "sensation seeking" trait, in Drug Abuse: Current Concepts and Research. Edited by Keup W. Springfield, IL, Thomas, 1972
2. Zuckerman M: Sensation seeking: The initial motive for drug abuse, in Etiological Aspects of Alcohol and Drug Abuse. Edited by Gottheil E, Druley TE, Skoloda TE, et al. Springfield, IL, Thomas, 1983
3. Milman DH, Anker JL: Patterns of drug usage among university students; multiple drug usuage, in Drug Abuse: Current Concepts and Research. Edited by Keup W. Springfield IL, Thomas, 1972
4. Anker JL, Milman DH: Patterns of nonmedical drug usage among university students; student attitudes toward drug usage, in Drug Abuse: Current Concepts and Research. Edited by Keup W. Springfield IL, Thomas, 1972

5. Smart RG, Fejer D: Relationships between parental and adolescent drug use, in Drug Abuse: Current Concepts and Research. Edited by Keup W. Springfield, IL, Thomas, 1972

6. Zuckerman M: Sensation Seeking: Beyond the Optimal Level of Arousal. Hillsdale, NJ, Erlbaum, 1979

7. Zuckerman M, Bone RN, Neary R, et al: What is the sensation seeker? Personality and experience correlates of the Sensation Seeking Scales. J Consult Clin Psychol 39:308–321, 1972

8. Zuckerman M, Kolin EA, Price L, et al: Development of a Sensation Seeking Scale. J Consult Psychol 28:477–482, 1964

9. Zuckerman M: Theoretical Formulations, in Sensory Deprivation: Fifteen Years of Research. Edited by Zubek JP. New York, Appleton-Century, 1979

10. Zuckerman M, Buchsbaum MS, Murphy DL: Sensation seeking and its biological correlates. Psychol Bull 88:187–214, 1980

11. Zuckerman M: Dimensions of sensation seeking. J Consult Clin Psychol 36:45–52, 1971

12. Zuckerman M, Eysenck SBG, Eysenck HJ: Sensation seeking in England and America: Cross-cultural, age and sex comparisons. J Consult Clin Psychol 46:139–149, 1978

13. Zuckerman M: Sensation seeking and sports. Personality Ind Differences 4:285–292, 1983

14. Zuckerman M, Neeb M: Demographic influences in sensation seeking and expressions of sensation seeking in religion, smoking and driving habits. Personality Ind Differences 1:197–206, 1980

15. Blackburn R: Sensation seeking, impulsivity and psychopathic personality. J Consult Clin Psychol 33:571–574, 1969

16. Emmons TD, Webb WW: Subjective correlates of emotional responsivity and stimulation seeking in psychopaths, normals and acting-out neurotics. J Consult Clin Psychol 42:620–625, 1974

17. Zuckerman M, Neeb M: Sensation seeking and psychopathology. Psychiatry Res 1:255–264, 1979

18. Perderson L, Magaro PA: Personality styles and psychopathy. J Clin Psychol 38:320–324, 1982

19. Kish GB: Reduced cognitive innovation and stimulus-seeking in chronic schizophrenia. J Clin Psychol 26:170–174, 1970

20. Zuckerman M: Sensation seeking and risk taking, in Emotions in Personality and Psychopathology. Edited by Izard CE. New York, Plenum, 1979

21. Nerviano J: Common personality problems among alcoholic males: A multivariate study. J. Consult Clin Psychol 44:104–110, 1976

22. Skinner HA, Jackson DN, Hoffmann H: Alcoholic personality types: Identification and correlates. J Abnorm Psychol 83:658–666, 1974

23. Zuckerman M, Sola S, Masterson J, et al: MMPI patterns in drug abusers before and after treatment in therapeutic communities. J Consult Clin Psychol 43:286–296, 1975

24. Zuckerman M, Neary RS, Brustman BA: Sensation Seeking Scale correlates in experience (smoking, drugs, alcohol, "hallucinations" and sex) and preference for complexity (designs). Proc 78th Ann Conv Am Psychol Assoc 5:317–318, 1970

25. Zuckerman M, Bone RN, Neary R, et al: What is the sensation seeker? Personality and experience correlates of the Sensation Seeking Scales. J Consult Clin Psychol 39:308–321, 1972

26. Segal BS, Huba CJ, Singer JF: Drugs, Daydreaming and Personality: A Study of College Youth. Hillsdale, NJ, Erlbaum, 1980

27. Schwarz RM, Burkhart BR, Green B: Turning on or turning off: Sensation seeking or tension reduction as motivational determinants of alcohol use. J Consult Clin Psychol 46:1144–1145, 1978

28. Kilpatrick DC, Sutker PB, Smith AD: Deviant drug and alcohol use: The role of anxiety, sensation seeking and other personality variables, in Emotions and Anxiety: New

Concepts, Methods and Applications. Edited by Zuckerman M, Spielberger CD. Hillsdale, NJ, Erlbaum, 1976
29. Malatesta VJ, Sutker PB, Treiber FA: Sensation seeking and chronic public drunkenness. J Consult Clin Psychol 49:292–294, 1981
30. Kissen B: Alcohol as it compares to other addictive substances, in Drug Abuse: Current Concepts and Research. Edited by Keup W. Springfield, IL, Thomas, 1972
31. Loper RG, Kammeier ML, Hoffman H: MMPI characteristics of college males who later become alcoholics. J Abnorm Psychol 82:159–162, 1973
32. Jones MC: Personality correlates and antecedents of drinking patterns in adult males. J Consult Clin Psychol 32:2–12, 1968
33. Jones MC: Personality antecedents and correlates of drinking patterns in women. J Consult Clin Psychol 36:61–69, 1971
34. Solomon RL, Corbitt JD: An opponent process theory of motivation: Temporal dynamics of affect. Psychol Rev 81:119–145, 1974
35. Perone M, DeWaard RJ, Baron A: Satisfaction with real and simulated jobs in relation to personality variables and drug use. J Applied Psychol 64:660–668, 1979
36. Goodwin DW: The genetics of alcoholism, in Etiological Aspects of Alcohol and Drug Abuse. Edited by Gottheil E, Druley KA, Skolada TE. Springfield, IL, Thomas, 1983
37. Buchsbaum MS, Silverman J: Stimulus intensity control and the cortical evoked response. Psychosom Med 30:12–22, 1968
38. Buchsbaum MS, Haier RJ, Johnson J: Augmenting and reducing: Individual differences in evoked potentials, in Physiological Correlates of Human Behavior, v 3. Edited by Gale A, Edwards JA. London, Academic Press, 1983
39. Zuckerman M, Murtaugh TM, Siegel J: Sensation seeking and cortical augmenting-reducing. Psychophysiol 11:535–542, 1974
40. Lukas JH: Human augmenting-reducing and sensation seeking. Psychophysiol 19:333–334, 1982 (abstract)
41. von Knorring L: Visual averaged evoked responses and platelet monoamine oxidase in patients suffering from alcoholism, in The Biological Effects of Alcohol. Edited by Begleiter H. New York, Plenum, 1980
42. Como P: The relationships among orienting and defensive reflexes, augmenting-reducing of the cortical evoked potential and disinhibitory sensation seeking. Doctoral dissertation, Univ of Delaware, 1984
43. Coursey RD, Buchsbaum MS, Frankel BL: Personality measures and evoked responses in chronic insomniacs. J Abnorm Psychol 84:239–249, 1975
44. Coger RW, Dymond AM, Serafetinides EA., et al: Alcoholism: Averaged visual evoked response amplitude-intensity slope and symmetry in withdrawal. Biol Psychiatry 11:434–443, 1976
45. von Knorring L: Visual evoked responses in patients suffering from alcoholism. Neuropsychobiol 2:233–238, 1976
46. Ludwig AR, Cain RB, Wikler A: Stimulus intensity modulation and alcohol consumption. J Studies Alcohol 38:2049–2056, 1977
47. Buchsbaum MS, Ludwig AM: Effects of sensory input and alcohol administration on visual evoked potentials in normal subjects and alcoholics, in Biological Effects of Alcohol. Edited by Begleiter H. New York, Plenum, 1980
48. Pfefferbaum A, Roth W, Tinklenberg J, et al: The effects of ethanol and meperidine on auditory evoked potentials. Drug Alcohol Dependence 4:371–380, 1979
49. von Knorring L, Perris C: Biochemistry of the augmenting-reducing response in visual evoked potentials. Neuropsychobiol 7:1–8, 1981
50. Major LF, Murphy DL: Platelet and plasma amine oxidase activity in alcoholic individuals. Brit J Psychiatry 132:548–554, 1978
51. Pandey GN, Dorus E, Shaughnessy R, et al: Reduced platelet MAO activity and vulnerability to psychiatric disorders. Psychiatry Res 2:315–321, 1980
52. Wiberg A, Gottfries CG, Oreland L: Low platelet monoamine oxidase activity in human alcoholics. Med Biol 55:181–186, 1977

53. Sullivan JL, Stanfield CN, Dackis C: Low platelet monoamine oxidase activity in chronic alcoholics. Am J Psychiatry 134:1098–1103, 1977
54. von Knorring L, Oreland L: Visual averaged evoked responses and platelet monoamine oxidase activity as an aid to identify a risk group for alcoholic abuse. A preliminary study. Prog Neuro-Psychopharmacol 2:385–392, 1978
55. Murphy DL, Wright C, Buchsbaum MS, et al: Platelet and plasma amine oxidase activity in 680 normals: Sex and age differences and stability over time. Biochem Med 16:254–265, 1976
56. Murphy DL, Belmaker RH, Buchsbaum MS, et al: Biogenic amine related enzymes and personality variations in normals. Psychol Med 7:149–157, 1977
57. Schooler C, Zahn TP, Murphy DL, et al: Psychological correlates of monoamine oxidase in normals. J Nerv Ment Dis 166:177–186, 1978
58. Perris C, Jacobsson L, Knorring L von, et al: Enzymes related to biogenic amine metabolism and personality characteristics in depressed patients. Acta Psychiatrica Scand 61:477–484, 1980
59. Schalling D. Edman G, Osberg M: Impulsive cognitive style and inability to tolerate boredom, in Biological Bases of Sensation Seeking, Impulsivity, and Anxiety. Edited by Zuckerman M. Hillsdale, NJ, Erlbaum, 1983
60. von Knorring L, Oreland L, Winblad B: Personality traits related to monoamine oxidase (MAO) activity in platelets. Psychiatry Res 12:11–26, 1984
61. Redmond DE Jr, Murphy DL, Baulu J: Platelet monoamine oxidase activity correlates with social affiliative and agonistic behaviors in normal rhesus monkeys. Psychosom Med 41:87–100, 1979
62. Coursey RD, Buchsbaum MS, Murphy DL: Platelet MAO activity and evoked potentials in the identification of subjects biologically at risk for psychiatric disorders. Brit J Psychiatry 134:372–381, 1979
63. Murphy DL: Technical strategies for the study of catecholamines in man, in Frontiers in Catecholamine Research. Edited by Usdin E, Snyder S. Oxford, Pergamon, 1973
64. Nies A, Robinson DS, Lamborn KR, et al: Genetic control of platelet and plasma monoamine oxidase activity. Arch Gen Psychiatry 28:834–838, 1973
65. Buchsbaum MS: Average evoked response and stimulus intensity in identical and fraternal twins. Physiol Psychol 2:365–370, 1974
66. Fulker DW, Eysenck SBG, Zuckerman M: The genetics of sensation seeking. J Personality Res 14:261–281, 1980
67. Zuckerman M: A biological theory of sensation seeking, in Biological Bases of Sensation Seeking, Impulsivity and Anxiety. Edited by Zuckerman M. Hillsdale, NJ, Erlbaum, 1983
68. Zuckerman M, Ballenger JC, Post RM: The neurobiology of some dimensions of personality, in International Review of Neurobiology, v 25. Edited by Smythies JR, Bradley RJ. New York, Academic Press, in press
69. Zuckerman M: Sensation seeking: A comparative approach to a human trait. Behav Brain Sci 7:413–471, 1984
70. Ballenger JC, Post RM, Jimerson DC, et al: Biochemical correlates of personality traits in normals: An exploratory study. Personality Ind Differences 4:615–625, 1983
71. Kalant, H: Animal models of alcohol and drug dependence: Some questions, answers and clinical implications, in Etiological Aspects of Alcohol and Drug Abuse. Edited by Gottheil E, Druley KA, Skoloda TE. Springfield IL, Thomas, 1983
72. Ellingboe J: Effects of alcohol on neurochemical processes, in Psychopharmacology: A Generation of Progress. Edited by Lipton MA, DiMascio A, Killam KF. New York, Raven Press, 1978

21

Alcohol, the Magic Elixir: Stress, Expectancy, and the Transformation of Emotional States

G. ALAN MARLATT

The purpose of this chapter is to provide a comparison of two alternative hypotheses about the reinforcing effects of alcohol: tension-reduction vs. arousal-enhancement. Research on the biphasic reaction to alcohol suggests that alcohol may have both arousal-enhancing and tension-reducing effects, but that the initial excitatory effects precede the inhibitory effects. Research on the biphasic response is reviewed, followed by a discussion of cognitive mediating factors that may underlie the arousal-enhancing effects of alcohol. Studies investigating outcome expectancies for the effects of alcohol in individuals with different drinking histories are examined in detail. In the final section, the outcome-expectancy of alcohol as a "magic elixir" capable of transforming emotional states, along with implications for differentiating between moderate drinking and addictive drinking, are discussed.

A decade ago, I wrote a paper entitled, "Alcohol, stress, and cognitive control" (1), in which I reviewed the currently available literature on the

Preparation of this paper is supported in part by grants AA03489 and AA05591 from the National Institute on Alcohol Abuse and Alcoholism.

relation between stress and alcohol consumption in humans. After a critical analysis of research findings derived from the Tension Reduction Hypothesis of the reinforcing effects of alcohol, I proposed an alternative hypothesis based on the notion that alcohol, at least in terms of its initial effects in human consumption, may serve to *enhance* arousal rather than to decrease it. This immediate arousal-enhancement effect may, in turn, serve as the experiential basis for positive outcome-expectancies for the initial effects of alcohol. Alcohol, viewed from this perspective, takes on the properties of a magic elixir, a substance that can enhance arousal, mood, or affect. Just as the alchemists of centuries past sought out an elixir that would transform lead into gold, so do many of today's problem drinkers turn to alcohol as an elixir to transform negative emotional states into positive ones.

This paper serves as an update and extension of my 1976 paper (1). The first section is devoted to a discussion of these two alternative hypotheses about the reinforcing effects of alcohol, the tension reduction hypothesis (TRH) and the arousal enhancement hypothesis (AEH). One important point to be advanced in this discussion is that alcohol may have *both* arousal-enhancing (excitatory) effects and tension-reducing (inhibitory) effects, but that the excitatory effects *precede* the inhibitory effects in a biphasic response. It is hypothesized that outcome expectancies are more likely to be influenced by these immediate positive effects than by delayed negative effects. Possible cognitive mediating factors that may underlie the arousal-enhancement effects of alcohol are discussed in the second section of this paper. A brief review of current research on outcome expectancies for alcohol's effects follows. In the final section, a theoretical model of alcohol dependence based on a vicious cycle of mood transformation is presented, along with implications for prevention, cognitive-behavioral therapy, and relapse prevention.

THE BIPHASIC RESPONSE TO ALCOHOL: IMPLICATIONS FOR OUTCOME EXPECTANCIES

The origins of the TRH are well documented in the literature (cf. 1, 2, 3) and will not be reviewed in detail here. Masserman's pioneering work with alcohol as a preventive agent of experimental neuroses in cats (4, 5) served as the impetus for the initial development of the TRH. Consistent with Masserman's own psychoanalytic interests and the "translation" of psychodynamic motivational principles into Hullian drive-reduction theory (6, 7), alcohol was thought to be reinforcing through its tension-reducing effects (much as eating behavior was considered by Hull and his followers to be reinforced via the reduction in the hunger drive).

In a follow-up to Masserman's work, Conger (8) hypothesized that alcohol facilitated approach behavior in rats subjected to an approach-avoidance conflict (a conflict situation similar to the experimental neurosis paradigm developed by Masserman). Conger attempted to demonstrate in his research that the effect of alcohol was to weaken avoidance behavior (lower the fear gradient), thereby permitting the animal to approach the goal (food) that had been previously associated with punishment. Conger (9) also provided the first clear statement of the TRH as applied to drinking in humans.

At that time, tension was defined as the fear or avoidance associated with the approach-avoidance conflict. Alcohol was thought to be reinforcing because of its effects on the *reduction* of fear or tension, presumably mediated by ethanol's pharmacological depressant or tranquilizing properties. A corollary of the TRH is that people consume alcohol because of its expected tension-reducing effects. A number of theoretical papers appeared in the 1950s and 1960s that further extended the TRH to the analysis of problem drinking and alcoholism (e.g., 10, 11).

The validity of the TRH as a unitary model of alcohol's reinforcing properties appears to be as outmoded today as in Hullian learning theory in contemporary psychology. Evidence in support of the TRH, both with animal and human research, is mixed and inconclusive (3, 12, 13). The role of cognitive mediation and information processing, largely overlooked by animal behaviorists such as Hull and Skinner, has received increased attention in recent theories of learning and motivation. The introduction of cognitive factors such as expectancy and causal attribution opens the door to an understanding of how the individual *subjectively perceives alcohol* and its expected effects on cognitive, affective, and behavioral processes.

Prior to the recent interest by cognitive theorists in the subjective perception of alcohol (as viewed phenomenologically by the drinker), the primary goal in research deriving from the traditional TRH has been to determine the objective or "real" effects of alcohol as measured empirically by the scientific observer. In other words, the primary aim of the scientist was to assess the effects of alcohol on response systems that could be reliably assessed by objective observers—such as the resolution of approach-avoidance conflict (assessed in terms of degree of approach to the goal box), or changes in physiological measures of tension (assessed by EMG monitoring or associated measures of stress).

Since most early research on the TRH was conducted with animals, and because verbal self-reports were considered by many learning theorists (especially those in the operant camp) to be both unreliable and invalid measures in human research, the subjective/phenomenological side of the coin was rarely the subject of empirical study. In some ways, the search for the objective "truth" about alcohol's effects reminds me of the old joke about the "drunk" who lost his car keys one night. When asked why he was restricting his search to the area under a streetlight, he replied, "The light's much better here." Even though the search for the effects of alcohol may seem to be facilitated through the use of objective behavioral and physiological measures, the "key" to unlocking the door in this puzzle may lie elsewhere, perhaps in the "darker" area of subjective experience.

Along with the recent emergence of cognition and other subjective experiences as potential determinants of behavior, there has occurred a switch in emphasis from the "back end" of the stimulus-response relation (focus on the response and its reinforcing consequences as determinants of subsequent behavior) to the "front end" (focus on expected outcomes as the functional stimulus or determinant of behavior). As an example of this change in focus, consider the case of a man who reaches for the sugar to put in his morning coffee. Unbeknownst to him, his son has filled the sugar bowl with salt as an April Fools' joke. Until he discovers otherwise (after taking his first sip), the father's behavior is guided by the assumption that the "salt" (objectively defined) is actually "sugar" (subjectively perceived). The subjective outcome expectancy (that sugar will sweeten the coffee), not the objectively "real" substance (salt), serves as the functional stimulus for the ensuing response.

The same argument can be applied to alcohol consumption: outcome expectancies for the effects of alcohol lie in the "eye of the beholder." For some beholders, alcohol is believed to possess highly attractive powers; for others, it is seen in a much more negative light, regardless of objective evidence as to its "real" effects. The way in which we evaluate alcohol and label it as good or bad (positive or negative outcome expectancies) determines much of our behavior toward it. A nonalcoholic placebo drink that is believed by the observer to contain alcohol (via experimental deception) will be perceived as "real" alcohol in the same way as salt was perceived to be sugar in the previous example. How we subjectively label and evaluate any stimulus will determine our response to it.

I once heard a story told by Jerome Franks that serves to further illustrate this point. Apparently, there were three baseball umpires who were discussing their criteria for distinguishing a strike from a ball. The first umpire, an objective realist, said emphatically, "I calls 'em the way they *are!*" The second umpire, a subjective phenomenologist, said quietly, "I calls 'em as I *sees* 'em." Finally, the third umpire turned to the others and said, "They ain't *nothing* until I calls 'em!" The same may apply to how we evaluate and label alcohol: the effects of alcohol take on meaning and guide our behavior to the extent that we give them labels and evaluate the effects (outcome expectancies). The same might be said of *theories* about alcohol and its effects; if the theory predicts tension reduction, for example, then that is what we look for and expect to find in our empirical studies.

Outcome expectancies are themselves determined by a multitude of factors. Expectancy effects for alcohol are presumably influenced by the following factors:

1. Cultural and personal beliefs about alcohol and its effects that vary from one society to another (14).
2. Personal experience with alcohol and past and present drinking habits, often couched in the form of post-hoc attributions about alcohol as a cause of various psychological and physical outcomes.
3. The setting or situation in which alcohol is consumed—individuals drinking alone, for example, evaluate the effects of alcohol differently compared to when they are drinking in an interpersonal setting (e.g., 15).
4. The "set" or expectancy about beverage content (alcohol vs. placebo) and dose level (amount of alcohol believed to be in the drink), as illustrated by research utilizing the balanced-placebo design (16) or studies that have varied information about the nature of the drug received (e.g., 17).
5. The pharmacological/physiological effects of alcohol, including individual differences in sensitivity, tolerance, metabolism, and genetic predisposition—such as the Oriental "flush" response to alcohol (18). Among these physical drug effects, perhaps the most central to the development of outcome expectancies is the biphasic response to alcohol.

Over the past few years, evidence has been accumulating that alcohol exerts a biphasic effect as a function of time and/or dose. In a review of relevant research on this topic, Mello (19) concluded that "alcohol acts as a stimulant at low doses and its depressive functions are evident only at higher concentrations" (p. 789). This conclusion is confirmed in a number of empirical reports that studied the effects of relatively low and high doses of alcohol on central nervous system functioning (20, 21). Low doses of alcohol appear to increase heart rate and skin conductance, whereas higher doses serve to depress these measures of physiological arousal (22). The effects of alcohol on motor and perceptual performance also suggest that alcohol facilitates responsiveness at low blood-alcohol levels and inhibits or retards performance only at higher dose levels (e.g., 23), suggesting that there may be an inverted-U-shaped function between blood-alcohol level and measures of performance. Dose and time factors are closely correlated in these studies, since one always proceeds from a low dose to a higher dose over time. Similarly, biphasic responses to alcohol have been identified for both the ascending limb (enhanced arousal) and the descending limb (depressive effects) of the blood-alcohol curve, even though the same absolute blood-alcohol level is involved in both the upswing and downswing segments (24).

What underlies the biphasic response to alcohol? Solomon and his colleagues have noted that a biphasic response may be common to a variety of affective, hedonic, or emotional states, including responses to psychoactive drugs (25, 26). These investigators postulate that the elicitation of a particular affective state automatically triggers a response of the opposite affective tone—an "opponent process" system designed as a homeostatic balancing mechanism to protect the organism from emotional extremes. Along similar lines, Siegel (27, 28) has argued that these protective homeostatic responses can be conditioned to psychoactive substance cues. Such conditioned compensatory responses, elicited by drug cues, are often opposite in hedonic quality to the pharmacological effects of the drug itself. It is as if the body, through past association with the effects of a particular drug, attempts to offset or compensate for the drug's pharmacological effect by responding in an direction opposite to that of the drug. Thus, for example, the body's compensatory response to a depressive drug such as alcohol may be an anticipatory *increase* in arousal, to compensate for the depressive effects of alcohol on the nervous system. The initial compensatory increase in physiological arousal, followed by a delayed depressive effect, may constitute the two-phase mechanism underlying the biphasic response to alcohol.

Outcome expectancies for the effects of alcohol or other psychoactive drugs may be "shaped" by the biphasic physiological response. Even though alcohol is a depressive drug in terms of its effects at higher doses or over time, people often speak of wanting to get "high" from booze—not to experience a depressed psychophysical state (although some alcoholics do state that they wish to get "wiped out" by drinking). The initial increase in arousal associated with the compensatory response to alcohol may be one of the motivating factors in social drinking. A person who returns home after a hard day's work and consumes a couple of martinis before dinner will experience an affective boost in energy or arousal, one that temporarily relieves the state of fatigue or physical exhaustion. One of the main assumptions of the present argument is that the initial increase in arousal or excitation, perhaps mediated by a conditioned compensatory response to alcohol cues, forms the basis of positive outcome expectancies for alcohol's effects.

Expectancies of reinforcement are shaped by the temporal *immediacy* of alcohol's effects, despite delayed consequences of a contrary hedonic quality. These positive expectancies remain robust over time, even though the organism's physiological responsivity to alcohol changes over time as tolerance increases, especially in heavy or problem drinkers. Unlike the process of metabolic or behavioral tolerance to alcohol, outcome expectancies do not show an increased tolerance effect over time. It is not unusual, therefore, that many heavy drinkers continue to harbor expectations of alcohol's effects that are markedly out of line with the actual physiological effects. In a series of studies by Mendelson and his colleagues (29, 30), for example, alcoholics were asked to describe their initial expectancies about the effects of alcohol on their feelings and moods prior to a scheduled period of drinking in a research ward setting. Almost all of the subjects anticipated that alcohol would make them feel more relaxed, more comfortable, and less depressed. These expected effects were the direct opposite of the actual dysphoric effects of prolonged drinking reported by subjects during the intoxication phase of the study.

Such mismatches between the expected and experienced effects of alcohol are not uncommon among problem drinkers. Why do such mismatches occur, and what is their significance in terms of understanding problem drinking? The material in the following section reviews a number of cognitive mechanisms that may mediate the maintenance of positive outcome expectancies despite "objective evidence" to the contrary.

COGNITIVE MEDIATORS OF
AROUSAL-ENHANCEMENT EFFECTS
OF ALCOHOL

Although the exact nature of the physiological mechanisms underlying the biphasic reaction is still a matter of debate and conjecture, a number of theories have been advanced concerning the effects of alcohol on cognition that seem to provide a "fit" with the biphasic reaction. Such postulated mechanisms include alcohol's effects on perceived personal "power," on memory and information-processing, and on self-awareness. Explanations that focus on the nonpharmacological effects of alcohol (e.g., alcohol as a cue or signal for "time out") are also relevant. Each of these hypothesized mechanisms will be discussed briefly in this section.

The work of McClelland and his associates on the effects of alcohol on personal cognition and fantasy provides one explanatory mechanism that may account for alcohol's initial reinforcing effects. In a wide-ranging series of studies involving male social drinkers, McClelland and his colleagues (31) concluded that the consumption of alcohol leads to increased fantasies of power. In these studies, heavy-drinking men who were given alcohol were administered selected cards from the Thematic Apperception Test (TAT) to provide a measure of thematic fantasies. Many studies reported in their book suggest that after two or three drinks, drinkers show an increase in "social power" fantasies (power for the good of others or a cause); in larger amounts, alcohol increased fantasies of "personal power" (self-aggrandizement, without concern for others). On the basis of these findings, McClelland concluded that "men drink primarily to feel stronger. Those for whom personalized power is a particular concern drink more heavily" (p. 334). There seems to be a consistency between the hypothesis that alcohol facilitates fantasies of power and the evidence indicating that alcohol consumption elicits an initial state of increased physiological arousal. Perhaps the physiological "rush" (increased heart rate and other indices of arousal) is subjectively experienced by the drinker as a surge of energy or power.

A second potential mediator of alcohol's reinforcing effects is the various effects of ethanol on information-processing and memory. Recent research strongly suggests that the consumption of alcohol (particularly at higher dose levels) interferes with the transfer of information in short-term memory to long-term memory storage (32). This deficit is especially relevant to the understanding of alcohol-induced memory "blackouts" in which the drinker, although capable of responding in a relatively normal fashion on the basis of short-term memory capacity, shows a subsequent loss of long-term memory for events that occurred under the influence.

In a related point, some investigators have hypothesized that alcohol interferes with the individual's ability to respond to the anticipated *consequences* of their actions. In one such study, for example, Zeichner and Pihl (33) reported that subjects given alcohol showed an unresponsiveness to the contingent feedback from a confederate subject while they were interacting in a "teacher-learning" task. In the learning task, sub-

jects delivered bogus electric shocks of variable intensity to the confederate, who, in turn, responded with a tone blast (delivered to the subject
via earphones), the loudness of which was matched to the prior shock
level set by the real subject. Subjects who were in the nonalcohol placebo
condition adjusted their shock levels to lower levels in response to the
confederate's contingent responses. On the other hand, subjects who
received alcohol continued to set higher levels of shock over trials, regardless of the confederate's contingent and escalating responses. This
inability to respond to contingencies may be mediated by the deleterious
effects of alcohol on memory storage—perhaps the subjects given alcohol "forget" the pattern of contingent consequences because it does not
become stored in permanent memory.

It may be the case, therefore, that alcohol serves to decrease fear or
tension not because of its pharmacologically tranquilizing effects on anxiety, but because alcohol interferes with the ability to retrieve and hence
act upon one's prior knowledge of potentially negative consequences of
excessive consumption. In other words, alcohol may reduce the *expectancy* of negative consequences rather than reducing the existing level of
tension or fear. The inhibitory influence of expected delayed negative
outcomes (e.g., of physical discomfort, social disapproval) may be *disinhibited* by alcohol's effects on memory storage and retrieval. Perhaps it is
this disinhibiting effect that accounts for the release of energy (enhanced
approach gradient) and the "freeing" effects of alcohol in the initial
"high" of intoxication. Freed from the pressures of past painful memories and the anxious anticipation of future negative consequences, the
heavy drinker experiences a narrowing of attention to the "here and
now"—an increased responsivity to immediate external cues to the ex-
clusion of other past or future events.

A related hypothesis has been advanced by Hull and his associates (34,
35, 36), who have argued that alcohol serves to impair the processing of
higher-order cognitive processes related to the self. Specifically, Hull has
hypothesized that alcohol interferes with the coding of self-awareness
(i.e., self-criticism and self-consciousness). More specifically, alcohol is
said to interfere with

> encoding processes fundamental to a state of self-awareness, there-
> by decreasing the individual's sensitivity to both the self-relevance
> of cues regarding appropriate forms of behavior and the self-eva-
> luative nature of feedback about past behaviors. Insofar as the latter
> form of information can provide a source of self-criticism and nega-
> tive affect, alcohol as an inhibitor of self-aware processing is pro-
> posed to provide a source of psychological relief. (34, p. 586)

It is this "psychological relief" or decrease in negative self-evaluation that serves as a "sufficient condition to induce and sustain alcohol consumption" (34, p. 589). Hull's theory and empirical data cited in support of his model have recently been critically reviewed by Wilson (37).

Finally, other theorists have pointed out that alcohol is often consumed in convivial settings, often associated with feelings of relaxation, social enjoyment, and a "time out" from the pressures of ordinary life and work. Drinking during the "happy hour" coincides with the end of the workday and a release from normal responsibilities, a state of relative exuberance and perceived freedom from the cares and woes of day-to-day existence. Some social psychologists and anthropologists have put forth the notion that the signal or cue properties of alcohol (alcohol as a discriminative stimulus signaling the availability of social reinforcement) exert a greater impact than the pharmacological effects of the drug (38). Through repeated association, we come to associate drinking-time as "fun-time" and we respond to situational cues (the setting, time, and personal company one is in).

Anthropological studies show that beliefs about alcohol and its disinhibiting effects sometimes exert a greater influence than the physiological effects of alcohol. In one study of the inhabitants of the Truk Islands, Marshall (39) showed that young males became visibly intoxicated and engaged in a wide variety of "drunken" behaviors after merely *sniffing* an empty liquor bottle (these youths were not aware that actual consumption of liquid alcohol was required to get drunk); the wild acting-out tactics of these "weekend warriors" were exonerated by the village elders, who attributed their "intoxication" to the effects of alcohol. Similar examples are provided by MacAndrew and Edgerton (14) in their analysis of cross-cultural differences in reactions to drinking and drunken comportment. In our own society, alcohol cues often play a similar role, acting as discriminative stimuli that signal the "appropriateness" of aggressive or sexual acting out (e.g., barroom brawls or cocktail lounge seductions).

There is a double payoff for the drinker who shows a disinhibition effect after drinking: (a) the person is able to indulge in an activity (e.g., aggressive or sexual responding) associated with immediate gratification; and (b) the person is able to avoid or be exonerated from delayed negative reactions (such as guilt or social disapproval) by "disclaiming authorship" for the disinhibited behavior. "I was drunk and didn't know what I was doing when I hit you," goes the typical excuse. Alcohol can also be used as an excuse *prior to* engaging in difficult or challenging acts, as well. Jones and Berglas (40) have described the use of alcohol as a "self-handicapping strategy" to offset anticipated problems in future performance. Taking a drink or two before a stressful situation (e.g., taking an exam or going on a date with a new potential partner) may provide the drinker with a built-in excuse in case things do not work out well: "It wasn't my fault; it was because I was drinking."

Research utilizing the balanced-placebo design supports the salience of nonpharmacological contributions to the effects of drinking (16, 41). Four groups are compared in this design: expect alcohol/receive alcohol; expect alcohol/receive placebo; expect placebo/receive alcohol; and expect placebo/receive placebo. The design permits the investigator who is administering alcohol or placebo to independently vary the expectation or belief that a drink contains alcohol with the actual alcohol content of the drink consumed. In research using this design, it has been found that expectancy effects predominate for behaviors involving some form of disinhibition (e.g., increased sexual or aggressive responding), such that subjects who are expecting to consume alcohol show disinhibited responsiveness, regardless of the actual alcohol content of the drinks. Alcohol itself, however, has a deleterious effect on nonconflict behaviors such as motor performance and reaction time, regardless of the expectancy set (42, 43).

OUTCOME EXPECTANCIES IN DIFFERENT DRINKING POPULATIONS

Research with the balanced-placebo design, discussed previously, involves the manipulation of expectancy by varying instructions (set) about the content of the beverage to be consumed. Presumably, if subjects are told they will be consuming an alcoholic beverage, this instructional set will elicit outcome expectancies concerning the anticipated effects of consuming alcohol; expectation of consuming a nonalcoholic drink, on the other hand, will not elicit alcohol outcome expectancies. This procedure does not, however, assess or manipulate the *content* of these outcome expectancies.

What do we know about the outcome expectancies that subjects bring with them to the drinking setting? Research reviewing alcohol-related expectancies prior to the present decade has been reviewed elsewhere (1, 44). In one early study of the emotional effects of alcohol, for example, Russell and Mehrabian (45) asked college students to describe how they would feel after drinking a moderate amount of alcohol (two drinks) and a heavy amount (six drinks). It was found that a moderate amount of alcohol was expected to produce pleasure, dominance, and moderate arousal, and a large dose was expected to cause moderate pleasure, submissiveness, and nonarousal.

In the present decade, several groups of investigators have studied alcohol outcome expectancies in different populations of drinkers. Goldman, Brown and colleagues at Wayne State University have conducted a series of studies utilizing the Alcohol Expectancy Questionnaire (AEQ). On the basis of interviews with a wide range of drinkers who were asked to describe any positive effects of drinking, the 90-item true-false AEQ was first developed and then administered to a large group of college students (46). For each item, subjects were asked to rate their degree of agreement indicating their belief that a moderate amount of alcohol (a "couple" or a "few" drinks) would produce a particular effect. A factor analysis of the AEQ yielded a six-factor solution approximating 51.3% of the overall variance. These factors, along with representative questionnaire items are as follows:

Factor 1. Portrays alcohol as a "global, positive transforming agent" (pp. 422–423). Sample items: "Alcohol seems like magic," and "Drinking makes the future seem brighter." On the AEQ, 67% of items had a significant loading on this general transformation factor.

Factor 2. Indicates that subjects expect alcohol to enhance both social and physical pleasure (e.g., "Drinking adds a certain warmth to social situations," "Having a few drinks is a nice way to celebrate special occasions").

Factor 3. Represents an enhanced sexual experience and performance dimension (e.g., "After a few drinks, I am more sexually responsive").

Factor 4. Corresponds to a dimension of arousal with facets of power and aggression (e.g., "I feel powerful when I drink, as if I can really influence others to do as I want").

Factor 5. Conceptualized as a dimension of increased social assertiveness (e.g., "If I have a couple of drinks, it is easier to express my feelings").

Factor 6. Corresponds to relaxation and tension reduction (e.g., "Alcohol decreases muscular tension").

According to the authors, the first two global expectancy factors account for a large portion of the variance, indicating "the degree to which alcohol is viewed by humans as a potent, even 'magical' drug" (p. 425).

Analyses indicated that particular expectancies were associated with differences in drinking patterns among the subjects tested: "less exposure to alcohol and limited consumption were associated with more general, positive expectancies . . . , whereas longer exposure and heavier consumption were paired with expectancies of sexual enhancement and arousal and aggressive behavior" (p. 423). Sex differences were also found; females were more likely to expect generally positive experiences when drinking, and males were more apt to expect arousal and potentially aggressive behavior.

Subsequent research by the Wayne State group has provided further information about alcohol outcome expectancies. In one study of outcome expectancies in adolescents (47), it was found that well-developed expectancies exist prior to any significant personal experience with alcohol consumption (age 12–14 years), suggesting that alcohol expectancies appear to be based upon social learning factors rather than pharmacological experience with alcohol. The expectancies remained strikingly consistent throughout adolescence, despite increasing use of alcohol as the adolescents became older. In a subsequent study, adolescent outcome expectancies were pitted against demographic and drinking history variables in the prediction of adolescent drinking (48). The results

> showed that expectancies at least equalled and even added to the predictive power of the background variables. Specifically, adolescents who drank in a frequent, social manner expected alcohol to enhance their social behavior, whereas adolescents who reported alcohol-related problems expected an improvement in their cognitive and motor functioning. (p. 249)

Finally, in a recent study by the Wayne State group (49), outcome expectancies of adult alcoholics were compared with those given by college students and hospitalized medical patients. Results indicated that the alcoholics were found to maintain stronger alcohol expectancies, even when demographic differences between groups were controlled for. The typical expectancy profile for alcoholics indicated more global, positive expectancies, increased interpersonal assertiveness, and more physical and social pleasure than the other populations tested. Alcoholics also maintained *less* expectations of tension reduction than their nonabusing peers. From this study, it appears that expectancies of magical transformation are more associated with drinking problems and alcoholism than are expectancies of tension reduction.

In a related paper, Rohsenow (50) differentiated between personal experiences (how alcohol is expected to affect the self) and general expectancies (how alcohol is expected to affect others). Rohsenow hypothesized that these two sets of expectancies arise from different sources: general expectancies reflect cultural beliefs and stereotypes, whereas personal expectancies derive from personal, family, and peer experiences with alcohol. In a modification of the AEQ developed by the Wayne State group, Rohsenow added items on cognitive and motor impairment (the original AEQ included only positive outcomes) and asked college student drinkers to fill out two versions of the questionnaire to assess both personal and general expectancies. Results showed that subjects expected *others* to be more strongly affected by alcohol than themselves for every questionnaire scale. A comparison between heavy and light drinkers showed that light drinkers expected themselves to experience significantly less social and physical pleasure from alcohol than others, whereas medium and heavy drinkers expected both themselves and others to experience virtually the same amount of pleasure. Medium and heavy drinkers both expected themselves to experience significantly more social and physical pleasure, sexual enhancement, aggressiveness, expressiveness, and relaxation after drinking than did the light drinkers, but did not differ significantly in the impairment, carelessness, or global positive effects they expected after drinking.

As with the Wayne State group, Rohsenow also found a significant sex effect on self-expectancies: women expected significantly less global positive effect, social and physical pleasure, and relaxation, and significantly more impairment from alcohol than men. As Rohsenow points out, women may expect more impairment from alcohol than men because (a) women reach a higher blood-alcohol content than men at the same dose level; and (b) there are greater social sanctions against drinking in women than men.

The studies reported above provide support for a general positive transformation effect as a result of drinking moderate amounts of alcohol. Although this supports the notion of an arousal-enhancement effect as the initial response to drinking at low-dose levels, it provides no information about the second phase of biphasic effect associated with higher dose levels. To correct for this shortcoming, and to balance positive and negative outcome expectancies, researchers in our laboratory developed an outcome expectancy questionnaire consisting of 37 bipolar items rated on a 5-point scale (e.g., relaxed/tense, careless/careful, happy/sad) that is administered in two phases corresponding either to the effects of a moderate amount of alcohol (Phase 1) or a large amount ("too much alcohol"—Phase 2).

This questionnaire was administered to college students who varied in drinking history from abstainers to heavy drinkers (51). Responses were factor analyzed yielding a three-factor solution for both Phases 1 and 2. The factors were named (a) stimulation/perceived dominance (e.g., "active/passive," "restless/peaceful"); (b) pleasurable disinhibition (e.g., "happy/sad," "uninhibited/inhibited"); and (c) behavioral impairment (e.g., "clumsy/coordinated," "careless/careful"). Analyses of responses provide support for the biphasic model of alcohol effects as reflected in differential expectancies for light versus heavy drinking. All categories of drinkers, except abstainers, expected stimulating alcohol effects during Phase 1 and more neutral effects during Phase 2. Phase 2 was associated with relatively more impairment than Phase 1. As the authors conclude, the results of this study

> demonstrate that alcohol expectancies are systematically related to drinking experience and to phase of intoxication. Heavier drinkers reported expectancies of relatively greater stimulation/perceived dominance and pleasurable disinhibition during moderate intoxication, reflected in significant linear relationships between the amount of habitual drinking and expectancies in Phase 1 drinking. There was no relationship between drinking habits and expectancies of behavioral impairment. This pattern of results suggests that heavier drinkers expect greater positive effects from drinking and the same negative effects that lighter drinkers expect. (p. 719)

IMPLICATIONS FOR ALCOHOL DEPENDENCE AND RELAPSE

Research reviewed above indicates that positive outcome expectancies differentiate between heavy and light drinkers, but that negative outcome expectancies are generally similar in both groups. Individuals who expect that alcohol will serve as a global, positive transforming agent (including enhanced stimulation and pleasurable disinhibition) are more likely to be heavy and problem drinkers than those who harbor less favorable expectancies. Alcoholics are more likely to expect positive transformation effects of alcohol (getting "high") than tension-reduction effects, contrary to earlier theoretical models of the reinforcing effects of alcohol in dependent or addicted drinkers. Taken as a whole, these findings are consistent with the view advanced by Maisto and his colleagues (52), that drinking is a goal-directed activity, and that the higher the subjective probability that alcohol will serve a desired function, the more likely it is that drinking will occur.

The results of this research are also congruent with the argument advanced in my 1976 paper (1) that individuals are more likely to drink in "high-risk situations" involving stress, negative affect, and other unpleasant mood states to the extent that they expect alcohol to transform their subjective experience. Alcohol may thus be viewed as an effective antidote to stress and negative mood states, especially when alternative (and more constructive) means of coping are unavailable or unused. As stated in my 1976 paper:

> . . . the hypothesis that emerges is that the probability of drinking will vary in a particular situation as a function of (a) the degree of perceived stress in the situation; (b) the degree of perceived personal control the person experiences; (c) the availability of an adequate coping response to the stressful situation and the availability of alcohol; and (d) the person's expectations about the effectiveness of alcohol as an alternative coping response in the situation. (p. 291)

In other words, if the individual expects alcohol to be an effective transformational elixir, the probability that the person will consume alcohol increases in situations associated with stress and negative emotional states. In our own research program on determinants of relapse in alcoholics and in other addictive behavior problems, we have found that over half of all initial lapses following abstinence-oriented treatment for alcoholism occur when the person reports experiencing negative emotional states, including interpersonal conflict situations (e.g., arguments with others) (53, 54). We have also found that providing the individual with an alternative coping response to drinking (e.g., expression of negative feelings) will reduce the probability of consuming alcohol (55). Taken together, these findings and the foregoing theoretical model provide a means of distinguishing between moderate and addictive/excessive alcohol use.

One way to distinguish between moderation and addiction is to focus on the affective consequences or changes in emotional state associated with drinking. Of particular interest in this regard is the *change* of affect or hedonic tone induced by alcohol relative to the emotional tone experienced prior to drinking. It is hypothesized that *moderation* is characterized by drinking that serves to enhance or maintain a prior neutral or positive emotional state. *Addiction* or alcohol dependence, on the other hand, is characterized by the individual's attempt to alleviate or transform a prior negative emotional state. The various transformations of affect associated with addictive vs. moderate drug use is illustrated by the hypothetical model presented in Figure 1.

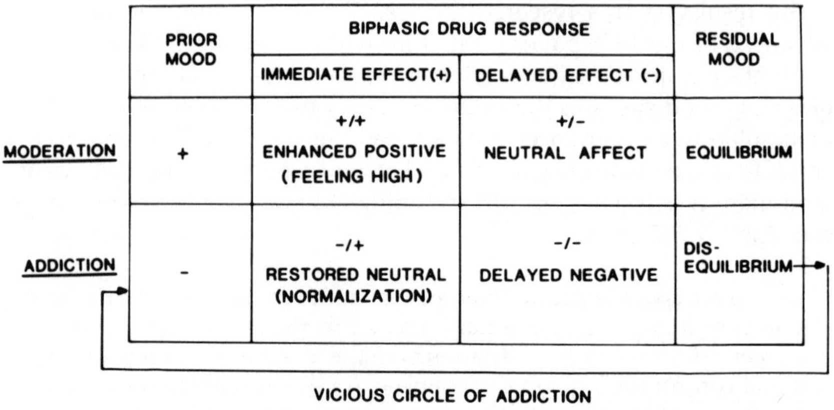

	PRIOR MOOD	BIPHASIC DRUG RESPONSE		RESIDUAL MOOD
		IMMEDIATE EFFECT(+)	DELAYED EFFECT (-)	
MODERATION	+	+/+ ENHANCED POSITIVE (FEELING HIGH)	+/- NEUTRAL AFFECT	EQUILIBRIUM
ADDICTION	-	-/+ RESTORED NEUTRAL (NORMALIZATION)	-/- DELAYED NEGATIVE	DIS-EQUILIBRIUM

VICIOUS CIRCLE OF ADDICTION

Figure 1. Moderation versus addiction in the transformation of affective state: hypothetical model.

In Figure 1, three stages of affect of hedonic quality are portrayed: affect or mood prior to drug use, and changes in mood that are associated both with the initial and delayed effects of the biphasic response that follow use of the drug or activity. The upper half of the diagram illustrates the effects of moderate use and the lower half depicts addictive use.

In moderate use, the individual chooses to engage in drug use only when the prior mood state is affectively neutral or positive (+). As an example, consider someone who is in a celebratory mood (+) at a wedding reception where champagne is being served. The initial effects of two or three glasses of champagne consumed under these circumstances would most likely be marked by increased euphoria or enhanced positive feelings (+). Taken together, the prior positive mood state enhanced by the initial effects of alcohol (the first stage of the biphasic response) produces a double-positive "high" (+/+). If the person continues to moderate intake, thereby titrating a pleasurable blood-alcohol level, the delayed negative effects of drinking (-) will be minimal, perhaps limited to a mild feeling of fatigue or malaise associated with the second stage of the biphasic response. These negative aftereffects will be offset or neutralized by the combined positive effects of the prior mood state and the initial excitatory phase of the biphasic response. The end state following this drinking episode should be basically neutral (+/-) as a result; the final product is one of emotional balance or equilibrium. Moderation leaves no negative aftereffects. On the next drinking occasion, the individual is more likely to initiate use when experiencing a neutral or positive mood.

In the case of addictive use, however, the transformation of affect follows quite a different course. Addiction, from this perspective, represents an attempt on the part of the user to transform or cope with a prior negative mood state. Prior to use, the addicted individual is likely to be experiencing dysphoric feelings (−) arising from either a stressful life situation (high-risk situation) and/or the delayed effects of heavy prior alcohol use (e.g., physical discomfort, hangover). Alcohol appears to offer instant relief (positive outcome expectancy) because of its initial positive effects (first phase of the biphasic response).

To illustrate, consider a businessman who goes out to a business luncheon meeting with some clients. Due to the residual effects of the past night's heavy drinking (ongoing hangover), he looks forward to his first martini as a little "hair of the dog" to alleviate physical discomfort. In addition, he is feeling some insecurity and doubt about his ability to secure a contract with his clients (high-risk situation) and he believes that a drink or two will fortify his confidence and lubricate the negotiations. His mood state prior to drinking is clearly negative (−). After downing his first martini, our friend may experience some temporary relief via the initial excitatory effects of alcohol (consumed prior to eating in order to maximize its effects). The degree of positive effect will be minimized to some extent, however, by the degree of tolerance involved. Heavy drinkers with pronounced tolerance may attempt to overcome this limiting factor by increasing drug dosage (ordering a "special" or double martini). Since the prior mood state is negative (−), the overall impact of the initial positive drug effect may be little more than a normalizing effect in which the person experiences a transformation from a negative to a neutral state. Our businessman may report feeling better after his second martini because the alcohol transformed his mood "upward" from a negative state to one of emotional neutrality (−/+).

The enhanced negative state (now neutral) is short-lived, however, due to the delayed negative effects associated with the biphasic response. After lunch is over, our businessman may begin to feel tired, restless, and unable to concentrate on his work as the delayed effects of his luncheon martinis intensify. As indicated in Figure 1, the cumulative effect is hedonically dysphoric (−/−) and leads to a continued desire for alcohol as a means of providing temporary relief. The end state, in contrast with the equilibrium of moderation (+/−), is one of disequilibrium or imbalance (−/−).

The negative aftereffects often linger on and provide the affective backdrop (−) for the next occasion of drug use. The person in our example looks forward to his happy hour at the end of the day as the next opportunity to alleviate his continuing distress; he "craves" a drink (positive outcome expectancy) as a means of escaping or avoiding these unpleasant feelings. Guilt and concern about his increasing dependence upon alcohol provide further fuel for this ongoing dysphoric state. A vicious cycle characterizes the addictive pattern; the disequilibrium experienced after one drinking occasion sets the stage for repeated use as an attempt to restore balance. Any short-term relief is quickly dispelled by the delayed negative effects which in turn give rise to another attempt to gain relief. The addicted individual is thus caught in a trap of his or her own making: the expected solution (more drugs) exacerbates the initial problem.

How can we help the person escape from this addictive trap? Future research is needed to assess the extent to which maladaptive (addiction-prone) expectancies can be modified in high-risk drinkers (56). Unlike genetic susceptibility or physiological differences in alcohol metabolism, factors considered to be beyond modification or change in most cases, cognitive expectancies represent processes that can be altered through education and cognitive-behavioral therapy. Future educational and prevention programs in the alcohol field may profit from the research findings reported in this review by focusing on attempts to alter maladaptive expectancies for alcohol as the magic elixir.

REFERENCES

1. Marlatt, GA: Alcohol, stress, and cognitive control, in Stress and Anxiety (vol 3). Edited by Sarason IG, Spielberger, CD. Washington, DC, Hemisphere, 1976
2. Cappell, H: An evaluation of tension models of alcohol consumption, in Research Advances in Alcohol and Drug Problems (vol 2). Edited by Gibbins Y, Israel H, Kalant RE. New York, Wiley, 1975
3. Higgins, RL: Experimental investigations of tension-reduction models of alcoholism, in Experimental Studies of Alcoholism. Edited by Goldstein G, Neuringer C. Cambridge, Ballinger, 1976
4. Masserman JH, Jacques MG, Nicholson MR: Alcohol as a preventive of experimental neuroses. Quart J Stud Alc 6:281–299, 1945
5. Masserman JH, Yum KS: An analysis of the influence of alcohol on experimental neuroses in cats. Psychosom Med 8:36–52, 1946
6. Dollard J, Miller NE: Personality and Psychotherapy. New York, McGraw Hill, 1950
7. Hull CL: Principles of Behavior. New York, Appleton, 1943
8. Conger JJ: The effects of alcohol on conflict behavior in the albino rat. Quart J Stud Alc 12:1–29, 1951
9. Conger JJ: Alcoholism: Theory, problem and challenge. Quart J Stud Alc 17:296–305, 1956
10. Kepner E: Application of learning theory to the etiology and treatment of alcoholism. Quart J Stud Alc 25:279–291, 1964

11. Kingham RJ: Alcoholism and reinforcement theory of learning. Quart J Stud Alc 19:320–330, 1958
12. Cappell H, Herman CP: Alcohol and tension reduction: A review. Quart J Stud Alc 33:33–64, 1972.
13. George WH, Marlatt GA: Alcoholism: The evolution of a behavioral perspective, in Recent Advances in Alcoholism (vol 1). Edited by Galanter M. New York, Plenum, 1983
14. MacAndrew C, Edgerton RB: Drunken Comportment. Chicago, Aldine, 1969
15. Pliner P, Cappell H: Modification of affective consequences of alcohol: A comparison of social and solitary drinking. J Abnorm Psychol 83:418–425, 1974
16. Marlatt GA, Rohsenow DR: Cognitive processes in alcohol use: Expectancy and the balanced placebo design, in Advances in Substance Abuse (vol 1). Edited by Mello NK. Greenwich, CT, JAI Press, 1980
17. Schachter S, Singer JE: Cognitive, social, and physiological determinants of emotional state. Psychol Rev 69:379–399, 1962
18. Mizoi Y, Ijiri Y, Tatsuno Y, et al: Relationship between facial flushing and blood acetaldehyde levels after alcohol intake. Pharmacol Biochem Beh 10:303–311, 1979
19. Mello NK: Some aspects of the behavioral pharmacology of alcohol, in Psychopharmacology: A Review of Progress. Edited by Efron DH. Washington, DC, Public Health Service Publication No 1836, 1968
20. Grenell RG: Effects of alcohol on the neuron, in The Biology of Alcoholism (vol 2). Edited by Kissin B, Begleiter H. New York, Plenum, 1972
21. Himwich HE, Callison DA: The effects of alcohol on evoked potentials of various parts of the central nervous system of the cat, in The Biology of Alcoholism (vol 2). Edited by Kissin B, Begleiter H. New York, Plenum, 1972
22. Knott DH, Beard JD: Effects of alcohol ingestion on the cardiovascular system, in Encyclopedic Handbook of Alcoholism. Edited by Pattison EM, Kaufman EK. New York, Gardner, 1982
23. Moskowitz H, DePry D: Differential effect of alcohol on auditory vigilance and divided attention tasks. Quart J Study Alc 29:54–63, 1968
24. Jones BM, Vega A: Cognitive performance measured on the ascending and descending limb of the blood alcohol curve. Psychopharm 23:99–114, 1972
25. Solomon RL: The opponent-process theory of acquired motivation: The costs of pleasure and the benefits of pain. Amer Psychol 35:691–712, 1980
26. Solomon RL, Corbit JD: An opponent-process theory of motivation: Temporal dynamics of affect. Psychol Rev 81:119–145, 1974
27. Siegel S: Morphine tolerance as an associative process. J Exp Psych: Animal Behav Processes 3:1–13, 1977
28. Siegel S: Classical conditioning, drug tolerance, and drug dependence, in Research Advances in Alcohol and Drug Dependence. Edited by Smart R. New York, Plenum, 1983
29. McGuire MT, Mendelson JH, Stein S: Comparative psychosocial studies of alcoholic and non-alcoholic subjects undergoing experimentally-induced ethanol intoxication. Psychosom Med 28:13–25, 1966
30. Tamerin JS, Weiner S, Mendelson JH: Alcoholics' expectancies and recall of experiences during intoxication. Amer J Psychiat 126:1697–1704, 1970
31. McClelland DC, Davis WN, Kalin R, et al: The Drinking Man. New York, Free Press, 1972
32. Birnbaum IM, Parker ES (eds): Alcohol and Human Memory. Hillsdale NJ, Lawrence Erlbaum, 1977
33. Zeichner A, Pihl RO: Effects of alcohol and behavior contingencies on human aggression. J Abnorm Psych 88:153–160, 1979
34. Hull J: A self-awareness model of the causes and effects of alcohol consumption. J Abnorm Psych 90:586–600, 1981
35. Hull J, Levenson R, Young R, et al: The self-awareness-reducing effects of alcohol consumption. J Personal Soc Psych 44:461–473, 1983

36. Hull JG, Reilly NP: Self-awareness, self-regulation, and alcohol consumption: A reply to Wilson. J Abnorm Psych 92:514–519, 1983
37. Wilson GT: Self-awareness, self-regulation, and alcohol consumption: An analysis of J. Hull's model. J Abnorm Psych 92:505–513, 1983
38. Levison PK, Gerstein DR, Maloff DR (eds): Commonalities in Substance Abuse and Habitual Behavior. Lexington, MA, DC Heath, 1983
39. Marshall M: Weekend Warriors. Palo Alto, CA, Mayfield, 1979
40. Jones EE, Berglas S: Control of attributions about the self through self-handicapping strategies: The appeal of alcohol and the role of underachievement. Personal Soc Psych Bull 4:200–206, 1978.
41. Rohsenow DJ, Marlatt GA: The balanced placebo design: Methodological considerations. Addictive Beh 6:107–122, 1981
42. Miller ME, Adesso V, Fleming JP, et al: The effects of alcohol on the storage and retrieval processes of heavy social drinkers. J Exp Psych Human Learning and Memory 4:246–255, 1978
43. Vuchinich RE, Sobell MB: Empirical separation of physiological and expected effects of alcohol on complex perceptual motor performance. Psychopharm 60:81–85, 1978
44. Donovan DM, Marlatt GA: Assessment of expectancies and behaviors associated with alcohol consumption. J Stud Alc 41:1153–1185, 1980
45. Russell JA, Mehrabian A: The mediating role of emotions in alcohol use. J Stud Alc 36:1508–1536, 1975
46. Brown SA, Goldman MS, Inn A, et al: Expectations of reinforcement from alcohol: Their domain and relation to drinking patterns. J Consult Clin Psych 48:419–426, 1980
47. Christiansen BA, Goldman MS, Inn A: Development of alcohol-related expectancies in adolescents: Separating pharmacological from social-learning influences. J Consult Clin Psych 50:336–344, 1982
48. Christiansen BA, Goldman MS: Alcohol-related expectancies versus demographic/background variables in the prediction of adolescent drinking. J Consult Clin Psych 51:249–257, 1983
49. Brown SA, Goldman MS, Christiansen BA: Do alcohol expectancies mediate drinking patterns of adults? J Consult Clin Psych 53:512–519, 1985
50. Rohsenow DJ: Drinking habits and expectancies about alcohol's effects for self versus others. J Consult Clin Psych 51:752–756, 1983
51. Southwick L, Steele C, Marlatt A, et al: Alcohol-related expectancies: Defined by phase of intoxication and drinking experience. J Consult Clin Psych 49:713–721, 1981
52. Maisto SA, Connors GJ, Sachs P: Expectation as a mediator in alcohol intoxication: A reference level model. Cognitive Ther Res 5:1–18, 1981
53. Marlatt GA, Gordon JR: Determinants of relapse: Implications for the maintenance of behavior change, in Behavioral Medicine: Changing Health Lifestyles. Edited by Davidson PO, Davidson SM. New York, Brunner/Mazel, 1980
54. Marlatt GA, Gordon JR: Relapse Prevention: Maintenance Strategies in the Treatment of Addictive Behaviors. New York, Guilford, 1985
55. Marlatt GA, Kosturn CF, Lang AR: Provocation to anger and opportunity for retaliation as determinants of alcohol consumption in social drinkers. J Abnorm Psych 84:652–659, 1975
56. Fromme K, Kivlahan DR, Marlatt GA: Alcohol expectancies, risk identification, and secondary prevention with problem drinkers. Adv Behav Res Ther 8:237–251, 1986

Index